MONOGRAPHS OF THE PHYSIOLOGICAL SOCIETY

Editors: H. Davson, A. D. M. Greenfield,
R. Whittam, G. S. Brindley

Number 22 THE PHYSIOLOGY OF LACTATION

MONOGRAPHS OF THE PHYSIOLOGICAL SOCIETY

Volumes marked * are now out of print.

THE PHYSIOLOGY OF LACTATION

A. T. COWIE and J. S. TINDAL

M.R.C.V.S., Ph.D., D.Sc.   B.Sc., Ph.D.,

National Institute for Research in Dairying,
Shinfield, Reading, Berks

LONDON
EDWARD ARNOLD (PUBLISHERS) LTD

© A. T. COWIE and J. S. TINDAL, 1971

First published, 1971
by Edward Arnold (Publishers) Ltd.,
41 Maddox Street,
London, W1R 0AN

ISBN: 0 7131 4186 7

Printed in Great Britain by
The Camelot Press Ltd., London and Southampton

PREFACE

In the last thirty years there has been no dearth of reviews on the physiology of lactation. Research progress has, however, been rapid and since it is some ten years since an extensive review appeared we believe there is justification for the present monograph. This book is intended for the advanced student in physiology but we believe the bibliography is sufficiently extensive that it may also prove of value to the research worker who is about to explore some aspect of the subject. Citations of original studies are, in the main, confined to papers appearing in the last ten years; otherwise the reader is referred to existing reviews for further information and references.

No attempt has been made to deal with the biochemistry of milk synthesis which is now a vast field in its own right and would warrant a separate treatise.

The late Professor S. J. Folley, F.R.S., was involved in the planning of this book. His original intention of contributing one of the chapters was thwarted by deteriorating eyesight and his untimely death occurred just as we completed our writing and as he was about to write a foreword. We gratefully acknowledge his valuable help and advice. We also thank our colleagues Dr. Isabel A. Forsyth and Dr. G. S. Knaggs for much help and critical discussion.

We record with pleasure the help of Miss Joan K. Swinburne, Mrs. Daphne E. Adler, Mrs. Anna Knaggs and Mrs. Laura A. Blake in preparing the typescript and bibliography. For permission to reproduce various figures, individually acknowledged in the captions, we are much indebted to the following workers: Professor Dr. W. Bargmann, Professor H. A. Bern, Dr. Jacqueline D. Cleverley, Professor E. Cobo, Dr. R. Denamur, Dr. J. L. E. Ericsson, Dr. A. L. R. Findlay, Dr. Isabel A. Forsyth, Dr. M.

Griffiths, Professor K. H. Hollmann, Dr. T. Johke, Dr. G. S. Knaggs, Professor C. H. Li, Dr. J. L. Linzell, Dr. F. Neumann, Mr. K. C. Richardson, Dr. Gutta I. Schoefl, Dr. Y. J. Topper and Mr. A. Turvey; to the editors of the following journals: the *American Journal of Obstetrics and Gynecology*, *Archives of Biochemistry and Biophysics*, *Endocrinologia Japonica*, *German Medical Monthly*, *Journal of Cell Biology*, *Journal of Endocrinology*, *Journal of Physiology*, *Journal of Ultrastructure Research*, *Journal of Zoology*, *Nature*, *Zeitschrift für Zellforschung und mikroskopische Anatomie* and to the following publishers: Academic Press, American Association for the Advancement of Science, Butterworth & Co. Ltd., Cambridge University Press, William Heinemann Medical Books Ltd., Longmans, Green & Co. Ltd., Pergamon Press Ltd., the Royal Society, the University of Pennsylvania Press and the Society for Endocrinology.

Reading, 1970   A. T. C.
                                                 J. S. T.

Considerable advances have been made in the field since the manuscript was completed. We have noted some of these in a series of six addenda, one for each chapter, which are grouped together just before the index. Items in these are indexed under their respective addendum number.

The help given by Miss Barbara Koster of Edward Arnold (Publishers) Ltd. in the preparation of the book is gratefully acknowledged.

Reading, 1971   A. T. C.
                                                 J. S. T.

CONTENTS

PHYSIOLOGY OF THE MAMMARY GLAND

Historical introduction

WE do not propose to dig deeply into the history of lactational physiology but we shall mention a few reviews and bibliographies which may serve as guides to anyone wishing to trace in greater depths the development of this branch of physiology.

The first documented review of the anatomy and physiology of the mammary gland is that by von Haller (1765, 1778), which includes sections on the comparative anatomy of the mammary gland, the nature of the milk ducts, the vascular and neural connexions to the gland, milk secretion, physiological relationship between the mammary glands and the uterus, and the physical and chemical nature of the milk constituents. A more recent source book is the *Bibliographia Lactaria* of Rothschild (1901) and its two supplements (1901, 1902) which list in chronological order, and with bibliographic details, publications on lactation in the widest sense of the term, sections being devoted to the milks of different species, methods of milk analysis, the physiology and pathology of the mammary gland, milk products, breast-feeding, artificial milks for infants, milk hygiene and milk-borne diseases, and related topics; in all, there are some 11,200 references ranging from the 16th to the beginning of the 20th centuries. Recently, Simon (1968) has reviewed much of the 19th-century literature on the physiology of lactation and has quoted extensively from the original papers. In the period under review, from 1800 to 1928, Simon recognizes three phases of research emphasis. In the first forty years or so of the 19th century, studies were mainly directed towards the morphology of the mammary gland and to the direct examination of milk; this period also saw much controversy about the origin of milk; was it derived from blood or from chyle? The second half of the 19th century saw the application of the light microscope to the study first of the nature of milk and later, as histological and cytological techniques were developed, to the study of the mammary gland itself. These studies gave rise to numerous theories on the nature of the cellular mechanisms involved in the synthesis of milk constituents within the alveolar cell and their excretion into the lumen of the alveolus; controversy over these mechanisms continued over a century and even now may not be quite dead (see also Mayer & Klein, 1961). Also towards the end of this second phase of mammary physiology the role of the nervous system as the possible regulator of mammary function was being investigated. The third or endocrine phase as recognized by Simon began with the present century and with the birth of endocrinology and during it much progress was made in the identification and elucidation of the hormonal complexes involved in the control of the growth of the mammary gland and in the regulation of its function. Stepping beyond the arbitrary limits of Simon's review the phases of research interest overlap; the second quarter of the present century saw a great upsurge in biochemical studies on mammary function, extension of hormonal investigations and a redirection of interest towards the nervous system and its role in the neuroendocrine control of mammary function. Early in the second half of this century came the application of the electron microscope to the study of mammary cytology and the resulting solution of some of the problems raised a century before by the introduction of the light microscope.

From time to time in the various sections of this monograph further reference will be made to some of the above historical facets of the physiology of the mammary gland. Finally, in closing this brief introduction we would mention two further reviews which deal not so much with the history of lactational physiology but with aspects of lactational physiology in history. *The exploitation of the milk-ejection reflex by primitive peoples* by Amoroso & Jewell (1963) and *The milk-ejection reflex: a neuroendocrine theme in biology, myth and art* by Folley (1969b) will provide a fascinating introduction to the current studies in this field reviewed in Chapter 5.

ANATOMY OF THE MAMMARY GLAND

Descriptions of the gross anatomy of the mammary glands of man and domestic animals are to be found in the standard text-books of anatomy although some of the diagrams and figures are of poor quality and have been much copied from generation to generation of text-books.

The serious student of the anatomy of the breast will find it interesting to consult Cooper's *Anatomy of the Breast* which appeared in 1840 and which contains a remarkable series of coloured illustrations of the fine structure of the breast. Indeed, this book covers a much wider field than the title implies and includes sections on the physiology and biochemistry of the mammary gland and clinical observations on the 'draught' (milk ejection) which are still of interest today; also included is a section on comparative anatomy with observations and illustrations concerning the mammary glands of the cow, goat, ewe, mare, rhinoceros, rabbit, hare, guinea-pig, cat, bitch, sow and porpoise—the high fat content (23%) of the milk of the porpoise and the presence of large central mammary ducts in this species which serve as cisterns are recorded. Atkins (1968) has recently commented as follows on this remarkable book: 'It was only the gross anatomy which was available for study by Sir Astley Cooper. His meticulous research led him to describe the anatomy of the skin, the nipple, the areola, the duct system, the fat, the fibrous tissue (Cooper's suspensory ligaments), the blood vessels and the nerves, together with the general form of the breast and its beautiful adaptation to function in a manner which could not be bettered and which, in the succeeding years, has required only trivial modification. Although, in general, the gross anatomy of the breast has little relevance to clinical considerations, there is one exception to this which has assumed importance in the modern treatment of certain cancers of the breast by the local infusion of cytotoxic drugs, namely the anatomy and distribution of the arterial supply, and in this field Sir Astley's account is detailed and accurate.' We may add that there are some fine figures depicting the lobules of alveoli prepared by injecting coloured waxes into the galactophores of the lactating gland, which are reminiscent of the display of the sectors of the rabbit mammary gland which can be obtained by the equally elegant but perhaps more physiological technique of

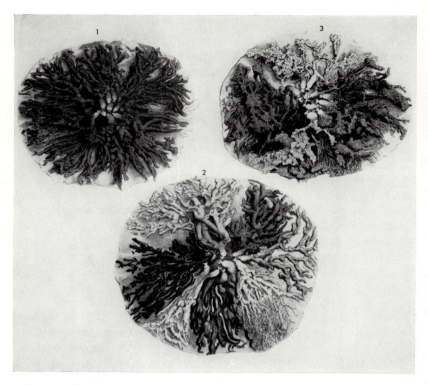

FIG. 1.1. Ducts and glandules of the human breast—a photograph of Plate VI from Cooper (1840). Cooper injected coloured waxes through the galactophores into the duct system and the ducts were subsequently displayed by repeated maceration and dissection of the breast. The original plate is in colour. The captions are as follows:

'Fig. 1. Lactiferous tubes or ducts injected with red wax, showing their radiated direction, and, in some places, their interramification.

Fig. 2. Mammary ducts injected with red, yellow, black, green and brown, and seen less intermixed than the former.

Fig. 3. Ducts injected more minutely with yellow, red, green, blue and black. This preparation shows two additional circumstances:—First, the glandules from which the ducts begin are seen filled with wax. Secondly, at the lower part of the preparation the separated ducts are seen passing above and beneath each other, to render the breast a cushion; while at the upper part the ducts are single.'

(From Cooper, Sir Astley P., 1840, *On the Anatomy of the Breast*. London: Longman, Orme, Green, Brown and Longmans.)

injecting prolactin into the galactophores as first practised by Lyons (1942) a century later (Figs. 1.1 and 2.3).

A clinical study of the growth changes of the nipple during pregnancy by Hytten & Baird (1958) shows that the diameter of the areola and of the nipple increases during pregnancy. The nipple also becomes more mobile or protractile, a characteristic which makes it more easily grasped by the baby thereby facilitating breast feeding. It appears from this study that the benefits ascribed in the past to antenatal treatment of the nipple are mainly normal physiological changes (see also Hytten & Leitch, 1964).

For the comparative anatomist there are two main sources of information and references; there is first the monograph *The Comparative Anatomy of the Mammary Glands* by Turner (1939) and secondly the more recent edition (1952) of part of this monograph dealing with the mammary glands of the cow, ewe, goat, sow, mare, elephant and marine mammals, entitled *The mammary gland, 1. The anatomy of the udder of cattle and domestic animals*. Since these books were published there have appeared studies of the mammary glands of several species, previously little investigated, which will now be described.

Sub-class Prototheria

Order Monotremata

Family Tachyglossidae. The early studies on the mammary apparatus of echidna (*Tachyglossus*) have been reviewed by Bresslau (1920) and Raynaud (1961, 1969) but recently much new information has been published (see review by Griffiths, 1968; and Griffiths, McIntosh & Coles, 1969). The echidna has two mammary glands located on either side of the abdomen. The lactating glands each consist of some 100–150 separate lobules each with its own duct opening to the exterior at two small areas, the *areolae*, on the ventral skin surface (Figs. 1.2, 5.1 and 5.2). The areolae are about 6 mm long and 2–3 mm wide. There are no teats or nipples, but the terminal duct of each lobule opens into a small invagination of the skin surrounding a hair whose follicle is situated in the areola; sebaceous glands associated with the hair follicle also open into the same skin invagination. The presence of these mammary hairs led to the erroneous guess that milk was imbibed by the young licking it off the hairs but as Griffiths (1968) has shown

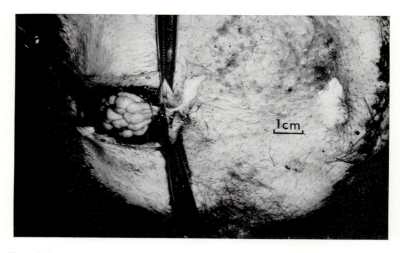

FIG. 1.2. Areolar region in the pouch of echidna (*Tachyglossus aculeatus aculeatus*). One of the mammary glands has been exposed and the club-shaped lobules are clearly visible. This echidna had been injected 7·75 min previously with oxytocin and milk is welling up from the areola and the mammary hairs (from Griffiths, M., 1968. *Echidnas*. International Series of monographs on pure and applied biology, zoology division, edited by Kerkut, G. A., vol. 38. Oxford: Pergamon Press).

milk is imbibed by sucking and the echidna possesses an efficient milk-ejection mechanism (see p. 192). In echidna carrying pouch young the areolae are situated on each side of the mid line on the dorso-lateral surface of the pouch or incubatorium. This pouch develops at the start of the breeding season and the areolae are located about midway between its cranial and caudal ends. The erroneous belief which was current for many years that the echidna had two slit-like pockets on either side which contained the areola has been discussed and explained by Bresslau (1920).

Before and during the early part of the breeding season the mammary glands are small and the lobules consist of solid cords of cells arranged as coils. The stimulus of pregnancy and incubation of an egg in the pouch is generally, but not invariably, necessary for the canalization of the cords, so that they become ducts, and for the growth of true alveoli. In the echidna in full lactation the mammary gland measures about 60×35 mm. In the male the gland consists of tiny lobules not exceeding 5 mm in length.

Family Ornithorhynchidae. In *Ornithorhynchus* the mammary glands resemble those of the echidna, there are two glands made up of some 150–200 lobules, each lobule opening through its own duct on the skin surface on the areolar area. No incubatorium develops in *Ornithorhynchus*.

Sub-class Metatheria

In marsupials the mammary glands are normally situated in the pouch or marsupium but in the Didelphidae (opossums) the pouch may be incomplete and be represented by a pair of lateral folds (e.g. in *Caluromys*) or may even be absent (e.g. in *Marmosa* and *Monodelphis*). The mammary ducts of marsupials, unlike those of the Monotremata, collect together and lead to the surface through a teat or nipple as in the Eutheria. The number of galactophores within the teat varies with the species, e.g. six in *Dasyurus*, 20 in *Megaleia*. The number of mammary glands varies greatly in the various families and there is even some variation between individuals of a species; in the Didelphidae there is usually an odd number of glands (ranging from 5 to 25) whereas in the higher families of marsupials the number is from 2 to 10. The disposition of the teats is very variable, there are frequently two longitudinal rows with a number of teats forming secondary rows or disposed irregularly, an unpaired median teat being often present. The macropod marsupials (kangaroos) may be nursing two generations of young simultaneously and the suckled glands will be at quite different stages of development (see p. 102, also review by Sharman, 1970). Unlike eutherian mammals the male marsupial lacks rudimentary teats and mammary glands (Sharman, 1970). Further information on the mammary glands of metatherian mammals will be found in the reviews by Turner (1939) and Raynaud (1969).

Sub-class Eutheria

As already noted the reviews by Turner (1939, 1952) provide information and references to anatomical studies of the mammary glands of a variety of eutherian mammals; some further information may be found in the review by Raynaud (1969). We shall therefore restrict our comments to subsequent studies.

Order Insectivora

Superfamily Macroscelidoidea. McKerrow (1954) has described the mammary glands of *Elephantulus myurus jamesoni* (Chubb). There are two pairs of glands, one pair thoracic, the other pair abdominal in position. Very little parenchymal growth occurs until the onset of the first pregnancy.

Order Primates

Sub-order Prosimii. Ahmed & Kanagasuntheram (1965) have described the mammary glands of the lesser bush baby (*Galago senegalensis senegalensis*). Usually there appear to be three pairs of mammary glands, the nipples extending along a line from the lower part of the axilla reaching towards the groin; in one specimen, however, a pair of considerably smaller nipples, which were nevertheless functional, were situated between the usual second and third pairs. In a specimen of slow loris (*Nycticebus coucang coucang*) also studied by these investigators there were only two pairs of nipples, pectoral in position.

Sub-order Anthropoidea. Speert (1948) has studied the normal growth of the mammary gland of the rhesus monkey (*Macaca mulatta*) through the foetal, postnatal, adolescent and adult stages. Speert stresses the wide individual variations in the growth of the mammary gland in both male and female monkeys under the same physiological conditions.

Order Rodentia, sub-order Hystricomorpha

Superfamily Chinchilloidea. The mountain viscacha or mountain chinchilla (*Lagidium*) has mammary glands located high upon the sides of the thorax (Dobson & DeViney, 1967).

Superfamily Octodontoidea. The coypu (*Myocastor coypus*) has its mammary glands located on its dorsal surface. The nipples have three galactophores (Dobson & DeViney, 1967; Long, 1969).

Order Cetacea

Slijper (1966) and Harrison (1969) have briefly described the mammary glands of whales, dolphins and porpoises. Cetaceae have two mammary glands which do not normally protrude, although in full lactation they produce some elevation of the body surface; they are elongated, narrow, flat organs on either side of the ventral mid-line extending from a point just cranial to the anus to a point just short of the umbilicus. The nipples are situated on either side of the female genital slit, males having a pair of rudimentary nipples in slits cranial to the anus. The ducts from the mammary lobules lead into a central lactiferous duct (first described by Cooper in 1840, see above) which is markedly distended in the nipple region—this central duct is probably comparable to the gland cistern in the ruminant mammary gland.

Order Pinnipedia

The few anatomical studies of the mammary glands of sea-lions, walruses and seals have recently been reviewed by Harrison (1969). In the Otariidae (Eared seals), Odobenidae (Walrus) and in two genera of phocids—*Erignathus* (Bearded seal) and *Monachus* (Monk seal)—there are two pairs of mammary glands, one pair cranial, the other pair caudal to the umbilicus; other phocids have only one pair of caudal mammary glands. The mammary glands lie beneath the blubber and occupy extensive areas on each side of the ventral abdominal wall. The nipples are said to become erectile during nursing but at other times they are hidden by the pelage.

HISTOLOGY AND CYTOLOGY OF THE MAMMARY GLAND

Light microscopy

In Prototheria the mammary gland is usually described as a tubular gland, branched and entwined like a sweat gland (see Raynaud, 1969). According to Griffiths (1968), in the non-lactating gland the lobules consist of solid cords of cells in which a lumen is rarely seen. At the beginning of the breeding season the mammary glands begin to differentiate and grow (and seem to do so independently of pregnancy), the cords becoming hollow tubules in which there is some secretion. In the fully lactating gland the lobules are swollen club-shaped structures composed of hundreds of typical alveoli which communicate with centrally located ductules leading into larger ducts each of which terminates at a sinus. Each sinus opens to the exterior through a duct of large calibre which ends in an invagination of the skin surface surrounding a mammary hair. From Griffiths's (1968) studies there appear to be no striking differences in the histology of the lactating mammary gland of the echidna which would distinguish it from the lactating gland in metatherian or eutherian mammals (Fig. 1.3).

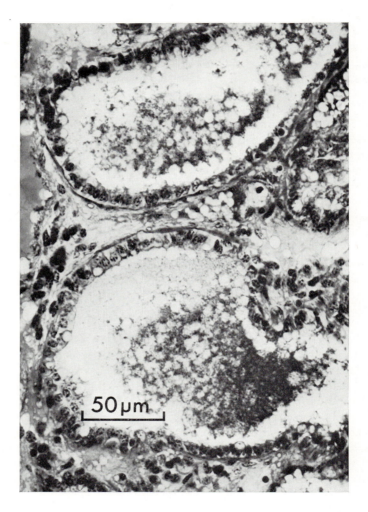

FIG. 1.3. Section of actively secreting alveoli in mammary gland of echidna (from Griffiths, M., 1968, *Echidnas*. International series of monographs in pure and applied biology, zoology division, edited by Kerkut, G. A., vol. 38. Oxford: Pergamon Press).

In Metatheria and Eutheria the fully developed mammary gland is a compound lobulo-alveolar gland divided into lobes and lobules by connective and elastic tissues.

Alveolar cells

The histological and cytological studies on the mammary gland from the inception of histological techniques in the middle of the 19th century to the first reports on the electron microscopic studies in 1959 have been reviewed in considerable detail by Mayer and Klein (1961). Another recent detailed review of mammary cytology is that by Ehrenbrand (1964).

Richardson (1947) comments that although structural investigation of the mature alveoli in pregnancy and during lactation have been pursued for over a century there are few examples in the histology and cytology of glandular tissues in which so much disagreement has occurred as to the nature of the secretory cycle. The vexed question concerned the manner of excretion from the cell cytoplasm into the lumen of the alveolus of the milk constituents after their synthesis within the alveolar cell. Three different mechanisms had been invoked, first the constituents passed through the intact cell membranes, secondly the cell membrane ruptured irregularly to release the larger secretory masses such as the fat; or thirdly, the apical cytoplasm became detached, pinched off or decapitated, leaving the cell to undergo a rapid phase of regeneration. Richardson (1947) attributes many of the discrepancies in the published observations to unsatisfactory histological techniques. For example the all too common habit of cutting out blocks of tissue from the mammary gland before fixation causes shifting and extrusion of stored secretion while the sudden release of pressure results in elastic recoil of the stroma and distortion of the alveoli. Richardson stresses that fixation by vascular perfusion and hardening the gland *in toto* are essential steps before isolating small blocks of parenchyma for embedding. Even with proper fixation artefacts arising from sectioning the tissue may make the interpretation of individual sections difficult unless serial sections are available. It is also important to know whether the gland was fixed while it was distended with milk or whether it had recently been milked out. The importance of this factor was dramatically illustrated by Richardson (1947) by fixing by intravascular perfusions one mammary gland in the distended condition immediately after its surgical removal from a goat, while the other gland was similarly fixed after it had been milked out (Fig. 1.4). By this procedure it was thus possible to examine the effects of milking on structural changes occurring in the alveoli in the one animal under con-

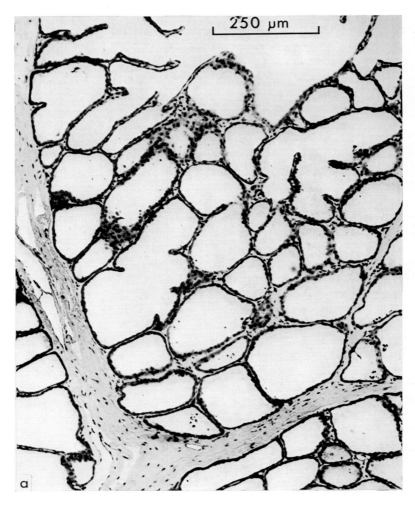

250 μm

a

FIG. 1.4 (a) Part of a lobule from the left half of a goat's udder fixed by intravascular perfusion while distended with milk.

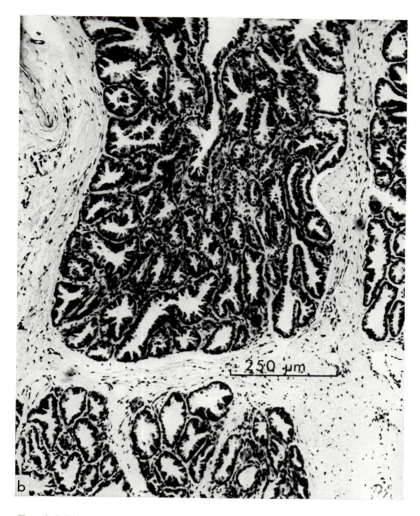

FIG. 1.4 (b) Part of a lobule from the right half of udder of the same goat which was milked out before intravascular fixation. Note the contracted lobules with collapsed alveoli and ducts lined with thick folded epithelium (from Richardson, K. C., 1949, *Proc. R. Soc.* B **136**, 30–45)

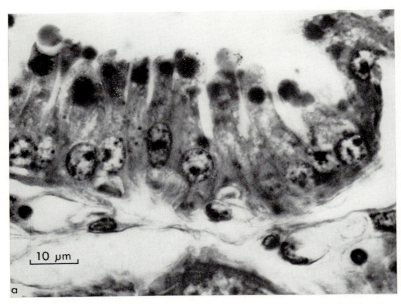

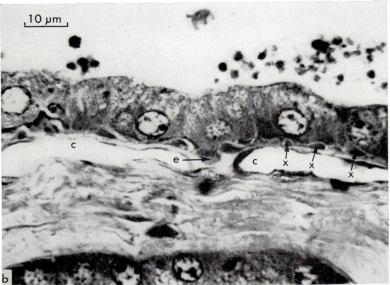

F_{IG}. 1.5.

trolled conditions. A marked shrinking of the lobules was observed when the gland was emptied and the inter-lobular septa were widened to the extent of being easily visible to the naked eye in a large horizontal section through the gland; the alveolar epithelium thickened about three-fold, the cells becoming tall and columnar in shape and projecting irregularly into the lumen. The alveolar walls became wrinkled and the alveoli elongated with a cleft-like lumen. The ducts remained open but were narrower and had thicker and more folded walls than the ducts in the distended gland.

Soon after the removal of milk from the alveoli the secretory products begin to accumulate in the cytoplasm in the form of fat droplets of relatively large size together with less conspicuous granular protein. As more and more milk is secreted into the alveolus the cells become stretched and much reduced in height. Among the best photomicrographs of mammary epithelium obtained with the light microscope are those of Richardson showing the change in shape and structure of the alveolar cells when the alveolar lumen fills up with secretion resulting in the stretching and compression of its cellular walls (Fig. 1.5). Not however until the advent of the electron microscope was the nature of the excretory mechanisms satisfactorily revealed (see p. 27).

Myoepithelial cells

Another problem in mammary histology and a source of controversy and discussion for many years was the nature of the stellate or basket cells which lie on the surface of the alveolus, i.e. between the base of the alveolar cells and the basement membrane. One of the earliest mentions of these cells is by Henle in

FIG. 1.5. (a) Section of alveolar epithelium of lactating goat soon after milking, i.e. when alveoli are empty. Note the tall epithelial cells containing fat droplets in their apical cytoplasm (preparation by Mr. K. C. Richardson, from Folley, S. J., 1952, in *Marshall's Physiology of Reproduction*, 3rd edn, edited by Parkes, A. S., vol. 2, chap. 20. London: Longmans, Green).

(b) Section of alveolar epithelium of a lactating goat just before milking, i.e. when alveoli are distended. Note the flattened epithelial cells. The processes of myoepithelial cells cut transversely appear as small oval or triangular bodies (X) indenting the basal epithelial membrane. In the centre, between two capillaries (C), an extension (E) of the secretory cell cytoplasm appears to be pinched between two myoepithelial processes (from Richardson, K. C., 1949, *Proc. R. Soc.* B **136**, 30–45).

1866 who noted the presence of stellate cells on the acini of the parotid and mammary glands. In 1868 Boll described in more detail and illustrated with drawings the multi-polar 'basket' cells in the tear and salivary glands while Langhans in 1873 gave a description of the stellate cells surrounding the alveoli in the human mammary gland. Kolessnikow (1877) and later Sticker (1899) reported the presence of stellate and spindle-shaped cells on the alveoli of the bovine mammary gland. A contractile function for these cells was postulated by Lacroix (1894) who, after studying them in thick sections of human and cat mammary glands which had been fixed in a mixture of osmium tetroxide, picric acid and silver nitrate, made a very shrewd guess as to their function: 'il est permis de se demander si ces cellules en panier n'ont pas une importance capitale dans le mécanisme de l'excrétion glandulaire. Si l'on reconnaît, en effet, à ces cellules des propriétés contractiles, on conçoit le rôle qu'elles doivent jouer dans l'expulsion des produits de la sécrétion accumulés dans la lumière des acini et des conduits excréteurs. Par le resserrement des mailles de ce

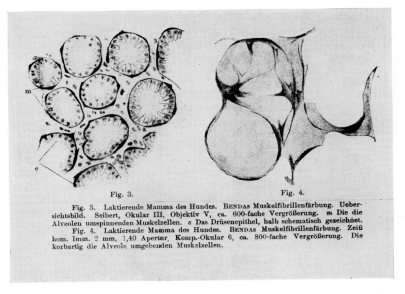

Fig. 3.   Fig. 4.

Fig. 3. Laktierende Mamma des Hundes. BENDAS Muskelfibrillenfärbung. Uebersichtsbild. Seibert, Okular III, Objektiv V, ca. 600-fache Vergrößerung. *m* Die die Alveolen umspinnenden Muskelzellen. *c* Das Drüsenepithel, halb schematisch gezeichnet.
Fig. 4. Laktierende Mamma des Hundes. BENDAS Muskelfibrillenfärbung. Zeiß hom. Imm. 2 mm, 1,40 Apertur, Komp.-Okular 6, ca. 800-fache Vergrößerung. Die korbartig die Alveole umgebenden Muskelzellen.

FIG. 1.6. Drawing from Bertkau (1907) of myoepithelial cells in the mammary gland of the lactating bitch (from Bertkau, F., 1907, *Anat. Anz.* **30**, 161–180).

vaste réseau, elle peuvent d'un seul coup réduire dans des proportions considérables la capacité totale des cavités glandulaires." In these early studies the most interesting illustrations of these cells are the drawings by Bertkau (1907) who studied the mammary glands of lactating women and bitches and *inter alia* noted that while the cells enmeshed the alveoli they were longitudinally dispersed over the mammary ducts (Fig. 1.6). Comparison of Bertkau's sketches with the photographs obtained forty years later by Richardson (Fig. 1.7) leave little doubt that the 'basket' or myoepithelial cells in the mammary gland had been clearly recognized by these early investigators. Also as we have noted their contractile properties had been postulated, several authors regarding them as similar to smooth muscle cells. There followed a period of some thirty years when little attention was paid to the myoepithelial cells apart from a few pathologists who were interested in their metaplastic activities in mammary tumours (for references see Linzell, 1952). In 1939 Turner reviewed some of the early descriptions of the myoepithelial cells and re-emphasized their possible role in milk ejection; later Swanson & Turner (1941) re-investigated the presence of these cells in the cow mammary gland and considered them to be smooth muscle cells spaced at intervals around the alveoli. While the description by Swanson & Turner agreed with earlier studies their photomicrographs were neither clear nor convincing and the confusion between myoepithelial cells and smooth muscle cells deepened. In 1949 a major advance was made by Richardson who studied thick silver-impregnated sections (75–100 μm) of goat mammary gland, obtained clear photomicrographs of the myoepithelial cells and was able to distinguish between myoepithelial and smooth muscle cells. Richardson observed an abundant network of myoepithelial cells (Fig. 1.8) covering the stromal surface of the epithelium of the alveoli, ducts and cisterns whereas smooth muscle was present only in scattered interlobular bundles closely associated with the blood vessels. The term 'myoepithelial' had long been used to describe these cells (e.g. by Arnold, 1905), because they were of epithelial origin but possessed some of the structural appearance of smooth muscle, but there, as Richardson emphasized, no real evidence of their contractile activities. In his study, however, Richardson noted structural changes in the myoepithelium of contracted as compared with distended alveoli,

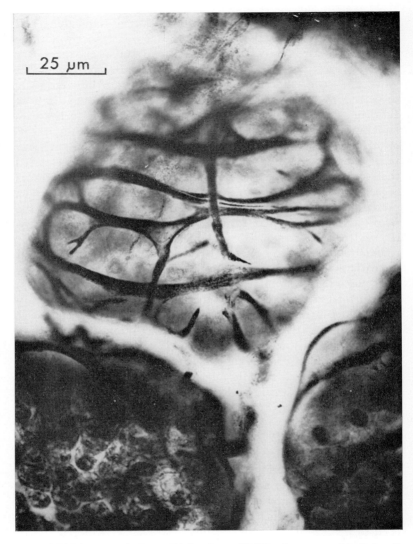

FIG. 1.7. Photograph from Richardson (1949) of a myoepithelial cell with nucleus and branching processes on a contracted alveolus in the mammary gland of a lactating goat (from Richardson, K. C., 1949, *Proc. R. Soc.* B **136**, 30–45).

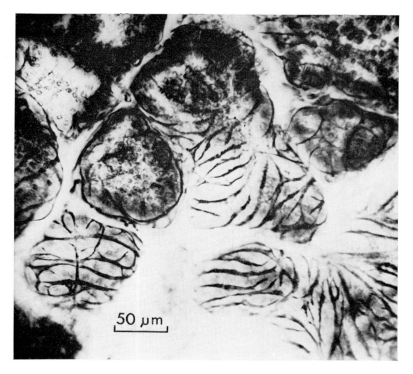

Fig. 1.8. Part of mammary lobule from a lactating goat showing the disposition of myoepithelial cells on contracted alveoli. After milking, the mammary gland was fixed by intravascular perfusion and the tissue silver impregnated by the technique of Richardson (1949). (Photograph by courtesy of Mr. K. C. Richardson.)

these changes, moreover, considered in conjunction with the general orientation of the myoepithelial cells and the precise relationship between these cells and the folds of the secretory epithelium of contracted alveoli, were fully consistent with the assumption that myoepithelium was the contractile tissue of the mammary gland which responded to oxytocin. Myoepithelial cells were also observed in the human mammary gland (Richardson, 1951). Linzell (1952), also using a silver-impregnation technique, confirmed Richardson's observation in the goat and man and further demonstrated the presence of the myoepithelial cells in the mammary gland of the cat, dog, rabbit and rat. Circumstantial evidence supporting a contractile role for these cells was further provided by direct microscopical examination of the mammary glands of living mice, rats, rabbits and guinea-pigs by Linzell (1955) who studied the contraction of the alveoli in response to the topical application of minute doses of pure oxytocin.

The outer cell layer of immature mammary ducts has, in the past, been referred to as myoepithelium, particularly by pathologists, irrespective of whether the cells at all resembled the elongated longitudinally-orientated myoepithelial cells of the lactating gland; presumably this habit was based on the assumption that the outer cell layer on the ducts became transformed into myoepithelium (see Richardson, 1949; Linzell, 1955). To avoid confusion it would seem desirable to restrict the term to the fully differentiated stellate or spindle-shaped cells as seen in the lactating gland.

The presence of alkaline phosphatase in the myoepithelial cells and in the capillary endothelium of the mammary gland of the rat has been demonstrated histochemically by both light and electron microscopy (Dempsey, Bunting & Wislocki, 1947; Silver, 1954; Holmes, 1956; Arvy, 1961; Bässler, Schäffer & Paek, 1967; Bässler & Brethfeld, 1968; Bässler & Paek, 1968). Because the efficacy of the silver-impregnation technique is at times uncertain, Silver (1954) suggested that staining for alkaline phosphatase was a more useful method for demonstrating myoepithelial cells. Grünefeld (1964), however, in a study contrasting the effectiveness of silver-impregnation techniques, of Benda's myo-fibril stain and of alkaline phosphatase techniques in the staining of myoepithelium in goat and cow mammary tissue, concluded that care must be exercised in the use of alkaline phosphatase techniques lest capillary networks be mistakenly identified as myoepithelium.

Lobulo-alveolar system

The architecture of the lobulo-alveolar system of the human mammary gland has been described in some detail by Dawson (1933, 1934, 1935), Geschickter (1945), Dickson & Hewer (1950), Dabelow (1957) and Bonser, Dossett & Jull (1961).

In the cow mammary gland the parenchyma is arranged in a series of leaves lying more or less parallel to the surface of the gland (Ziegler & Mosimann, 1960). The arrangement of the alveoli and fine ducts has been investigated by three-dimensional reconstructions based on serial sections by Weber, Kitchell & Sautter (1955) and Ziegler and Mosimann (1960). The lobular units are elongated and flattened, about 1·5 mm long, 1 mm wide and 0·5 mm in thickness; the intralobular duct may be variously branched, dividing into 2 to 6 branches which extend for variable distances before redividing into several successive orders of smaller branches. Evidence of secretory activity was present in the entire intralobular duct system which generally consisted of a single layer of epithelium. In the cow a lobule may contain up to 200 alveoli; the majority of the alveoli open individually into their respective terminal intralobular ducts but some open in groups of 2 or 3 into a duct, while in a few instances large aggregates of up to 20 alveoli open into a terminal intralobular duct. Some of the more peripheral branches of the intralobular duct system have sacculated structures like alveoli interposed in their course.

Stroma

The stroma supports and protects the parenchyma and in the fully developed mammary gland divides it into lobes and lobules. The proportion of fatty to connective tissues in the stroma varies with the species; in the mouse and rat it is mainly composed of adipose tissue, in the goat and cow there is a considerable proportion of connective tissue, while in man it is mostly connective tissue. The stroma surrounding the developing alveoli has a more delicate structure than in the other zones—this is the so-called 'mantle tissue'—it is more cellular, the collagenous fibres are less dense and ground substance is more abundant (see review by Mayer & Klein, 1961). Elastic tissue occurs in the udder of the virgin heifer in thin bands lying between the collections of ducts; in the lactating cow much more elastic tissue is present in the mammary gland both between lobules and between lobes; it is not present within lobules (Prusty, 1958).

Nipple or teat

The structure of the nipple of the human mammary gland has been reviewed and described by Dabelow (1957) and Bonser, Dossett & Jull (1961). The terminal mammary ducts or galactophores which open on the nipple are lined by a stratified squamous epithelium and the keratin produced by the lining cells forms a plug which seals the nipple in the resting gland. Proximally each galactophore communicates with a lactiferous sinus which is a sac-like structure lying beneath the areola. At the point of junction the stratified squamous epithelium changes abruptly to columnar epithelium. There are about twenty lactiferous sinuses.

In the dense connective tissue of the nipple and areola there is a complex network of smooth muscle fibres both within and around the base of the nipple which have a multitude of fine attachments to the corium; also encircling the periphery of the areola is a further network of muscle fibres with attachments to the skin and which send connecting fibres to the network in the nipple. The main function of these networks of muscle fibres is the erection of the nipple (see Dabelow, 1957).

Turner (1952) has reviewed studies on the structure of the teat of the cow. The teat or streak canal at the tip of the teat leading from the exterior into the teat cistern is lined with a stratified squamous epithelium like that of the skin with which it is continuous. At the junction of the teat canal and teat cistern the stratified squamous epithelium changes abruptly to the two-layered epithelium of the teat cistern (see also Adams, Rickard & Murphy, 1961).

Histochemical studies have been made on the epithelium of the bovine teat canal with reference to the possible presence of antimicrobial substances in the keratin. The presence of lipid-containing cells located within the epidermis has been observed and it was believed that these lipids migrated into the keratin layer (Adams *et al.*, 1961; Hubben, Morse & Mealey, 1966). Biochemical studies suggested, moreover, that antimicrobial activity was associated with the non-esterified fatty acids in the keratin (Adams & Rickard, 1963) but a later study showed that certain cationic proteins present in the keratin layer were also antimicrobial (Hibbit, Cole & Reiter, 1969). A recent electron microscopic study of the teat-canal epithelium, however, does not entirely support the existence of any specific secretory activity of the epidermal cells (see p. 34).

Functional accessory glandular tissue may occur in the form of small 'periductal lobules' in the wall of the teat sinus and even in the wall of the teat canal (Weber, Wyand & Phillips, 1957). In the teat wall there is an outer network of smooth muscle arranged longitudinally while in the deeper portions the fibres are arranged circularly and intermingle with bundles of collagen and elastic fibres. At the outlet of the teat the circular muscle is said to be unusually heavy forming a sphincter for the teat canal. However, despite the distinct muscular sphincter shown in some published diagrams, a study of histological sections of the region of the tip of the teat reveals no well defined sphincter, although a loose network of smooth muscle fibres is present (Fig. 1.9). Discussing

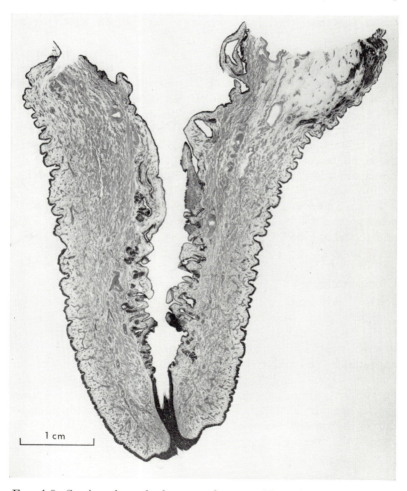

FIG. 1.9. Section through the teat of a cow. Note the thick stratified squamous epithelium lining the teat canal and the absence of any well-defined sphincter muscle around the teat canal. The section is 40 μm thick and is stained with haematoxylin. (By courtesy of Mr. A. Turvey.)

the mechanisms involved in the closure of the teat canal, Pounden & Grossman (1950) concluded that the circular muscle fibres alone were unlikely to be responsible for maintaining the closure of the teat canal, and that the folds of the mucosa at the inner end of the teat canal—the Fürstenberg rosette—and the elastic fibres around the teat canal participated in the closure. In dry cows the teat canals may be closed by firm plugs of desquamated epithelial cells.

Measurements of the teat canal in the living cow by radiographic methods give an average length of 10·8 mm and distal and proximal diameters of 0·40 mm and 0·77 mm respectively; this study, however, provided no evidence that the Fürstenberg rosette acted as a closure mechanism (McDonald, 1968).

The nipple and areola of the guinea-pig show marked changes in the alkaline phosphatase content of the dermis during pregnancy; the significance of this is obscure (Bujard, 1966) but is probably associated with changes in oestrogen levels (Lansing & Opdyke, 1950).

Further references to the structure of the nipples and teats of other species will be found in the reviews by Turner (1939, 1952) and Raynaud (1969).

Ultrastructure

Major advances in the study of the cytomorphology of the mammary gland have been made in the last decade with the aid of the electron microscope. We shall now give a brief description of the ultrastructure of the fully lactating mammary gland; there appear to be no striking species differences in ultrastructure of the mammary glands and the general description given below is based on various publications on the mammary ultrastructure of nine species listed in Table 1.1. Further references to the ultrastructure during the various phases of the growth of the gland will be given later in the appropriate sections.

Mammary duct cells

The superficial cell layer of the intralobular ducts consists of electron dense cells (luminal dark cells) and a small number of clear cells; the basal layer comprises clear cells and myoepithelial

Table 1.1. References to the ultrastructure of the mammary gland in several species

Species	References
Man	Langer & Huhn (1958), Waugh & van der Hoeven (1962), Wellings & Roberts (1963), Ehrenbrand (1964), Toker (1967), Bässler (1968, Bässler & Schäfer (1969*a*, *b*)
Cow	Feldman (1961), Chandler, Lepper & Wilcox (1969)
Pig	Adamiker & Glawischnig (1967)
Rabbit	Hollmann (1966), Girardie (1967*a*, *b*), Hollmann & Verley (1967), Verley & Hollmann (1967), Girardie (1968), Bousquet, Fléchon & Denamur (1969)
Dog	Sekhri & Faulkin, Jr. (1967)
Golden Hamster	Bargmann, Fleischhauer & Knoop (1961), Bargmann & Welsch (1969)
Guinea-pig	Howe, Richardson & Birbeck (1956), Stockinger & Zarzycki (1962), Zarzycki (1964), Girardie (1967*a*, *b*, 1968), Schoefl & French (1968)
Rat	Bargmann & Knoop (1959), Bässler (1961), Bässler, Schäfer & Paek (1967), Girardie (1967*a*), Hollmann & Verley (1967), Verley & Hollmann (1967), Bässler (1968), Bässler & Brethfeld (1968), Girardie (1968), Helminen & Ericsson (1968*a*, *b*, *c*), Kurosumi, Kobayashi & Baba (1968), Schoefl & French (1968), Murad (1970)
Mouse	Hollmann (1959), Wellings, DeOme & Pitelka (1960), Wellings, Grunbaum & DeOme (1960), Bargmann, Fleischhauer & Knoop (1961), Wellings & DeOme (1961, 1963), Wellings & Philp (1964), Miyawaki (1965), Fiske, Courtecuisse & Haguenau (1966), Girardie (1967*a*, *b*), Hollmann & Verley (1967), Sekhri, Pitelka & DeOme (1967*a*, *b*), Stein & Stein (1967), Verley & Hollmann (1967), Schoefl & French (1968), Wellings & Nandi (1968), Pitelka, Kerkof, Gagné, Smith & Abraham (1969)

cells. The luminal layer of cells appear to be secretory (see Toker, 1967).

The presence of a well organized filamentous component in the division furrows in dividing cells of the end buds of the growing mammary ducts of the mouse has recently been described (Scott & Daniel, 1970).

B

Alveolar cells

As already noted the shape of the alveolar cells depends on the state of distension of the alveolus. The cells are firmly joined to one another by junctional complexes at the intercellular boundary just below the luminal surface although the junctional complexes are not always well defined; the lateral surface of the alveolar cell adjoining the next cell is almost straight. From the free surface of the cells, i.e. the luminal surface, arise numerous microvilli which may reach a length of 1 μm. These microvilli may not be evenly distributed over the free surface but they can be closely packed, for example in the mouse gland there may be some 25/sq μm forming a brush border with a large surface area. A certain amount of filamentous substance adheres to the free surface expecially around the microvilli. The basal region of the alveolar cells abuts on the myoepithelial cells or the basement membrane and shows folding of the cell membrane to produce numerous irregularly shaped cytoplasmic processes forming a labyrinthine system of clefts between the cell membrane and basal lamina (Ehrenbrand, 1962; Adamiker & Glawischnig, 1967; Bargmann & Welsch, 1969). These cytoplasmic processes are best seen in those cells which are near capillaries and may well be concerned in the uptake of substances from the extracellular spaces. The nuclei of the alveolar cells are large, rounded or oval and may be somewhat indented but never lobed. A characteristic feature of the secretory alveolar cell is the highly developed granular endoplasmic reticulum or ergastoplasm in the form of membranes, covered with ribosomes, frequently running parallel to one another and extending from the cell base to the upper part of the cell; these membranes may be arranged concentrically around mitochondria. The Golgi apparatus is well developed and is usually located in the supranuclear zone. It consists of peripheral vesicles, lamellae of smooth-surfaced membranes forming flattened sacs arranged in parallel fashion, often in the form of a crescent-like stack and around the stack many small vesicles and a few vacuoles. Mitochondria are dispersed in the cytoplasm in large numbers and vary considerably in size and shape. Electron-microscopic studies have provided little evidence for direct involvement of the mitochondria in the transformation of material into secretory products although they are likely to be indirectly involved.

The electron microscope has given particularly useful information on the secretory functions of the alveolar cell. While light
microscopy had readily permitted the detection of fat globules
within the alveolar cytoplasm the mode of excretion of these fat
globules into the alveolar lumen could not be resolved (see p. 15).

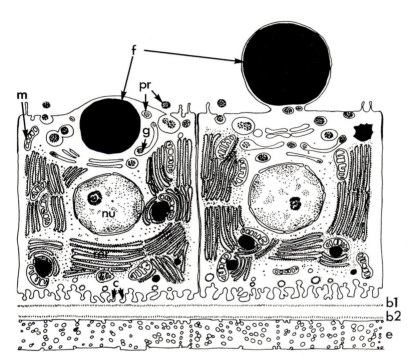

FIG. 1.10. Schematic representation of alveolar cells in the mammary
gland.

nu = nucleus   rer = rough endoplasmic reticulum
m = mitochondrion   g = Golgi apparatus
pr = protein granules in the Golgi cisterns and in the alveolar lumen
f   = fat droplets—on the right a fat droplet is being pinched off
c   = cytoplasmic processes at base of cell
b1 = basal lamina of the epithelium
b2 = basal lamina of adjacent capillary
e   capillary endothelium
(from Bargmann, W. & Welsch, U., 1969, in *Lactogenesis: the Initiation of
Milk Secretion at Parturition*, edited by Reynolds, M. & Folley, S. J.,
pp. 43–52. Philadelphia: University of Pennsylvania Press).

The smallest and most recently formed fat droplets appear in the basal region of the alveolar cell, and these droplets increase in size as they pass towards the apex of the cell (Fig. 1.10). It is generally believed that fat is synthesized within the rough endoplasmic reticulum although Kurosumi, Kobayashi & Baba (1968) dispute this view since they observed the constant presence of accumulations of tubular, vesicular or vacuolar elements of the smooth endoplasmic reticulum in the vicinity of the small fat droplets in the basal cytoplasm. Bargmann & Welsch (1969) have, however, failed to confirm these observations concerning the smooth endoplasmic reticulum nor do the observations of Kurosumi *et al.* (1968) accord with the observations of others, especially those of Stein & Stein (1967) who demonstrated, in an electron-microscopic autoradiographic study, that after esterification of the fatty acids into glycerides in the rough endoplasmic reticulum, an *in situ* aggregation of lipid occurs with the appearance of fat droplets. Bargmann & Welsch (1969) also comment that the close association of the fat droplet with bowl-shaped mitochondria may be significant and find a parallel with the shape of the mitochondria in the cells of brown adipose tissue.

The mechanism of release of the fat globules into the alveolar lumen has also been clarified. When the fat droplet reaches the cell apex it causes the plasmalemma to bulge and to lose its microvilli. As protrusion continues the fat droplet surrounded by an envelope of plasma membrane becomes pinched off from the cell body, the plasma membrane forming a gradually constricting neck between the apex of the cell and the globule (Fig. 1.11). As the constriction narrows varying amounts of cytoplasm containing protein granules and sometimes organelles may be included within the fat globule envelope (Stockinger & Zarzycki, 1962; Stein & Stein, 1967; Sekhri, Pitelka & DeOme, 1967*a*; Girardie, 1968; Helminen & Ericsson, 1968*a*; Kurosumi *et al.*, 1968; Wellings, 1969). The constricted neck of membrane eventually becomes closed off and ruptures and the globule surrounded by plasma membrane falls free into the lumen. About 1% to 5% of the fat globules may have portions of cytoplasm attached (Wooding, Peaker & Linzell, 1970). The diameter of the fat droplets lying free in the lumen may range from 1–18 μm. The apex of the cell remains virtually sealed off and seldom is there any evidence of the free escape of organelles such as mitochondria into the lumen.

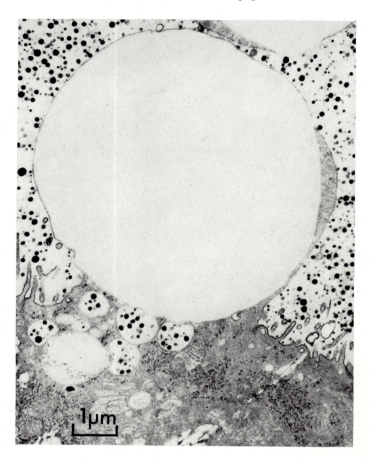

Fig. 1.11. Electron micrograph of apical portion of alveolar cell of mammary gland from a lactating rat showing fat globule becoming pinched off (from Bargmann, W., 1964, *Germ. med. Mon.* **9**, 309–313).

Patton & Fowkes (1967) have presented biochemical evidence in support of the role of the plasmalemma in enveloping the fat globule and they have also provided a rationale for the biophysics of the process—the envelopment of the droplet being due to London–Van der Waals forces estimated to achieve an attraction force of several atmospheres at distances between the membrane and droplet of about 2 nm. Keenan, Morré, Olson, Yunghans &

Patton (1970) also conclude that there is little doubt that the milk-fat globule membrane originates directly from the plasmalemma although some structural re-arrangement of the membrane constituents occurs for, while the membrane is relatively stable in the predominantly aqueous environment of the cytoplasm, it is

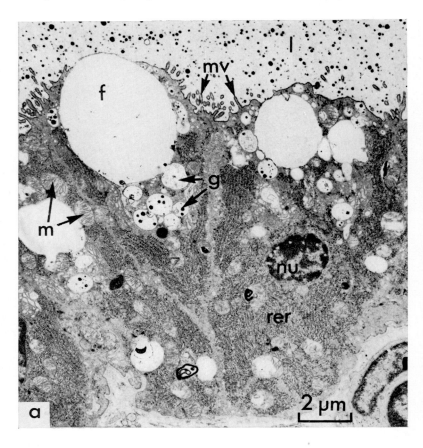

Fig. 1.12 (a) Electron micrograph of alveolar cells of mammary gland from lactating rat.

nu = nuclei   rer = rough endoplasmic reticulum
m = mitochondria   mv = microvilli
g = Golgi apparatus containing protein granules
f = fat droplet   l = lumen containing protein granules

(from Bargmann, W., 1964, *Germ. med. Mon.* **9**, 309–313).

likely that it will undergo a re-arrangement when it comes in contact with the less polar and more hydrophobic fat droplet.

Clearly there must be a considerable loss of plasmalemma from the alveolar cells as fat droplets are excreted and Patton & Fowkes (1967) have suggested that the plasma membrane may be, at least in part, replenished from the membranes of the vacuoles containing the protein granules when these vacuoles open to the surface (see below). Further references to the structure of the fat-globule membrane will be found in the reviews by Prentice (1969) and Storry (1970).

The milk protein appears as a finely granular material within the flattened sacs and vacuoles of the Golgi apparatus (Fig. 1.12*a*). This finely granular material varies in granule size from 10 to 30 nm (Wellings, 1969), but when examined under higher magnification these fine granules are seen to consist of small particles about 1·5–2·0 nm in diameter and while this size may correspond to the diameter of the casein molecule great caution is necessary in evaluating these sub-units as refraction phenomena might simulate particles of this size (Bargmann & Welsch, 1969). The finely granular material itself aggregates to form chains of granules or 'micelles'—the mature protein granules or droplets (Fig. 1.12*b*). The origin of the smallest particles still requires clarification. It is generally believed that specific proteins are synthesized in the rough endoplasmic reticulum and that they progress by a route at present unknown to the inner spaces of the Golgi apparatus where a particular portion is concentrated to form milk protein granules (Wellings & Philp, 1964). These granules along with other materials enclosed in vacuoles move towards the apex of the cell, the vacuoles come to rest just below and in contact with the plasmalemma and finally open into the lumen. The vacuoles containing the protein granules are bordered by a triple-layered membrane about 10 nm thick (Helminen & Ericsson, 1968*a*) and as noted above this membrane may help to replace plasmalemma lost during the excretion of fat droplets. The size of the mature protein granules or droplets varies with the species, and the following approximate diameters are given by Bargmann (1964) man: 30 nm; cow: 80–120 nm; rat: 150–300 nm; mouse: 100–250 nm.

Although the protein granules were first clearly revealed by electron microscopy they can be seen under the light microscope if sections of the mammary gland are cut on the ultramicrotome

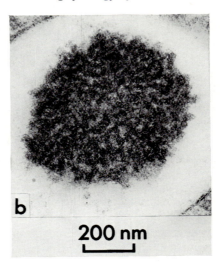

FIG. 1.12. (b) Electron micrograph of part of Golgi cistern in the alveolar cell of mammary gland from a lactating rat showing a mature protein granule composed of aggregated fine granular material (from Bargmann W., & Welsch, U., 1969, in *Lactogenesis: The Initiation of Milk Secretion at Parturition*, edited by Reynolds, M. & Folley, S. J., pp. 43–52. Philadelphia: University of Pennsylvania Press).

(0·25–1·0 μm thick) and stained with toluidine blue–pyronine (Hollmann & Verley, 1966).

While the protein granules are normally shed into the lumen of the alveolus, Hollmann (1966) has observed in the lactating rabbit that occasionally granules fuse within the vacuole which may then lose its membrane thus liberating the protein aggregate into the cytoplasm; protein granules may also find their way into the intercellular spaces and even into the perialveolar connective tissue. Hollmann was unable to decide whether the granules reached these sites by way of the lumen or from vacuoles opening into the side or base of the alveolar cells, but he considered that these processes represented a form of resorption of protein during normal lactation.

Evidence has been obtained for accepting the protein nature of these granules; first, they do not dissolve in fat solvent but they can be digested with trypsin (Wellings, Grunbaum & DeOme, 1960), secondly autoradiographic studies show that ^{3}H-leucine is concentrated in the Golgi apparatus during the formation of these granules (Wellings & Philp, 1964; Fiske, Courtecuisse & Haguenau 1966; Verley & Hollmann, 1966). Preliminary electron microscopic studies of the protein granules and fat globules in raw milk by the freeze etching technique have recently been reported (Buchheim, 1969, 1970a, b).

There has been some discussion as to whether the complex type of secretion as described above in alveolar cells should be termed 'apocrine' (Adamiker & Glawischnig, 1967; Kurosumi, Kobayashi & Baba, 1968; Wooding, Peaker & Linzell, 1970). We consider there is much in favour of the proposal of Bargmann & Welsch (1969) that the term 'apocrine secretion' should be abandoned, for it is associated with erroneous concepts of lipid formation which originated in the 19th century and we have therefore avoided its use.

Myoepithelial cells

The nucleus of the myoepithelial cell is elongated, its long axis being parallel to the basement membrane; it may be considerably indented and may present dense chromatin masses at its periphery. The cytoplasm has a low electron density and contains fine myofilaments which run parallel to the long axis of the cell processes and are inserted into the cell membrane (Bässler, Schäfer & Paek, 1967). Near the nucleus and on its upper (luminal) side the organelles are situated—Golgi apparatus, some mitochondria, some rough endoplasmic reticulum and lysosomes. After the injection of oxytocin the myoepithelial cells form dense fibrillar swellings at the cell base and the basal membrane of the myoepithelial cell is contracted into a series of corrugations at the insertions of the myofilaments. Owing to the compressive forces exerted on the alveolar cells part of the cell membrane of an alveolar cell may sometimes be extruded in a small prolapse-like structure between two adjacent myoepithelial cells (Bässler et al., 1967) (see also Fig. 1.5b).

Connective tissue

Zarzycki (1964) has described the ultrastructure of two types of fibroblasts in the stroma of the guinea-pig mammary gland. In one type the whole of the cytoplasm is filled with rough endoplasmic reticulum, in the other type the endoplasmic reticulum is poorly developed but slender fibrils are present in the peripheral parts of the cell, similar fibrils lying on bundles on the surface of the fibroblast extending into the intercellular substance. The intercellular substance contains large bundles of interlacing collagen fibrils. The first type of fibroblast is considered to indicate that the cell is actively synthesizing collagen, the second type with scant ergastoplasm may indicate that collagen synthesis has been completed and the cells are transforming into fibrocytes.

Teat

The ultrastructure of the bovine teat canal has been investigated by Chandler, Lepper & Wilcox (1969) with special reference to the role of the teat canal as a barrier against mammary infections. Specialization of cell connexions across the intercellular spaces of the basal epidermal cells were observed. The connecting processes between contiguous cells were numerous, appearing in section as thin projections curving in varying planes and intercalating strongly with each other in the form of desmosomal junctions. It is suggested that these connexions are an adaptation facilitating expansion and contraction of the canal relevant to sphincter function. The keratin layer appeared to be derived from epidermal cells as would any antibacterial substances it might contain, there being no evidence of any specific secretion.

Cytochemistry

Studies on the cytochemistry of the mammary gland have been well reviewed by Mayer & Klein (1961) and by Ehrenbrand (1964) and we shall refer in the main to subsequent studies.

Proteins

Immunofluorescent staining techniques have been used by Turkington (1969b) and by Young & Nelstrop (1969, 1970) to determine the cellular localization of casein and α-lactalbumin in the mammary glands of the lactating rat and mouse. Both proteins were detected in virtually all the secretory epithelial cells, thus supporting the concept that the expression of differential function in terms of these specific milk proteins is not segregated into specific cell types but is homogeneous among the secretory cells (Turkington, 1969b).

Mucopolysaccharides

In a histochemical study of the mucopolysaccharides of the stroma of the human breast, Ozzello & Speer (1958) observed that the intralobular connective tissue contained mainly acid mucopolysaccharides the concentration of which varied during the menstrual cycle, the highest levels being reached just before menstruation. The increases in acid mucopolysaccharides were coincident with increases in stromal cellularity and were considered to be associated with increased oestrogen levels. The interlobular stroma contained mostly neutral mucopolysaccharides which showed little change, suggesting that this part of the stroma has essentially a supportive function. Extensive histochemical studies of the mammary stroma of rats during the various stages of mammary growth and function have confirmed the role of oestrogens in inducing a rise in the concentration of acid mucopolysaccharides in the intralobular connective tissue (Bässler, Schulze & Schriever, 1970).

Iron

The presence of iron in the mammary epithelium has been known for many years (see review by Mayer & Klein, 1961) but the earlier cytochemical studies have now been supplemented by electron microscope studies and the following description is based on the observations of Bässler (1963), Ehrenbrand (1964), Miyawaki (1965) and Girardie (1967b). Iron has been detected in the mammary epithelium in virgin mice over the age of 30 weeks, and in the mammary epithelium of mice, rats, rabbits and guinea-pigs in late lactation and during mammary involution; it has also been detected in mammary tissues of man and dog. In general the amount of iron deposits increases with age and with multiparity. In histological sections iron is associated with the lipofucsin type of insoluble lipo-pigments while the electron microscope reveals ferritin-like particles free in the cytoplasm and also associated with membraneous or vacuolar structures, and with many of the small dense bodies which show acid phosphatase activity and may therefore be regarded as lysosomes. In mice these deposits of iron may remain for long periods in the mammary tissue if the animal does not again become pregnant but if pregnancy does occur then there is a marked reduction in the amount of iron during late pregnancy and lactation.

Iron-binding proteins of whey have been studied in human milk and in the milk of the cow, rat, rabbit, quokka (*Setonix brachyurus*) and echidna (*Tachyglossus aculeatus*) (for references see Blanc & Isliker, 1963; Baker, Shaw & Morgan, 1968; Jordan & Morgan, 1969). In human and bovine milk the iron-binding protein has been variously named 'red milk protein', lactotransferrin, lacto-siderophilin, ekkrinosiderophilin, and perhaps more commonly lactoferrin. In man, lactoferrin differs in amino-acid composition and in its immunological properties from transferrin—the iron-binding protein in plasma but also present in low concentration in milk—and it has a greater avidity for binding iron than trans-ferrin (see Blanc & Isliker, 1963; Schade, Pallavicini & Wisemann, 1969). Lactoferrin is, however, not specific to the mammary gland nor to milk for it can be found in most exocrine secretions, in the kidney, and in the spleen (Masson, Heremans & Ferin, 1968; Masson, Heremans, Schonne & Crabbé, 1969). In rabbit milk an iron-binding protein is present in high concentration but it is chemically and immunologically similar to the transferrin in rabbit blood, differing in composition by having only one sialic acid residue instead of two. It has been designated 'milk transferrin' (Baker, Shaw & Morgan, 1968). In addition to its role of binding iron, lactoferrin possesses bacteriostatic activity when not fully saturated with iron and has been described as a 'bacteriostatic paint' protecting mucosae from bacterial invasion (Masson, Heremans, Prignot & Wauters, 1966; Oram & Reiter, 1968; Masson, Heremans & Ferin, 1968). There is not much information about the role of lactoferrin in mammary physiology but Blanc & Isliker (1963) consider that the most likely route for the transfer of iron from plasma to milk is the direct wresting of iron from transferrin by lactoferrin. The content of iron in the milk would thus depend on the concentration of apolactoferrin (i.e. iron-deprived lactoferrin) in the alveolar cells, the greater its biosynthesis the more iron will be extracted from the plasma.

Girardie (1967b) considers that during mammary involution the destruction of lactoferrin in the alveolar cells by hydrolytic enzymes (e.g. acid phosphatase) liberates iron in the form of ferritin within the lysosomes. These stores of iron in the mammary gland can be again immobilized and their disappearance in pregnancy and early lactation can be explained on the basis of a resumed synthesis of apolactoferrin and the binding of the iron for transport into the milk.

In the rat and rabbit the iron-binding protein is not considered to aid iron transfer into the milk (Ezekiel, 1965; Baker, Shaw & Morgan, 1968).

Enzymes

Leucine aminopeptidase. Aminopeptidase activity occurs mainly in lysosomal particles and is probably an indication of lysosomal proteolytic potentiality (see Bitensky, 1967). In histochemical studies on the mammary tissues of the mouse, rat, guinea-pig, rabbit, dog, cow and man, leucine aminopeptidase has been variously reported as being present in the duct epithelium, alveolar epithelium and in the endothelium of the blood vessels— the more usual locations being the duct epithelium and sometimes the alveolar epithelium during pregnancy. There is, however, considerable disagreement in the various studies on its location and as to whether, in some species, its presence in mammary epithelium is merely an artefact due to diffusion from the blood vessels. While this enzyme may well have a proteolytic role during mammary involution its function in the mammary epithelium during pregnancy and lactation remains obscure (Talanti & Hopsu, 1961; Arvy, 1961; Girardie & Porte, 1965; Girardie, 1967b).

Acid phosphatase. Acid phosphatase—another enzyme associated with the lysosomal system—has been studied by histochemical methods by Miyawaki (1965) and Girardie (1967a, b) who reported its presence in the mammary gland of mouse, rat, rabbit, guinea-pig, dog and man. Electron-microscopic studies showed that the enzyme was associated with multivesicular and lysosome-like structures. Acid phosphatase is frequently present in small bodies rich in ferritin but usually absent from the larger ferritin-containing bodies; this behaviour may reflect its possible role in breaking down lactotransferrin.

Acid phosphatase also occurs in the myoepithelial cells.

Other enzymes. Bässler & Paek (1968), Bässler & Brethfeld (1968) and Simpson & Schmidt (1970) have reported cytochemical studies on other enzymes in the mammary gland of rats during mammary growth and lactation; these include glucose-6-phosphatase, adenosine triphosphatase, 5′-nucleotidase, glucose-6-phosphate-dehydrogenase, succinic dehydrogenase, lactate dehydrogenase and monoamine oxidase.

MAMMARY GLAND IN THE MALE

In man the mammary gland remains rudimentary, there are no alveoli but only a series of ducts which are lined by a two-layer epithelium. In some ducts there may be a breakdown of the superficial layer of cells with accumulation of debris in the lumen. The various histological studies on the male gland have been reviewed by Dabelow (1957). The ultrastructure of the male gland has been described by Bässler & Schäfer (1969*a*) who observed no signs of secretory activity in the epithelial cells although portions of cytoplasm appeared to be extruded into the lumen and the desquamation of whole superficial cells was observed (see p. 113).

CELLS IN MILK

The nature of the cells present in milk depends on the stage of lactation, the main difference being between colostral secretions and normal milk. Mayer & Klein (1961) have reviewed the many studies on the cytology of the mammary secretions and we shall therefore consider studies subsequent to their review.

Colostrum

Colostral secretions may occur under various circumstances (*a*) in the new-born i.e. witch's milk, (*b*) in some species during certain phases of the reproductive cycle, (*c*) at the end of normal pregnancy, (*d*) during weaning, (*e*) under conditions of hormone or drug administration for experimental or clinical purposes and (*f*) during endocrine disturbances. In general colostral secretion appears when a hormonal lactogenic stimulus acts on the secretory cells but is not followed by the removal of the secretions so formed. The secretion is thus stored in the gland and differs in chemical composition from milk and can be distinguished on cytological examination by the presence of the colostral corpuscles (the corpuscles of Donné). Colostrum also contains mononuclear cells —lymphocytes, macrophages (histiocytes) and desquamated epithelial cells: the presence of polynuclear cells is generally indicative of an inflammatory process. The colostral corpuscles first described by Donné in 1837 may reach a diameter of 40 μm, and since their discovery their origin has been an enduring source of controversy. They have been accorded leucocytic, epithelial and histiocytic origins (see reviews by Mayer & Klein, 1961; Simon, 1968). Mayer & Klein (1961) consider that their origin is histiocytic, i.e. they are derived from monocytes or histiocytes, and that they are responsible for the removal or partial removal of the lipids from the stagnant secretion within the gland. On the other hand, it has been postulated that they are responsible for the transport of fat into milk, i.e. they represent an aspect of fat excretion (Duran-Jorda, 1944). In a series of studies Okada (1956*a*, *b*, 1957, 1958*a*, *b*, 1959, 1960) concluded that most of the colostral corpuscles were of lymphoid origin but some were of neutrophil origin; he failed to obtain evidence of adsorption of milk fat by these cells and he considered that the fatty inclusions within them represented a fatty degeneration of the cells themselves and that the appearance of these cells in milk was associated with stimulation of the pituitary–adrenocortical system. Girardie, Gros, Le Gal & Porte (1964) using the electron microscope studied the corpuscles of Donné in the regressing mammary gland of the mouse and, having found no evidence to support the view that the cells were of mesenchymal origin or functioned as macrophages, they concluded that these cells were desquamated and necrosing alveolar epithelial cells. Further support for the epithelial origin of the colostral corpuscles came from both light (using 0·5 μm thick sections) and electron-microscopic studies on the mammary glands of mice, rats and rabbits by Verley & Hollmann (1967) (also Hollmann & Verley, 1967) who reached precisely the same conclusions as Girardie *et al.* (1964).

The proponents of the histiocytic origin of the corpuscles, however, have returned to give battle and in the last two years they have affirmed that the corpuscles are macrophages. Smith & Goldman (1968) studying human colostrum concluded that the cells were macrophages engorged with fat, noting that the cells were amoeboid and phagocytic both in fresh colostrum and in culture. They also observed the frequent close association of lymphocytes and macrophages (lymphocyte–macrophage inter-actions) which is deemed to be of immunological significance and they postulated that the ingestion of maternal cells in the colostrum by the neonate might affect its immunological status. In a later study on the *in vitro* culture of colostral cells Murillo & Goldman (1970) demonstrated the synthesis of immunoglobulins IgA and β_1C by the cells but there was no evidence for the synthesis of IgG and IgM; they considered that β_1C was in all probability produced by the macrophages. (The synthesis of IgA in rabbit mammary tissue cultured for short periods has recently been investigated by Lawton, Asofsky & Mage, 1970.) Independent studies by Lascelles and his colleagues have also led to the conclusion that colostral corpuscles are macrophages (Lee, McDowell & Lascelles, 1969; Lascelles, Gurner & Coombs, 1969). After infusion of colloidal carbon into the mammary glands of cows and ewes during involution clumps of carbon were observed in the cytoplasm of the colostral corpuscles, also in some typical macrophages but rarely in polymorphs, suggesting that the colostral corpuscles are the predominant phagocytic cells. Histological studies of these infused mammary glands showed the presence of carbon-laden colostral cells not only in the alveoli and ducts but in the interstitial spaces between alveoli, in the lymphatics within the mammary gland and in the regional lymph node. The authors conclude that the phagocytosis of fat by macrophages with its subsequent transport to the regional lymph node is the most important mechanism by which fat is removed from the involuting mammary gland. Lascelles and his colleagues also confirmed the avid phagocytic activity of human colostral corpuscles in culture, the corpuscles taking up fat globules, colloidal carbon and carbonyl iron when these substances were added to the culture medium; they were, however, unable to detect immunoglobulin on the surface of the colostral cells.

Also relevant to the question of the nature of the colostral corpuscles are further observations by Lee & Lascelles (1969*a*) who confirmed that fatty vacuolation and degenerative changes occur in the alveolar cells of the ewe mammary gland in the early stages of involution (see Chapter 4) and while these fat-laden degenerating alveolar cells with faintly staining nuclei might be found free in the secretion they could nevertheless be readily distinguished from the fat-laden macrophages or colostral corpuscles whose nuclei were deeply staining; moreover fat-laden macrophages were still plentiful in the secretion 32 days after milking had ceased when degenerating epithelial cells had virtually disappeared and the alveolar remnants and ducts were lined with regenerated epithelium.

It is evident that this century-old controversy of the origin of the corpuscles of Donné is not entirely resolved, the bulk of the experimental evidence seems to support the view that the corpuscles are macrophages which have ingested varying quantities of fat but it seems also true that, in some species at least, when colostrum is produced particularly in the involuting gland that desquamated and degenerating alveolar cells may also appear in the secretion and closely resemble the fat-laden macrophages. There is, however, little or no evidence to indicate that such alveolar cells are phagocytic.

Milk

The nature of the cells in milk has been studied mainly in the woman and cow with reference to the diagnosis of early mastitis, and this field has been reviewed by Cullen (1966). Studies by Okada (1960) on the cells in the milks of nine different domestic and laboratory animals suggest that the same types of cell occur in all the milks but that the proportions of the various types of cells vary considerably with the species and with the stage of lactation. There is some evidence in the cow that leucocytes may be removed from the blood by the mammary gland during milking but the physiological significance of this is not known (Paape & Guidry, 1969).

Numerous cell fragments, apparently derived from the alveolar cells, are present in milk (Paape & Tucker, 1966; Wooding, Peaker & Linzell, 1970).

INNERVATION OF THE MAMMARY GLAND

The mammary gland is of cutaneous origin and its innervation is the same as that of the contiguous skin. Particulars of the precise nerve supply of the mammary gland in the various species will be found in the standard text-books of human and veterinary anatomy and in the reviews by Turner (1939, 1952) and Linzell (1953). Recent studies on the nature of the innervation have been reviewed by Cross (1961*b*) and Findlay & Grosvenor (1969). The mammary nerves contain somatic sensory and sympathetic motor fibres but there is no evidence of the existence of a parasympathetic innervation. The sympathetic innervation supplies the smooth muscle of the blood vessels, of the teat, and the very limited smooth muscle on the ducts and in the cistern wall. Findlay & Grosvenor (1969) conclude that there is no evidence that the myoepithelial cells are innervated, although the nervous system does exert some measure of control over the resistance of the duct system, nor is there support for the existence of a neural substrate within the mammary gland sufficiently well-developed to act as an afferent link for reflex arcs activated by intramammary pressure changes within physiological ranges (see p. 217). It has been suggested, however, that very fine non-myelinated nerve fibres of the C type, which have a slow rate of conduction, may be present in mammary tissue. Such fibres would be extremely difficult to demonstrate even under the electron microscope (Linzell, 1971). The nature of the sensory nerve endings in the teat and nipple is discussed in Chapter 6.

CIRCULATORY SYSTEM OF THE MAMMARY GLAND

'It is worth recalling that the mammary glands are entirely skin structures. . . . Being found in various regions of the body in different mammals, the mammary glands share the blood, lymph, and nerve-supply of the skin of the area' (Linzell, 1961); and, as Cooper (1840) observed, 'it therefore appears that if the gland receives its supply of arterial blood, it matters little, as to the secretion, from what source it is derived'.

Anatomy

Details of the anatomy of the vascular supply and drainage of the mammary gland in the various species will be found in the reviews given by Turner (1939, 1952). More detailed information for the bovine udder is given by Swett & Matthews (1949) and Ziegler & Mosimann (1960); and for the laboratory animals by Linzell (1953).

Several trans-illumination techniques have been described for studying the microvasculature and microcirculation in the mammary glands of living mice (Glebina, 1940; Linzell, 1955; Warner, Reynolds & Henning, 1968) but have been little used.

The vasculature of the udder of the sheep has been described by Palić (1954) who studied the effects of unilateral ligature of the main supply artery on the arterial anastomoses between the two glands.

Linzell (1960*a*) has made important observations on the venous drainage of the ruminant mammary gland (goat, sheep and cow) which have relevance to reliable blood sampling and blood flow measurements in biochemical and physiological investigations (Fig. 1.13). The classical description of the venous drainage of the ruminant udder names three vessels, (1) the external pudic vein running from the base of the udder through the inguinal canal, (2) the caudal superficial epigastric vein (subcutaneous abdominal or 'milk' vein) running from the cranial border of the udder towards the thorax, and (3) the perineal which runs from the caudal border of the udder towards the vulva. Linzell (1960*a*) found valves in all the main veins in the mammary region of the sheep, goat, cow, mare and sow. In the virgin goat, ewe and heifer the valves were all competent and their direction is such that the external pudic carried all the mammary venous blood together with some blood from surrounding areas; the perineal and caudal superficial epigastric veins carried blood *towards* the mammary region and into the external pudic vein. Since the caudal superficial epigastric vein anastomoses with the cranial superficial epigastric vein there is a point where blood may flow in either direction; this in the virgin goat and sheep lay just behind the umbilicus, as cranial to this point the valves point forward while caudal to it the valves are backward-pointing; in the heifer the point of reversal was about the level of the front pair of teats. In goats and sheep that are pregnant, or lactating, or have lactated, the external pudic and the superficial epigastric veins become greatly enlarged and the valves in the caudal superficial epigastric veins in the mammary region become completely incompetent, the valves in the external pudic also become partially incompetent and permit back flow to occur; the valves in the perineal vein, however, usually remain competent. As a result of these valvular deficiencies when the animal is standing the flow in the caudal superficial epigastric and sometimes in the external pudic veins is in the reverse direction to the flow in the virgin female, so that some or all of the mammary blood leaves by way of the caudal superficial epigastric veins. When the animal lies down or is placed on its back the flow then reverts to the virgin condition. To ensure

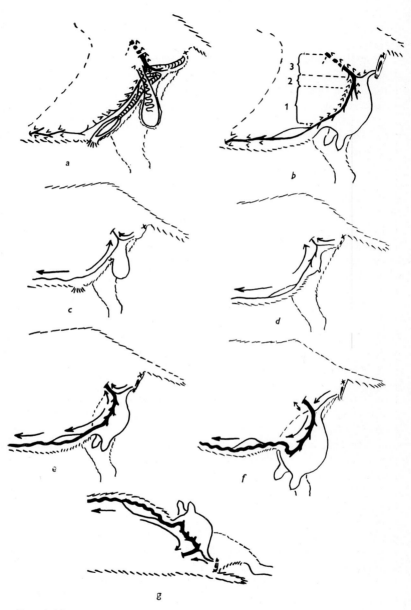

Fig. 1.13.

proper sampling of mammary blood or to measure total mammary venous flow in the conscious ruminant Linzell (1960a) recommends that the external pudic vein be manually compressed between the base of the udder and the inguinal canal, and that the perineal vein be compressed just below the vulva, thus ensuring that mammary blood leaves only by way of the caudal superficial epigastric vein and is not diluted by blood from non-mammary tissues.

Blood flow rates

In recent years there has been a need for an accurate but simple method of measuring blood flow through the mammary gland. The more usual procedures which have been used have been briefly discussed by Reynolds, Linzell & Rasmussen (1968). Initially blood flow was determined by use of the Fick principle from the mammary arterio-venous differences of a milk precursor in the blood, usually Ca or P and the quantity of the substance appearing in the milk in a given time; however, the method has grave limitations (see Folley, 1949). More satisfactory methods also based on the Fick principle have now been developed. In the goat and cow Rasmussen (1963, 1965) has measured mammary blood flow from the rate of appearance of antipyrine in the circulation after its injection into the duct system of the mammary gland; in goats, Reynolds (1964, 1965) has determined mammary blood flow by the uptake of inhaled N_2O from the blood by mammary tissue and the difference between arterio-venous concentrations of N_2O during the time required for the two concentrations to come to virtual equilibrium.

Another method of determining mammary blood flow is the thermodilution method developed by Linzell (1966a), based on the technique of Fegler (1957), which involves the injection of

---

FIG. 1.13. Position of valves in the veins of the ventral abdomen of the goat. (a) male goat: (b) female goat—1. valves which are always incompetent in multiparous females; 2. valves which are usually incompetent in older females; 3. valves which are sometimes partially incompetent in old females;
Usual direction of venous blood flow in:
(c) males of all ages; (d) virgin females; (e) primiparous females; (f) multiparous females; (g) females of all ages when held on the back
(from Linzell, J. L., 1960a, *J. Physiol.* **153**, 481–491).

cold saline into the vein and recording its passage downstream with a needle thermocouple.

Direct arterial blood flow measurements can be made by an electro-magnetic technique based on the principle that blood, an electric conductor, flowing between two poles of an electro-magnet cuts the lines of magnetic force and induces a current in electrodes which also lie across the blood stream; the current so produced is proportional to the flow of blood (Westersten, Herrold & Assali, 1960).

The antipyrine, N_2O and thermodilution techniques have the advantage that they can be repeatedly used in conscious lactating or non-lactating animals whereas the direct flow measurements involve surgical intervention for the implantation of the probe and the risk of eventual damage to the wall of the artery. Reynolds *et al.* (1968) compared the above four techniques used simultaneously in both anaesthetized and conscious goats. The continuous thermodilution method and the electro-magnetic method gave similar results, the N_2O method tended to give flow rates which were about 19% lower, while the antipyrine method overestimated flow rates by some 30%. The authors conclude that none of the four methods is ideal and that there is still room for improvements in techniques for blood flow determinations.

Reynolds (1969) using the continuous thermodilution method has determined the rate of mammary blood flow in goats from three weeks before to 3 weeks after parturition. The flows were relatively constant until 2–3 days before parturition, the day before parturition the flow had increased 70% and by a few hours before kidding it had increased 120% over the late pregnancy values; a further increase was noted just after parturition (180%), thereafter there was a gradual fall in the flow rate which, however, remained above the late pregnancy rate. These increases in blood flow rates preceded increases in mammary oxygen consumption so that the factor responsible for the increase in blood flow operates in anticipation of the energy needs of the lactating gland. Reynolds postulates that the increased blood flow to the mammary gland is associated with a marked decrease in blood flow to the uterus and there thus seems to be a reciprocal shifting of uterine and mammary circulations. Dramatic increases in mammary blood flow at the time of parturition have also been observed in cows (Kjaersgaard, 1968b).

In rats cardiac output and mammary blood flow increase significantly during lactation but at parturition cardiac output shows little change; the increases during lactation may well be associated with the increasing milk yields which reach peak values about day 12 (Chatwin, Linzell & Setchell, 1969).

Vascular changes in mammary engorgement

Vascular changes during mammary engorgement in lactating rats have been briefly described by Silver (1956). Some 36–48 hr after removal of the litter there was a marked reduction in the number of patent capillaries over the alveoli, after 110 hr when the alveoli were tending to collapse the capillaries again filled with blood. Lactation could be re-established only if suckling were recommenced within 110 hr, the capillary beds refilling shortly after the renewal of suckling.

Development of the vascular system

The growth of the vascular system of the mammary gland during pregnancy and lactation has been studied in the mouse by Turner & Gomez (1933) and in the mouse, rat, guinea-pig and rabbit by Dabelow (1934). Dabelow noted that the lobules of alveoli developed in relation to the already established vascular system of the fat pad so that the lobules and fat pad shared a common capillary network which enlarged as the parenchyma replaced the stroma. The development of the mammary capillaries in the bovine foetus is closely associated with the development of the fat pad (Chumakov, 1961).

A detailed study of the mammary vascular system in mice during pregnancy and lactation and under experimental conditions of hormone administration and hormone deficiencies has been reported by Soemarwoto & Bern (1958). They observed that a single mammary duct was usually supplied by capillary plexuses associated with several arterioles and venules. During the oestrous cycle no significant changes in the vascularity of the mammary glands of the virgin mouse were detected although there occurred a gradual increase in the richness of the vascularity with increasing age. In the first few days of pregnancy there was a marked increase in the capillary plexuses around the ducts but later these disappeared from the main ducts, by day 6 the capillary plexuses supplying the finer ducts and developing lobules were visible, their numbers increasing during the second and third weeks of pregnancy, the maximum number being reached by days 19–20 and thereafter maintained throughout lactation. There was an increase in capillary size during lactation. Ovariectomy combined with either adrenalectomy or hypophysectomy caused a severe regression of the vascular system, and duct plexuses were rarely seen. Intact female mice treated with oestrogen or adrenal steroids showed an increased mammary vascularity and more capillary plexuses were present than in untreated mice; when treated with oestrogen + progesterone or with prolactin (ovine) or growth hormone (bovine) the mice showed a vascularity of the mammary glands similar to that of the second week of pregnancy except that capillary plexuses were present on ductal as well as on lobulo-alveolar regions. Adrenocortical and anterior pituitary hormones required the presence of the ovary for any effects on the vascular system to be exerted. The various changes in the vascular bed occurred in close association with changes in the particular glandular structures (ducts or alveoli) and did not occur in their absence since removal of the mammary gland from the fat pad prevented any response in the vascular bed to hormonal stimulation although the bed of the adjacent or contralateral intact gland was stimulated.

Proliferation of the endothelial cells of arterioles and venules in the mouse mammary gland in early lactation has been demonstrated by Traurig (1967a) using ³H-thymidine and autoradiographic techniques.

Permeability of mammary blood vessels

The vascular permeability to particulate fat of the smaller blood vessels in the mammary gland which are lined with a continuous endothelium has been investigated by Schoefl & French (1968) in lactating rats, mice and guinea-pigs. Chylomicra and particles of an artificial fat emulsion were observed to concentrate on, and apparently stick to, the luminal surface of the vascular endothelium (Fig. 1.14). No evidence of penetration of the endothelium by the chylomicra was obtained but some of the artificial fat particles did appear to enter the cytoplasm of the endothelial cells. The evidence obtained favoured the views that the chylomicra were broken down by lipase action on, or very close to, the

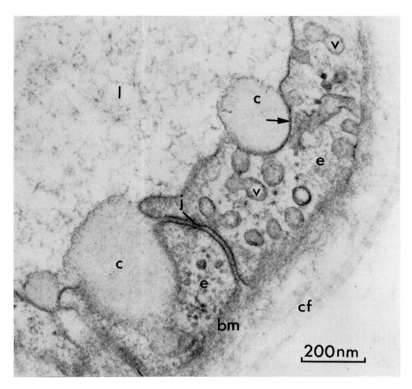

FIG. 1.14. Two chylomicra sinking into the cytoplasm of the endothelial cells of a small blood vessel in the mammary gland of a lactating rat 10 min after the intravenous injection of chyle. No gap is apparent (arrow) between lipid particles and cell membrane.

l = lumen   c = chylomicron
e = endothelium   bm = basement membrane
cf = collagen fibres   v = vesicle   j = junctional complex
(from Schoefl, G. I. & French, J. E., 1968, *Proc. R. Soc.* B **169**, 153–165).

luminal surface of the endothelium and that the fatty acids so released were rapidly transported across the endothelium.

Lymphatic system

Anatomy

Descriptions of the mammary lymphatic system in the various species have been reviewed by Turner (1939, 1952). More detailed studies of the anatomy and structure of mammary lymph nodes of the cow have been made by Hampl (1964, 1965*a*, *b*, 1967, 1968) and of the sheep by Hampl, Bartoš & Zedník (1967).

The lymphatic drainage of the human breast has been studied by vital dye staining and radiography. The direction of lymph flow is normally away from the nipple. The lymphatic trunks are contiguous to the dermis in the areolar area and tend to course deeper peripherally; in most cases drainage is specifically to the axilla (Halsell, Smith, Bentlage, Park & Humphreys, Jr., 1965; Kett, Varga & Lukács, 1970).

Because the mammary gland lymphatics form the major route for the removal of protein resorbed from the alveoli during mammary involution in sheep (Lascelles, 1962; Mackenzie, 1968), Lee & Lascelles (1969*b*) have recently made a detailed study of the distribution of the lymphatic capillaries and vessels in the mammary gland of the lactating ewe. The regional efferent lymphatic ducts were ligated to cause dilatation of the lymphatic system within the mammary gland, at autopsy the mammary gland was fixed by intravascular perfusion and the perfusate replaced with coloured latex or reconstituted blood so as to distinguish as far as possible the blood capillaries from the lymphatic capillaries. After hardening, the mammary gland was cut into slices and blocks prepared for histological examination. The lymphatic capillaries originated in the interalveolar spaces and drained into larger vessels passing in turn through the intralobular, interlobular, intralobar and interlobar connective tissues hence to radicles of the main afferent ducts.

Lymph flow

In 1959 Linzell (1959*b*) reviewed what scanty information there was available at that time on the lymph flow from the mammary gland. Since then a number of studies have been reported which indicate that, in ruminants at least, the rate of lymph flow from the mammary gland is relatively high. Studies in goats have been reported by Linzell (1960*b*), Reynolds (1962), Grachev & Gostev (1962) in which lymph has been collected for long periods, three weeks or longer, when daily flow rates from 150 to 840 ml. were obtained. Lascelles, Cowie, Hartmann & Edwards (1964) studied lymph flow in cows for periods up to 26 days: in non-lactating animals the flow rate ranged from 7 to 120 ml./hr per half-udder, i.e. two mammary glands, just before parturition and in early lactation the rate increased to 1300 ml./hr when as much as 25 l./day were collected from the half-udder; values of over 20 l./day were also reported from the half-udder of lactating cows by Peeters, Cocquyt & De Moor (1963, 1964) and up to 10 l./day by Kottman, Hampl & Pravda (1970). In sheep lymph flows of 1–50 ml./hr were noted by Lascelles & Morris (1961).

The act of milking is said to increase the rate of lymph flow in the goat (Grachev & Gostev, 1962) and in the cow (Peeters, Cocquyt & De Moor, 1963, 1964) but this was not observed by Linzell (1960*b*) in the goat nor by Lascelles *et al.* (1964) in the cow.

Studies on the composition of the lymph of the cow were first reported by Heyndrickx & Peeters (1958*a*, *b*) and by Heyndrickx (1959, 1961) who collected lymph from the mammary lymph ducts immediately after the animals had been killed. Linzell (1960*b*) in studies on the composition of mammary lymph in the goat obtained by cannulation of the lymph ducts noted that when lymph was collected under general anaesthesia the rate of flow was reduced and that significant changes occurred in the composition of the lymph compared with lymph collected from the conscious goat. Because of this observation Linzell queried the value of lymph samples collected post mortem for investigations on lymph composition; the validity of this criticism was later acknowledged by Verbeke & Peeters (1965).

The composition of the lymph collected from the mammary gland in the conscious goat and its relationship to plasma are similar to those of lymph from other organs. The main difference between mammary lymph and plasma is that the protein content of lymph is considerably less; the concentrations of electrolytes in lymph and plasma are very similar but strikingly different from those in milk. In short the composition of mammary lymph in normal lactation appears to result from diffusion of plasma from capillaries but with no back diffusion from mammary alveoli or ducts (Linzell, 1960*b*; Reynolds, 1962). In distension of the mammary gland, however, there is a marked movement of protein (Mackenzie, 1968) and of lactose (Kuhn & Linzell, 1970) from the alveoli into the lymph and probably of other milk constituents as well. Similar observations on the general composition of mammary lymph have been reported in the sheep (Lascelles & Morris, 1961) and in the cow (Lascelles *et al.*, 1964).

The amino acid composition of bovine lymph has been studied in samples collected both *in vivo* by cannulation and in post-mortem samples (Verbeke & Peeters, 1965). The concentrations of the individual free amino acids in the mammary lymph obtained *in vivo* were similar to those present in the cow's plasma but in the post-mortem samples of lymph the concentrations of many amino acids were 2–4 times higher. The composition of the mammary lymph may be of importance relative to studies on the uptake of milk precursors as determined from arterio-venous differences. Clearly if uptake is to be measured quantitatively from simultaneous measurements of blood flow and arterio-venous differences it is necessary to know what quantities of possible precursors are removed from the plasma and returned to the circulation by way of the lymph. Linzell (1960*b*) discusses the problem and considers that in most studies the quantities of precursor that pass to the lymph are small (e.g. about 2% of the Ca and 0·5% of the glucose) relative to the errors associated with measuring the mean uptake from the plasma—because of the high blood flow the arterio-venous differences are often small.

Skin temperature over the mammary gland

Thermographic techniques, in which the skin over the breasts is scanned by an infrared camera and a thermal image is recorded, are being developed for physiological (see p. 187) and diagnostic purposes (see Vuorenkoski, Wasz-Höckert, Koivisto & Lind, 1969; Feasey, James & Davison, 1970).

PROLACTIN AND RELATED MAMMOTROPHIC HORMONES

CHEMISTRY

Prolactin

Isolation and preparation

The lactogenic activity of the anterior pituitary was first demonstrated by Stricker & Grueter in 1928 while they were studying the gonadotrophic effects of anterior pituitary extracts in rabbits. Subsequently Stricker (1951) reviewed the events leading to this important observation. Attempts by Stricker & Grueter to isolate the hormone concerned were unsuccessful but a few years later Riddle, Bates & Dykshorn (1933) prepared partially purified extracts and showed that the lactogenic response was associated with the recently discovered property of the anterior pituitary to stimulate the secretory activity of the pigeon crop sac. The other anterior pituitary hormones—gonadotrophins, growth hormone and thyrotrophic hormone—which at that time had been fairly well characterized—did not appear to participate in the response. Riddle and his colleagues designated this new hormone 'prolactin' (subsequently it has been variously given the names 'mammotrop(h)in', 'galactin', 'lactogen', 'lactogenic hormone' and perhaps most unsuited of all—'luteotrophin', see p. 63).

The pigeon crop response proved a useful method of assay and greatly facilitated the subsequent purification and isolation of the hormone. We do not propose to consider in great detail the various methods of preparation and purification of prolactin since there have been numerous reviews about the problems involved (e.g. Folley, 1952; Lyons & Dixon, 1966; Forsyth, 1967). The early isolation procedures were based on extracting the hormone from pituitary tissue into acid or alkaline solution, followed by extraction with ethanol or acetone and fractional precipitations. The methods were tedious as they required the recycling of the main product through a series of fractional precipitation steps, nevertheless a highly purified material was obtained and by 1936–7 Lyons had prepared from sheep pituitaries virtually pure prolactin—one of the first of the anterior pituitary hormones to be isolated in this state. Later an isolation procedure was developed by Cole & Li (1955) in which the purification was carried out by countercurrent distribution techniques (see review by Li, 1961).

In 1961 Ellis described an extraction procedure with ammonium sulphate for ox, sheep and pig pituitaries which provided in sequence extracts containing (1) mainly FSH, (2) LH & TSH, (3) GH and (4) prolactin. Ellis's procedure was subsequently used for the routine preparation of anterior pituitary hormones distributed by the Endocrine Study Section of N.I.H.* Jiang & Wilhelmi (1965) have further purified the prolactin-rich extract obtained by the Ellis procedure by extraction with alkaline ethanol followed by ethanol precipitation, dialysis and salt fractionation of the active material. This procedure gave excellent yields of highly active prolactin, and the ox and sheep prolactin so obtained could be still further purified by DEAE-cellulose chromatography. Rat prolactin has also been prepared by Ellis, Grindeland, Nuenke & Callahan (1969) by sequentially extracting rat pituitary glands with ammonium sulphate by a modification of the Ellis (1961) procedure to remove other anterior pituitary hormones, then extracting and precipitating the prolactin with ethanol and effecting further purification with gel filtration and chromatography on DEAE cellulose; this procedure yielded a rat prolactin assaying 28–37 i.u./mg (see also Ahmad, Lyons & Ellis, 1969).

In recent years the development of immunoassays for prolactin has given impetus to the development of new procedures suitable for isolating prolactin from small amounts of pituitary tissue since the development of an immunoassay in a given species usually requires the isolation of prolactin from that species. These new

* We take this opportunity of acknowledging the important part played in advancing endocrine research by the scheme which the Endocrine Study Section of N.I.H. started in 1956 for the distribution to investigators of highly purified pituitary hormones.

methods have been reviewed by Forsyth (1967) and include the isolation of prolactin from particulate fractions obtained from pituitary gland homogenates by differential centrifugation, e.g. rat prolactin (Hodges & McShan, 1970), rat and mouse prolactins have also been isolated from the sub-cellular fractions of pituitary tumours (see Kwa, van der Bent & Prop, 1967; Kwa, Verhofstad & van der Bent, 1967). Small quantities of purified prolactin can also be obtained by the use of starch gel or polyacrylamide gel electrophoresis and Groves & Sells (1968) prepared rat prolactin, assaying 15 i.u./mg, by extracting 20 rat pituitaries with ammonium sulphate followed by preparative polyacrylamide gel electrophoresis. Mouse prolactin has also been isolated directly from mouse pituitaries by disc electrophoresis in a polyacrylamide gel (Yanai, Nagasawa & Kuretani, 1968; Cheever, Seavey & Lewis, 1969). The mouse prolactin obtained by this method had a potency of 16 i.u./mg (Cheever *et al.*, 1969).

The preparation of internally labelled rat prolactin with ^{3}H and ^{14}C-lysine has been described by Catt & Moffat (1967); the pituitaries were incubated *in vitro* in the presence of the labelled amino acids and the prolactin isolated by preparative disc electrophoresis. Similar studies have been described using slices of bovine pituitaries incubated in a medium containing ^{3}H-DL-phenylalanine or ^{3}H-L-leucine with subsequent purification of the prolactin by the Ellis (1961) procedure followed by isoelectric precipitation and chromatography on DEAE cellulose (Rao, Robertson, Winnick & Winnick, 1967).

Tashjian (1969) has recently predicted that within the next decade it should be possible to use cell culture methods for manufacturing purposes to produce hormones in quantity.

Storage

It has been customary to store pituitaries awaiting extraction in acetone but fresh freezing appears to give the best preservation of the biological activity of prolactin (Desjardins, Sinha, Hafs & Tucker, 1965). Its electrophoretic behaviour, and subsequent staining properties may, however, be altered by deep-freezing possibly because free fatty acids, liberated by lipolysis of lipid esters, are absorbed by the prolactin (Lewis & Cheever, 1967; Nicoll, Parsons, Fiorindo & Nichols, Jr., 1969).

The use of toluene as an antimicrobial agent in pituitary extracts may give misleading results in studies using gel-electrophoresis as the prolactin band may be increased in intensity while the growth hormone band is reduced (Lewis & Cheever, 1967).

Heterogeneity

The sheep prolactin prepared by Cole & Li was at first considered to be monodisperse with a molecular weight of 24,200; it assayed at 35 i.u./mg and was essentially free from other anterior pituitary hormones. However, despite chemical and biological evidence of purity the application of further separation techniques disclosed polydispersity in the sense of a number of biologically active components rather than contamination by inactive materials. The phenomenon is apparently associated with reversible and irreversible polymer formation during certain stages of the isolation procedure, and also with the actions of proteolytic enzymes and with chemical degradation during preparation. While Li and his colleagues found that fractions consisting largely of monomer, dimer and polymer respectively showed no significant differences in amino-acid composition or biological activity, other workers have separated fractions differing in biological activity. The monomer has also been isolated by several other workers (for references see review by Forsyth, 1967). The determination of monomer molecular weights of proteins showing concentration-dependent association-dissociation behaviour presents some difficulties but the gel filtration method devised by Andrews (1966) is particularly suitable and this technique indicates a molecular weight of 20,000 for the monomer of sheep prolactin (see review by Forsyth, 1967, also Cheever & Lewis, 1969). Molecular weights of bovine, rat and mouse prolactins are 24,000, 23,000 and 23,000 respectively (Cheever & Lewis, 1969).

Amino-acid sequence of prolactin

The complete amino-acid sequence of sheep prolactin (Fig. 2.1) has been recently published by Li, Dixon, Lo, Pankov & Schmidt (1969); its empirical formula (198 amino-acid residues) being as follows: Lys_9 His_8 Arg_{11} Asp_{33} Thr_9 Ser_{15} Glu_{22} Pro_{11} Gly_{11} Ala_9 Cys_6 Val_{10} Met_7 Ile_{11} Leu_{22} Tyr_7 Phe_6 Trp_2. There are three disulphide bridges—between residues 4 and 11, 58 and 173, and between 190 and 198.

NH₂- Thr- Pro- Val- Cys- Pro- Asn- Gly- Pro- Asp- Cys- Gln- Val- Ser- Leu- Arg- Asp- Leu- Phe- Asp- Arg- Ala- Val- Met-
   1   5   10   15   20

Val- Ser- His- Tyr- Ile- His- Asn- Leu- Ser- Ser- Glu- Met- Phe- Asn- Glu- Phe- Asp- Lys- Arg- Tyr- Ala- Gln- Gly- Lys-
 25   30   35   40   45

Gly- Phe- Ile- Thr- Met- Ala- Leu- Asn- Ser- Cys- His- Thr- Ser- Ser- Leu- Pro- Thr- Pro- Glu- Asp- Lys- Glu- Gln- Ala-
 50   55   60   65   70

Gln- Gln- Thr- His- His- Glu- Val- Leu- Met- Ser- Leu- Ile- Leu- Gly- Leu- Arg- Ser- Trp- Asn- Asp- Pro- Leu- Tyr- His-
          75   80   85   90   95

Leu- Val- Thr- Glu- Val- Arg- Gly- Met- Lys- Gly- Val- Pro- Asp- Ala- Ile- Leu- Ser- Arg- Ala- Ile- Glu- Ile- Glu- Glu-
                100   105   110   115   120

Glu- Asn- Lys- Arg- Leu- Leu- Glu- Gly- Met- Glu- Met- Ile- Phe- Gly- Gln- Val- Ile- Pro- Gly- Ala- Lys- Glu- Thr- Glu-
           125   130   135   140

Pro- Tyr- Pro- Val- Trp- Ser- Gly- Leu- Pro- Ser- Leu- Gln- Thr- Lys- Asp- Glu- Asp- Ala- Arg- His- Ser- Ala- Phe-
 145   150   155   160   165

Tyr- Asn- Leu- Leu- His- Cys- Leu- Arg- Arg- Asp- Ser- Ser- Lys- Ile- Asp- Thr- Tyr- Leu- Lys- Leu- Leu- Asn-
 170   175   180   185

Cys- Arg- Ile- Ile- Tyr- Asn- Asn- Asn- Cys- COOH
 190   195   198

FIG. 2.1. Amino-acid sequence of the sheep prolactin molecule (from Li, C. H., Dixon, J. S., Lo, T. B., Pankov, Y. A. & Schmidt, K. D., 1969, *Nature, Lond.* **244**, 695–696).

c

Primate prolactin

Primate prolactin has not yet been isolated and its existence is still a matter of controversy. Application of the usual chemical and electrophoretic separation procedures to human and monkey pituitaries has not so far succeeded in separating growth hormone from prolactin. Human growth hormone, however, has itself intrinsic prolactin-like activities (see below) and while it has been possible to prepare fractions from human pituitary tissue which differ in their ratio of growth hormone to prolactin activity the significance of this is debatable; do the differing ratios represent a partial separation of two related but distinct molecular entities—human growth hormone and human prolactin, or do they arise from chemical degradation during purification of a single homogeneous protein with both activities intrinsic to it? (see reviews by Apostolakis, 1968; Forsyth, 1969; Lyons, 1969). However, evidence in favour of the existence of a human pituitary prolactin seems to be accumulating (see p. 66 and Addendum 2).

Primate growth hormone

Homogeneous primate growth hormone preparations exhibit prolactin-like activity which thus appears to be an intrinsic characteristic of human and simian growth hormone (Li, 1968; Peckham, Hotchkiss, Knobil & Nicoll, 1968). In passing it may be noted that non-primate growth hormone, apart from its mammotrophic action in some strains of mice, has no other prolactin-like effects (see review by Cowie, 1966).

Procedures for the purification of human growth hormone have been reviewed by Greenwood (1967*b*) and Li (1968); the method favoured for chemical studies involves saline extraction, ammonium sulphate fractionation, chromatography on cation exchanger, ethanol fractionation and finally exclusion chromatography on Sephadex, a yield of about 70 mg from 50 fresh pituitary glands being obtained.

For clinical studies much of the HGH has been prepared by the Raben (1959) procedure, which involves extraction of pituitary tissue by glacial acetic acid, removal of ACTH and intermedin by adsorption on oxycellulose, and ethanol precipitation of the active material, or by the procedures devised by Wilhelmi and his colleagues (Wilhelmi, 1961; Parlow, Wilhelmi & Reichert, 1965) which involve serial fractionation with ammonium sulphate. A simplified extraction procedure for obtaining HGH for clinical studies has recently been described by Mills, Ashworth, Wilhelmi & Hartree (1969).

Apostolakis (1965, 1968) (see also Apostolakis, Theile & Berle, 1969) has described a method, involving water extraction of acetone-dried human pituitaries followed by acetone and iso-electric precipitations and final purification by Sephadex chromatography, which is claimed to give preparations of unusually high activity when assayed by the pigeon-crop method (see p. 69).

Reports that patients treated with HGH may develop antibodies and cease to respond to the therapy have led to the suspicion that during some extraction procedures the hormone becomes chemically altered to the extent that the immunological system of the recipient regards the hormone as a foreign protein. Because of these immunological problems an isolation procedure using ultra-filtration has recently been described which does not expose the hormone to extremes of pH or of ionic strength or to organic solvents, and which is said to give an aggregate-free hormone in a good yield (8 mg/pituitary gland) which is highly active and exhibits a high degree of homogeneity (Lewis, Cheever & Seavey, 1969; Lewis, Parker, Okerlund, Boyar, Litteria & Vander Laan, 1969).

The biosynthesis of HGH internally labelled with ^{14}C (L-leucine-^{14}C or an L-amino acid-^{14}C mixture) by culturing foetal pituitaries *in vitro* has been described by Gitlin & Biasucci (1969).

The primary structure of HGH (Fig. 2.2) has been determined by Li and his colleagues (see Li, Dixon & Liu, 1969). Human growth hormone has a molecular weight of 21,500. The molecule consists of a single polypeptide chain, its empirical formula (188 amino-acid residues) is as follows: Lys_9 His_3 Arg_{10} Asp_{12} Asn_8 Thr_{10} Ser_{18} Glu_{17} Gln_9 Pro_8 Gly_8 Ala_7 Cys_4 Val_7 Met_3 Ile_8 Leu_{25} Tyr_8 Phe_{13} Trp_1. Disulphide bridges are formed by residues 68–162 and 179–186.

Comparison of the primary structures of HGH and sheep prolactin reveals three homologous segments in each molecule comprising approximately 45% of either peptide chain which strongly suggests their separate evolution from a common ancestor molecule (Bewley & Li, 1970).

Growth hormone from the pituitaries of rhesus monkeys has been prepared in a homogeneous form by Peckham (1967) by

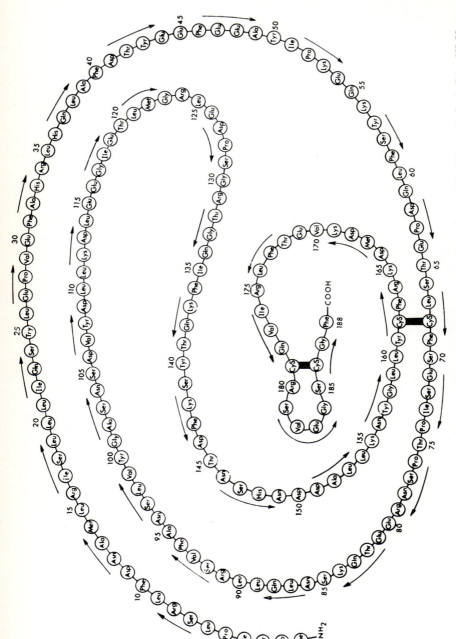

Fig. 2.2. Amino-acid sequence of the human growth hormone molecule (from Li, C. H., Dixon, J. S. & Liu, W-K., 1969, *Archs Biochem. Biophys.* **133**, 70–91). (See Addendum 2)

the sequential application of exclusion chromatography, ion-exchange chromatography on DEAE Sephadex with a single eluent and density gradient column electrophoresis. Its molecular size is similar to that of HGH.

Chorionic somato-mammotrophin (placental lactogen)

The early attempts to detect mammotrophic activities in the placentae of various species have been reviewed by Lyons (1958). At that time there was evidence for the presence in rat placentae of a prolactin-like substance and there were hints that a similar substance might be present in human placenta.

Man. A prolactin-like substance was isolated from the human placenta by Kurosaki (1961) and by Ito & Higashi (1961) (see also Higashi, 1961, 1962) and independently by Josimovich & MacLaren (1962). This substance was initially referred to as human placental lactogen but the term human chorionic somato-mammotrophin (HCS) has since been deemed more appropriate (Li, Grumbach, Kaplan, Josimovich, Friesen & Catt, 1968).

The various procedures for the isolation of HCS have been reviewed by Forsyth (1967). In general the procedures have been modifications of those used for HGH. Aqueous alkaline extraction of the placental tissue is usually followed by fractional precipitation with ammonium sulphate and further purification by chromatographic procedures. Highly purified preparations of HCS have been made but few if any have been homogeneous either because of association phenomena or because of chemical alteration during preparation. Catt, Moffat, Niall & Preston (1967) prepared HCS which was homogeneous on gel filtration, disc electrophoresis and analytical ultra-centrifugation but when the molecular weight was determined by equilibrium ultra-centrifugation some heterogeneity of molecular weight was apparent. The graphical estimate of the molecular weight of this preparation was 39,000 but the minimum molecular weight calculated from quantitative NH_2-terminal data was 21,500. Florini, Tonelli, Breuer, Coppola, Ringler & Bell (1966) and Catt, Moffat, Niall & Preston (1967) suggested that HCS might be a dimer composed of two HGH-like molecules. In reviewing the evidence, however, Forsyth (1967) considered that HCS might be a single polypeptide chain of molecular weight about 20,000 and subject to association phenomena. A recent study by Andrews (1969) on the gel-filtration behaviour of several highly purified preparations of HCS indicates that HCS does exist in dilute solution as a monomeric form similar to that of HGH; for the more homogeneous preparations he obtained a molecular weight of 18,600 to 20,400 while in the heterogeneous preparations an elution peak corresponding to a molecular weight of 38,000–40,000 was noted. Andrews concluded that HCS could exist as a monomer in dilute solution at physiological pH but that the dimer and higher aggregates are the stable forms. As will be noted later (see p. 64) there is some evidence that HCS must be in the dimer form to exhibit its biological activity (Breuer, 1969).

The biosynthesis of internally labelled HCS by the *in vitro* culture of placental tissue has been described by Gitlin & Biasucci (1969) and Suwa & Friesen (1969*a*, *b*).

The amino-acid sequence of HCS has not been fully established. Catt, Moffat & Niall (1967) determined the sequence of the first 17 residues from the NH_2-terminus, of these 11 are identical with those occupying the same position in the HGH molecule. Sherwood (1967; see also Sherwood in discussion to Friesen, Suwa & Pare, 1969) has confirmed the observations of Catt, Moffat & Niall (1967) and has found that similarities in the rest of the peptide chain are even more striking. There is no doubt that HGH and HCS share major similarities in amino-acid composition, in sequence and in the location of the two disulphide bonds (see also Parcells, Dahlgren, & Evans, 1968).

Other primates. A prolactin-like hormone is present in monkey placenta (Kaplan & Grumbach, 1964) but there has been little attempt to extract or characterize the material. Grant, Kaplan & Grumbach (1970) have studied crude chorionic somato-mammotrophin (MCS) obtained from monkey placenta by salt extraction and fractional precipitation with ammonium sulphate. Gel filtration studies showed two elution peaks corresponding to molecular weights of 25,000 and 50,000 but while this may indicate the presence of polymeric forms no evidence of dimer formation was obtained on further gel filtration of the extract.

The *in vivo* biosynthesis of MCS has been studied by Friesen, 1968 (also Friesen *et al.*, 1969) and it appears to be one of the major proteins synthesized by the monkey placenta.

Non-primates. Prolactin-like activity has been detected in the placenta of the rat (see Lyons, 1958; Wrenn, Bitman, DeLauder & Mench, 1966; Kinzey, 1968; Matthies, 1967, 1968; Desjardin, Paape & Tucker, 1968; Shani (Mishkinsky), Zanbelman, Khazan & Sulman, 1970) and of the mouse (Cerruti & Lyons, 1960; Kohmoto & Bern, 1970) but so far as we are aware the active material has not been isolated (see Addendum 2).

BIOLOGICAL ACTIVITIES OF THE LACTOGENIC HORMONES

Physiological studies

Prolactin (non-primate)

The mammotrophic (i.e. mammogenic and lactogenic) activities of prolactin and its pigeon-crop stimulating activity have been extensively reviewed by Lyons & Dixon (1966) and are further discussed elsewhere in this book. Prolactin, however, has numerous other activities in mammals; one of the better-known of these being its luteotrophic activity from which it has derived one of its names—luteotrophin. This designation is, however, unfortunate since only in a few species—rat, mouse and possibly ferret is this activity observed (see reviews by Lyons & Dixon, 1966; Bern & Nicoll, 1968; also Ahmad, Lyons & Ellis, 1969). It has been claimed that prolactin influences maternal behaviour in rats but the evidence for this is still controversial (see reviews by Lehrman, 1961; Riddle, 1963; also Zarrow, Grota & Denenberg, 1967).

In the male prolactin may be concerned in the growth of the accessory reproductive organs of mice, rats and possibly guinea-pigs but the physiological significance of these observations is not yet established (see review by Meites & Nicoll, 1966; also von Berswordt-Wallrabe, Steinbeck, Hahn & Elger, 1969). Prolactin may also participate in the regulation of androgen production by the interstitial tissue of the mouse testis (Bartke & Lloyd, 1970). Effects of prolactin on renal function and on lipid metabolism have been reported (see review by Apostolakis, 1968) as have growth-hormone like effects in animals and man (see review by Forsyth, 1967).

It is necessary to emphasize that caution is necessary in interpreting experimental observations since most studies have been carried out with ruminant prolactins and it may be desirable in many instances for confirmatory studies to be made using homologous prolactin (see reviews by Meites & Nicoll, 1966; Cowie, 1969b).

Prolactin (primate) (see p. 66 and Addendum 2)

Human growth hormone (HGH)
The mammotrophic activities of HGH are noted elsewhere in this book. In man its other activities include promotion of body growth, lipolytic effects and regulation of blood glucose homeostasis (for reference see review by Greenwood, 1967b, and a series of papers in the book edited by Pecile & Müller, 1968). In rats HGH exerts both growth-stimulating and luteotrophic activities (Hartree, Kovačić & Thomas, 1965) and it increases markedly DNA synthesis in rat costal cartilage (Murakawa & Raben, 1968).

Human chorionic somato-mammotrophin (HCS)
The mammotrophic activities of HCS are similar to those of HGH and are mentioned elsewhere in this book. In its other activities, however, it differs in some respects from HGH in being in general quantitatively less active. Although it is less active in its growth promoting and metabolic activities in man it may well exert important metabolic effects in the second half of pregnancy (see Grumbach, Kaplan, Sciarra & Burr, 1968). HCS is markedly less active in stimulating body growth and DNA synthesis in costal cartilage in rodents. It is luteotrophic in mice. HCS has the property, however, of potentiating the effects of HGH in experimental animals (for references see reviews by Forsyth, 1967 and Ringler, 1968). A recent observation of some interest is that when HCS is dissociated into monomeric form it has little or no stimulatory effect on DNA synthesis in cartilage suggesting that HCS must be in a dimerized form to exert its full hormonal activities (Breuer, 1969).

Immunological studies
Interest in the species specificity of lactogenic hormones has been considerable in recent years (see review by Geschwind, 1966) and immunological techniques have played a major role in studies in this field.

Although the antigenicity of sheep prolactin was first demonstrated over thirty years ago it is only during the last fifteen years that immunological properties of the lactogenic hormones have been widely investigated (see reviews by Hayashida, 1966; Forsyth, 1967; Greenwood, 1967*a*, *b*).

An antiserum to a lactogenic hormone allows a wide range of immunological, immunoelectrophoretic, radioimmunological, immunofluorescence and antihormonal experiments to be carried out. Such immunological studies can be used (a) to supplement the physico-chemical techniques in investigations on the occurrence of heterogeneity in purified hormones, (b) in cross-reaction studies to determine relationships between the different lactogenic hormones within a species and the relationships of the hormones between species for phylogenetic and clinical purposes, (c) to reveal the presence of impurities and contaminants (e.g. other hormones, serum proteins) in purified hormone preparations, (d) to reveal the presence of lactogenic hormones in tissue cells using antibody tagged with enzymes or fluorescing dyes, (e) to assay rapidly and accurately hormonal activity during the various stages of purification of lactogenic hormones and in body fluids and tissues in physiological and clinical studies and (f) to assess changes in the antigenicity of the hormone molecule after its partial hydrolysis or chemical modification by proteolytic enzymes or other chemical treatments.

Prolactin

There is serological cross-reaction between prolactins of the sheep, cow and goat, but not between sheep prolactin and pituitary extracts from rat, rabbit, dog, pig, guinea-pig, pigeon and man. Some of the more sensitive procedures such as micro-complement fixation have, however, revealed minor immunological similarities between the prolactins of species previously regarded as different, e.g. rat and sheep prolactin (for references see review by Forsyth, 1967). The antibiological activity of antiserum to sheep prolactin has been demonstrated in pigeons (see review by Forsyth, 1967) and more recently Saji & Crighton (1968) have shown that the antiserum will inhibit the local lactogenic response to prolactin injected into the galactophores of the pseudopregnant rabbit.

Since human prolactin has not yet been isolated no specific antiserum has been prepared against it. Pasteels (1969), however, has immunized rabbits against organ culture media containing what he terms 'human prolactin secreted *in vitro*' (HPSIV) and has obtained immune sera which will inhibit the crop-sac stimulating activity of HPSIV. These sera, as Pasteels notes, carry no claim to immunological specificity since they contain antibodies to other proteins present in the culture medium (see Addendum 2).

Human growth hormone (*HGH*)

Antiserum to HGH cross-reacts with monkey GH but not with growth hormones of non-primates but there are serological relationships between the growth hormones of various species (see review by Greenwood, 1967*b*). If there is a human prolactin, then existing evidence derived from organ culture studies (see p. 68) suggests that it and HGH will not cross-react. HGH does not cross-react with sheep prolactin nor with a trypsin digest of bovine GH (Sundaram & Sonenberg, 1969).

Human chorionic somato-mammotrophin (*HCS*)

The immunochemical studies on HCS have been reviewed by Forsyth (1967); while HCS and HGH share antigenic determinants they each have determinants not present in the other (see Sherwood, 1967). There is little cross-reaction between HCS and sheep prolactin or human chorionic gonadotrophin.

Monkey CS is immunologically more closely allied to HCS than to monkey GH (Grumbach & Kaplan, 1964).

THE PROBLEM OF THE SEPARATE IDENTITIES OF HUMAN GROWTH HORMONE AND HUMAN PROLACTIN

The use of standard chemical and electrophoretic separation procedures has not yet resulted in the isolation of separate growth hormone and prolactin activities from human and monkey pituitary glands (for references see Forsyth, 1969). Lyons, Li & Johnson (1960) showed that a human pituitary fraction which possessed growth-promoting activity was mammotrophic and lactogenic in the rat and also stimulated the pigeon crop sac. However, although human growth hormone (HGH) preparations were found to be equipotent with purified ovine prolactin when assayed by the intraduct rabbit mammary test (Fig. 2.3), the pigeon-crop stimulating activity of HGH was extremely weak (Forsyth,

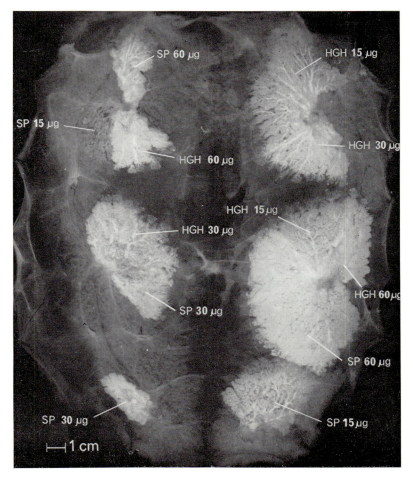

Fig. 2.3. The freshly dissected mammary glands of a pseudopregnant rabbit showing the lactogenic responses in those sectors of the mammary glands which 7 days previously had received injections of sheep prolactin (SP), assaying 21 i.u./mg, or human growth hormone (HGH) in doses of 15, 30 or 60 μg (in 0·3 ml. saline) into the mammary duct draining the respective sector. Both hormones have induced a similar degree of lacto-genesis. The non-injected sectors contain no milk and their lobulo-alveolar tissue shows only faintly (from Cowie, A. T. & Folley, S. J., 1970, in *Scientific Foundations of Obstetrics and Gynaecology*, edited by Philipp, E. E., Barnes, J. & Newton, M., pp. 423–432. London: Heinemann Medical Books. Photograph by courtesy of Dr. Isabel A. Forsyth).

Folley & Chadwick, 1965). It is of interest that human chorionic somato-mammotrophin (HCS) shares, with HGH, this property of high activity in the rabbit lactogenic test and low pigeon-crop stimulating activity (Forsyth & Folley, 1970), and it is possible that HGH and HCS play a role in the normal development of the breast and in lactation (for fuller discussion see Forsyth, 1969; Forsyth & Folley, 1970). Histological evidence has been presented for the presence of prolactin-secreting cells in the human pituitary (Pasteels, 1963) (see p. 79). In addition, studies with cultured human pituitary glands *in vitro* have shown that, under such conditions, while the titre of HGH in the incubation medium decreases with time, that of prolactin increases (see Pasteels, 1969) while polyacrylamide electrophoresis of a human pituitary tumour revealed the absence of HGH and the presence of prolactin (Peake, McKeel, Jarett & Daughaday, 1969). The two latter studies could be criticized on the grounds that the material under investigation was not produced by a normal pituitary *in situ* and that more convincing evidence might be obtained by assay of the blood of lactating women during or shortly after suckling. However, a further problem arises here, since Stephenson & Greenwood (1969) reported the presence of human chorionic somato-mammotrophin (HCS) in blood samples taken after suckling from lactating women six days post partum and from patients with galactorrhoea. Since, by definition, this could hardly have been HCS, they suggested that either it provided evidence for a human prolactin related immunologically to HCS, or that an artefact of radioimmunoassay was involved. In contrast to these findings, Spellacy & Buhi (1969) could not detect HCS during the early post partum period. More recently, Forsyth (1970) detected prolactin activity, by the *in vitro* lactogenic bioassay, in the blood of lactating women, and radioimmunoassay of the plasma samples showed that there was insufficient HGH present to account for the prolactin activity.

Recently evidence suggesting the independent secretion of growth hormone and prolactin by adenohypophyses of rhesus monkeys has been obtained from *in vitro* studies (Nicoll, Parsons, Fiorindo, Nichols, Jr. & Sakuma, 1970).

In conclusion, therefore, while HGH and HCS possess prolactin-like activity, and although a separate primate prolactin has yet to be demonstrated unequivocally, the evidence in favour of a distinct primate prolactin seems to be increasing (see review by Boot, 1970). (See Addendum 2.)

METHODS OF ASSAY

Methods for the biological assay of prolactin were reviewed recently by Forsyth (1967) and we shall, therefore, focus attention on the current state of the various assay techniques. Before discussing individual biological assay methods it should be pointed out that, in general, they suffer from a lack of sensitivity which limits their application for direct estimation of circulating levels of prolactin in body fluids. For this reason some of them are likely to be superseded in the near future by radioimmunoassay methods. A preparation of ovine prolactin was established as the Second International Standard for prolactin with a defined potency of 22 i.u./mg (Bangham, Mussett & Stack-Dunne, 1963).

Biological and chemical assays

Pigeon assay

The basis of this assay is the stimulation of the pigeon's crop-sac mucosa by exogenous prolactin. When the hormone is administered systemically, the method is relatively insensitive. Some improvement in precision was reported by using older pigeons and by injecting prolactin over a longer period (Bates, Garrison & Cornfield, 1963), practices which had been used in our laboratory for many years (see Clarke & Folley, 1953). Greater sensitivity is achieved by the local method of pigeon crop assay, introduced by Lyons & Page (1935), in which the hormone is injected intradermally. A problem with this latter technique has been to devise a satisfactory objective method for scoring the response of the crop sac. The methods used include the measurements of the diameter of the response (Grosvenor & Turner, 1958a; Pasteels, 1963), cutting out, drying and weighing the stimulated area (Kanematsu & Sawyer, 1963a) and the combination of the latter technique with a balanced incomplete block design (Forsyth & Hosking, 1969) which makes allowance for the variation which is considerable between birds but not significant between right and left crops of the same bird (Nicoll & Meites, 1963). Further modifications of the Kanematsu & Sawyer (1963a) method include the use of an instrument which applies a uniform degree of stretch to a hemi-crop to enable a standardized 4 cm disc of mucosa to be scraped from the site of local injection (Nicoll, 1967), a procedure which has also been applied to the systemic pigeon assay (Nicoll, 1969). Methods of assessing the crop sac response which utilize the uptake of ^{32}P or ^{3}H-methyl thymidine or the measurement of RNA and DNA levels have also been reported (Peruzy, Amoruso & Pavoni, 1963; Ben-David, 1967; Nicoll & Bern, 1968) since prolactin-induced stimulation of the crop sac mucosa is mediated via RNA and protein synthesis (Sherry & Nicoll, 1967). Cytological changes in the crop sac mucosa which occur in response to prolactin have been investigated at the ultrastructural level by Bässler & Forssmann (1964) and Dumont (1965).

When the pigeon crop sac is stimulated by prolactin, the response of the crop sac reflects an increase in the number of epithelial cells, which contain large numbers of fat droplets and which exhibit intense cytoplasmic basophilia. In contrast, the injection of human urine concentrates, serum and non-specific agents causes an epithelial thickening when injected over the crop but does not induce cytoplasmic basophilia (Bahn & Bates, 1956). Specific and non-specific responses can also be distinguished on the basis of the vascular structure of the stimulated area of the crop sac (Kurcz, 1966). Attempts to assay prolactin in human blood and urine by the pigeon-crop method have been discussed by Forsyth (1969) who concludes that such assays are unsatisfactory because of (a) non-specific responses, (b) methods of extraction which have not been adequately checked for recovery, (c) results that have seldom been confirmed, and lastly because the pigeon is not the most appropriate assay animal for a primate lactogenic hormone. Support for these contentions comes from a recent study in which the most commonly used method for extracting prolactin from blood prior to assay (Sulman, 1956; Simkin & Goodart, 1960) is shown to be totally unreliable (Kurcz, Nagy, Kiss & Halmy, 1969a, b). Although prednisolone has been reported to eliminate the non-specific inflammatory response of the pigeon crop sac to unextracted human plasma (Herlyn, Jantzen, Flaskamp, Hoffman & von Berswordt-Wallrabe, 1969) the use of this steroid appears to introduce other complications, since the values for the circulating levels of prolactin in the blood of lactating women reported by Herlyn *et al.* (1969) are unrealistically high when compared with values obtained by the *in vitro* lacto-genic assay (Forsyth, 1970 and personal communication).

Luteotrophic assay

The luteotrophic action of prolactin in certain species (see p. 63) has been exploited to form the basis of several assays. These depend on the ability of prolactin to prolong dioestrus in the intact mouse (Kovačić, 1962), to support deciduomata forma-tion in the hypophysectomized and in the intact mouse (Kovačić, 1963, 1965), and to induce hyperaemia of corpora lutea of ovulation in the mouse (Kovačić, 1968). However, this latter method, which Forsyth (1967) pointed out was the most practicable for routine use, has since been shown to be non-specific (Weller, Mishkinsky & Sulman, 1968). Wolthuis (1963*a*, *b*) devised a method using hypophysectomized immature female rats treated with pregnant mares' serum and human chorionic gonadotrophin. Prolactin causes an increase in luteal cell size which is measured as a dose-related decrease in the number of corpus luteum cell nuclei per unit area in histological preparations of the ovary. This method, although tedious, is specific and has been used to measure blood prolactin levels in the rat (Wolthuis, 1963*c*).

Lactogenic assay

The initial observation of Lyons (1942) that prolactin could induce localized milk secretion in sectors of the rabbit mammary gland (see Fig. 2.3) was confirmed by Meites & Turner (1947) and was subsequently developed into a semi-quantitative assay system (Bradley & Clarke, 1956; Chadwick 1963). It was found later that by combining results obtained in several rabbits it was possible to obtain potency estimates (Forsyth, Folley & Chadwick, 1965; Rivera, Forsyth & Folley, 1967). The culture of mammary gland explants *in vitro* has been developed for the semi-quanti-tative determination of prolactin. The end-point for such assay procedures, using tissue from the virgin mouse (Prop, 1963) or rat (Mishkinsky, Dikstein, Ben-David, Azeroual & Sulman, 1967) is alveolar growth. Cultured mammary tissue (Fig. 2.4) removed from the pseudopregnant rabbit has proved to be sufficiently sensitive to measure circulating levels of prolactin in blood (see also p. 68), assessed by the presence of secretion in the explants

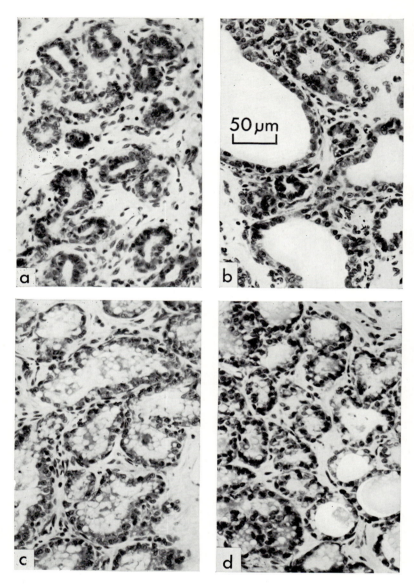

50 μm

Fig. 2.4

(Brumby & Forsyth, 1969; Forsyth, 1970 and review by Forsyth, 1971).

Electrophoresis

The separation of prolactin from other protein hormones by disc electrophoresis has formed the basis of an assay for prolactin. The isolation is performed by means of polyacrylamide disc electrophoresis and the optical density of the stained band of hormone forms the end-point of the assay. This technique has been used to monitor, semi-quantitatively, changes in level of pituitary hormones under various physiological conditions (Jones, Fisher, Lewis & VanderLaan, 1965; Lewis, Cheever & VanderLaan, 1965; Baker & Zanotti, 1966; MacLeod, Smith & DeWitt, 1966; Nicholson, 1970) and has been refined to the point where it may be considered as a quantitative method for prolactin assay (Kurcz, Nagy & Baranyai, 1969; Lewis, Litteria & Cheever, 1969; Nicoll, Parsons, Fiorindo & Nichols, Jr., 1969; Yanai & Nagasawa, 1969). As Nicoll *et al.* (1969) pointed out, although this method is not as sensitive as immunological procedures, in terms of efficiency and precision it is certainly comparable and has the advantage of being applicable to a wide variety of vertebrates after their prolactin bands have been identified.

Immunological assays

The use of serological procedures to study the purity and specificity of anterior pituitary hormones and to assay them in anterior pituitary tissue has been reviewed by Berson & Yalow (1964) and by Greenwood (1967*a*, *b*). For the assay of the hormones

---

FIG. 2.4. Sections of pseudopregnant rabbit mammary gland before and after culture in synthetic medium. (All sections at the same magnification, see (*b*), 7 μm thick, and stained with haematoxylin and eosin.)

(*a*). Mammary gland on day 11 of pseudopregnancy at time of explantation.

(*b*). Effect of culturing in the presence of insulin (5 μg/ml.) and corticosterone (1 μg/ml.) for 5 days.

(*c*). Effect of culturing in the presence of insulin (5 μg/ml.), corticosterone (1 μg/ml.) and sheep prolactin (0·5 μg/ml.) for 5 days. Note presence of fat droplets in alveolar cells and fat-laden secretion in the lumina.

(*d*). Effect of culturing in the presence of plasma from a lactating woman (10% of volume of medium), insulin (5 μg/ml.) and corticosterone (1 μg/ml.). Note presence of secretion and of fat globules.

(By courtesy of Dr. Isabel A. Forsyth.)

in blood, however, only two procedures have proved sufficiently sensitive. The first, the haemagglutination-inhibition technique, is based on the observation that red blood cells are agglutinated by immune serum when the immunizing antigen is conjugated or adsorbed on to the surface of the red blood cells; small amounts of antigen can then be detected by their ability to inhibit this agglutination (see reviews by Read, Eash & Najjar, 1962; Berson & Yalow, 1964). Experience has shown, however, that this method does not provide the sensitivity, specificity and accuracy achieved by the second procedure—radioimmunoassay—which has now virtually superseded the former.

Radioimmunoassay

The development of this procedure has been reviewed by Berson & Yalow (1962, 1964). Like other serological assays the procedure is based on the specificity of the reaction between antigen and antibody. It is possible to raise a specific antiserum to a protein or peptide hormone, such as prolactin, because the amino-acid sequence in one or more parts of the hormone molecule differs from species to species. This difference is detected by the immune-competent cells of the animal used for antiserum production and these cells produce specific antibodies. These antibodies in their turn recognize only prolactin molecules with closely similar amino-acid sequences to those responsible for eliciting the response. Two essentials are required for this assay; first a sufficiently purified hormone preparation from the species under study and one that can be conveniently labelled with a radioactive group or groups, secondly a suitable antiserum to the hormone. Radioiodine is generally used as a label, the chemistry of the iodination process being essentially the substitution of iodine into tyrosine groups.

The principles of radioimmunoassay are relatively simple. Labelled hormone binds to specific antibody to form a labelled antigen–antibody complex and the assay exploits the ability of unlabelled hormone in plasma or other solutions to compete with labelled hormone for limited antibody and thereby to inhibit the binding of labelled hormone. As a result of this competitive inhibition the higher the concentration of the unlabelled hormone the less radioactively-labelled hormone will be bound to the antibody, i.e. the ratio of antibody-bound to free labelled hormone will be decreased (see Fig. 2.5)

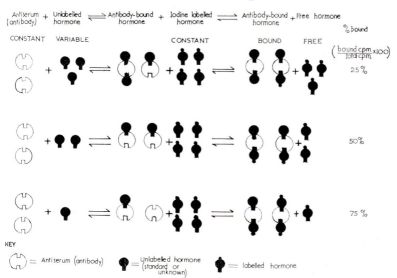

FIG. 2.5. Diagrammatic representation of radioimmunoassay technique for the assay of hormones.
(By courtesy of Dr A. S. McNeilly.)

Prolactin. The procedure may be illustrated by the method described by Bryant & Greenwood (1968) for the assay of sheep prolactin. A preliminary titration of the antiserum is carried out by incubating ^{131}I-labelled sheep prolactin (50 pg) with various dilutions of the antiserum (1 : 3000 to 1 : 536,000) and the percentage of the ^{131}I-labelled prolactin bound to antiserum is determined. The dilution of the antiserum which gives 50% binding of the prolactin is chosen for the assay. A series of standard sheep prolactin solutions (at the nanogram level) and a series of plasma dilutions are incubated with antiserum for 48 hr, ^{131}I-labelled sheep prolactin (50 pg) is then added to each dilution of standard and unknown and the incubation continued for a further 48 hr. The antibody-bound hormone is then separated from the free labelled hormone in the reaction mixture by chromatoelectrophoresis or by adsorbing the free labelled hormone on charcoal–dextran, then the radioactivities of the bound hormone and the free labelled hormone are measured for each reaction mixture. The ^{131}I-labelled prolactin which has been bound to antibody is calculated as a percentage (radioactivity of bound hormone, counts per min × 100/radioactivity of bound hormone + radio-activity of free hormone, counts per min) and is plotted against the amounts of standard added by using a logarithmic/linear plot; the amounts of ovine prolactin, or their immunological equivalents, in the test samples are calculated from this curve.

For separating the antibody-bound from the free hormone there are three main types of procedures based on:

(a) differential mobility of free and bound hormone, e.g. chromatography, electrophoresis, chromatoelectrophoresis, gel filtration;

(b) selective removal of antibody complex; e.g. double antibody technique, salt precipitation, solvent fractionation, solid-phase antibody technique;

(c) adsorption of free hormone, e.g. ion exchange, charcoal, silica, talc. References to papers dealing with the technical problems of radioimmunoassays including methods of labelling and separation of antibody-bound antigen from free labelled antigen will be found in the reviews by Hunter (1967, 1969), by Wright & Taylor (1967) and by Yalow & Berson (1969). It may also be cautionary to quote from a review by Greenwood (1967*a*) '. . . although the principles involved in radioimmunoassay are simple, it does not necessarily follow that it is simple to set up a valid assay for a particular hormone in plasma even when the techniques for that hormone have been published.' Some of the difficulties likely to be encountered have been discussed by Greenwood (1967*a*), Hunter (1967), Quabbe (1969) and Yalow & Berson (1969); these include damage to the hormone during iodination, subsequent radiation damage and damage during incubation, inefficient separation of bound and free hormone or partial dissociation of the bound complex during separation.

According to Bryant & Greenwood (1968) there is complete cross-reaction between sheep prolactin and goat pituitary extracts which permits the antiserum against sheep prolactin to be used for measuring goat prolactin. The cross-reaction between sheep and ox prolactin is, however, only partial, and it would seem preferable to prepare an antiserum for ox prolactin if ox prolactin is to be assayed.

Radioimmunoassays for prolactin have been described for the sheep (Arai & Lee, 1967; Bryant & Greenwood, 1968; McNeilly, 1971), for the goat (Bryant & Greenwood, 1968; Johke, 1969*a*, *b*;

Bryant, Linzell & Greenwood, 1970), for the cow (Johke, 1969 *a*, *b*; Karg, Hoffmann & Schams, 1969; Schams & Karg, 1969), for the rat (Kwa & Verhofstad, 1967; Kwa, Van der Gugten & Verhofstad, 1969; Niswender, Chen, Midgley, Meites & Ellis, 1969; Neil & Reichert, 1970), and for the mouse (Kwa, Verhofstad & Van der Bent, 1967).

It has not yet been possible to develop a radioimmunoassay for human prolactin since this hormone has yet to be isolated (see p. 58 and Addendum 2).

Human growth hormone (HGH). Haemagglutination-inhibition techniques were first used for the immunoassay of HGH but these have now been replaced by radioimmunological methods. The development of radioimmunoassay procedures for HGH has been reviewed by Greenwood (1967*a*). Initially the chromato-electrophoretic procedures for separating bound from free hormone were widely used but latterly a variety of separation procedures have been employed. One of the more ingenious is the use of disposable polypropylene or polystyrene incubation tubes which when coated with the antiserum act as a solid-phase antibody. After incubation the free labelled hormone is washed out, the bound labelled complex remains firmly attached to the wall of the tube and can be readily counted (Catt & Tregear, 1967, 1969).

Human chorionic somato-mammotrophin (HCS). HCS can be assayed by radioimmunological methods which have been reviewed by Forsyth (1967). Although there is a reaction of partial identity between HCS and HGH interference from HGH in the assay is not a practical problem. While it is possible to carry out the assay using antiserum to HGH, since HCS is present in much higher concentrations and the necessary dilution of the plasma rules out interference from HGH, it is preferable to use antiserum to HCS as this gives a greater sensitivity. Recently Leake & Burt (1969) and Crosignani, Nakamura, Hovland & Mishell, Jr. (1970) have shown that the solid-phase antibody technique yields satisfactory results in the radioimmunoassay of HCS.

Immunological versus biological assays

The use of immunological methods has greatly facilitated the assay of protein hormones in blood but it must be stressed that such assays measure *immunological* activity and while this may in most instances be similar to *biological* activity it is quite possible for biologically inactive fragments of a protein hormone to be present in the blood and for these to react with antibody and be measured as intact hormone; conversely biologically active fragments may not be measured by radioimmunoassay (see Greenwood, 1967*a*).

Because of such possible divergence between biological and immunological activities it is clearly desirable, whenever a biological assay of sufficient sensitivity is available, to carry out comparative assays on at least a proportion of the samples under investigation. The usefulness of such comparative assays is well illustrated by the observations of Forsyth (1969) relative to the curious detection by radioimmunological assay by Stephenson & Greenwood (1969) of the presence of chorionic somato-mammotrophin in the blood of non-pregnant lactating women (see p. 68).

Further references and particulars about radioimmunoassays will be found in the books edited by Wolstenholme & Cameron (1962), Weir (1967) and Margoulies (1969).

CELLULAR ORIGIN

Prolactin

The adenohypophysial cells which are responsible for secreting prolactin have been identified in a number of species and several comprehensive reviews of this subject are available (Pasteels, 1963; Herlant, 1965; Purves, 1966; Forsyth, 1967; Herlant & Pasteels, 1967; see also the book edited by Benoit & DaLage, 1963). Progress in this field was accelerated by the development of the tetrachrome staining method of Herlant (1960) which enabled two types of acidophil cell to be distinguished in the mammalian adenohypophysis. One type of cell stains with Orange G, exhibits little variation in different physiological states and is believed to be the source of growth hormone. The other type stains with erythrosin, exhibits marked variations in relation to different phases of the female reproductive cycle and to reserpine administration and is considered to be the source of prolactin (Pasteels & Herlant, 1962; Pasteels, 1963; Dubois & Herlant, 1968). The erthryosinophil prolactin-secreting acidophils have been denoted, like other pituitary cells, by a letter of the Greek alphabet. However, this system of nomenclature led to confusion and has virtually been abandoned (see review by Purves, 1966).

In addition to conventional histological methods, a specific immunofluorescent technique which utilizes antiserum to prolactin has been used to identify the prolactin-secreting cells in the pituitary of the rat and cat (Emmart, Spicer & Bates, 1963; Emmart, Bates & Turner, 1965), rat and rabbit (Shino & Rennels, 1966), sheep (Stokes & Boda, 1968) and ox (Nayak, McGarry & Beck, 1968), and has confirmed that prolactin and growth hormone are to be found in two distinct types of acidophil cell. Also, the highly specific peroxidase-antibody technique (Nakane & Pierce, 1967) has been used to investigate the prolactin-secreting cells and their distribution in the pituitary of the rat at both the light and electron microscope levels (Baker, 1970; Nakane, 1970). This technique also provided additional evidence for the presence of two types of acidophil. By treating both cell types immunochemically with different peroxidase substrates in the same histological section, the growth hormone and prolactin cells stained in contrasting colours and no cells appeared to contain both hormones (Baker, 1970).

Studies on the ultrastructure of pituitary cells have also advanced knowledge in this field (for reviews see Herlant, 1965; McShan, 1965). Of particular interest is the work of Pasteels (1963) who studied the process of the formation of secretory granules in rat pituitary and provided evidence for synthetic activity in the endoplasmic reticulum, condensation of secretory material into granules in the Golgi region, accumulation of these granules at the apex of the cell and their liberation by fusion of the membrane of the granule with the cell membrane. Under the electron microscope the prolactin-secreting cells are further distinguished by the large size of their secretory granules which have been variously reported as being from 400 to 700 nm in diameter (Hymer, McShan, & Christiansen, 1961; Pasteels, 1963; Dekker, 1968). The release of these secretory granules in response to suckling will be discussed later (see p. 265).

Primate prolactin

Cells of the human adenohypophysis, which, on the basis of their staining affinity to the prolactin-secreting cells of the rat, might be considered to be the source of human prolactin, are extremely rare in the normal gland. They are only present in appreciable numbers during pregnancy and lactation, or during *in vitro* culture of the gland (Pasteels, 1963, 1969; Goluboff & Ezrin, 1969). In the monkey pituitary, cells which are believed to be the source of prolactin have been identified by light micro-scopy in *Macacus sylvanus* and *Macacus irus* (Girod, 1964) and at both the light and electron microscope levels in *Macacus irus* (Yamashita, 1967).

Human chorionic somato-mammotrophin (HCS)

Human chorionic somato-mammotrophin is secreted by the syncytial cytoplasm of the villous trophoblast. Sciarra, Kaplan & Grumbach (1963) utilized the immunofluorescent technique to demonstrate the presence of HCS in the syncytiotrophoblast from the 12th week of gestation to term. This group also demon-strated the production of HCS *in vitro* by chorionic villi derived from a term, a 66-day and an 83-day placenta (Grumbach & Kaplan, 1964).

COMPARATIVE AND EVOLUTIONARY ASPECTS

Although the name 'prolactin' might suggest a virtually exclusive role for this hormone in the processes of secretion by mammary gland or crop sac, prolactin exerts many different actions through-out the vertebrates. Out of a total of forty-seven actions which have been claimed for prolactin, a few of the better-known ones will now be discussed briefly, in the course of which frequent reference will be made to the able and comprehensive review of this field by Bern & Nicoll (1968).

One of the most primitive actions of prolactin in the vertebrates appears to be an osmotic effect in fish, termed freshwater survival activity. This was discovered by Pickford & Phillips (1959), who reported that prolactin enabled hypophysectomized euryhaline fish to survive in freshwater. Blood osmotic pressure and electro-lyte concentrations were restored after hypophysectomy by pro-lactin injection and the effect is apparently exerted at both the branchial and the renal level (see review by Ball, 1969).

In the Amphibia, prolactin plays an important role in the growth of the larval stage. This was foreshadowed by Etkin & Lehrer

(1960) who reported that autotransplantation of the pituitary resulted in gigantic tadpoles. Although, in the mammal, this procedure is known to result in the secretion of prolactin alone by the transplanted hypophysis (see p. 253), in this and in a subsequent publication (Etkin, 1963), emphasis was placed more on the reduction of thyroid activity than on the presence of pro-lactin. However, it was shown later that injection of prolactin into tadpoles elicited an increase in body weight and tail length, and that this growth effect of prolactin occurred after hypophy-sectomy (for references see Bern & Nicoll, 1968). The current view, originally proposed by Etkin (1963) and elaborated by H. A. Bern and colleagues (see Bern & Nicoll, 1968), is that prolactin is secreted autonomously by the tadpole hypophysis until portal connexions are established with the hypothalamus (see p. 256). During this period of unrestrained prolactin secretion growth of larval structures is stimulated. As hypothalamic dominance of the adenohypophysis develops, elevated thyroxine levels are able to promote resorption of larval structures because of diminished circulating prolactin levels.

In addition to its larval growth-promoting activity, prolactin exerts what is called water-drive activity in the adult terrestrial amphibian. Thus, the land-living stage of the eft will return prematurely to water after injection of mammalian prolactin (see Bern & Nicoll, 1968 for references).

The two major actions of prolactin in the bird are the stimulation of crop 'milk' formation in pigeons and doves, and the formation of the brood patch in certain species to facilitate incubation of the eggs. For the latter action, prolactin generally synergizes with oestrogen, an effect which is analagous to its action in promoting mammary growth (see p. 115), although it is of interest that in the phalaropes, where the male alone incubates, prolactin synergizes with androgen (see Bern & Nicoll, 1968 for references).

The mammogenic and lactogenic effects of prolactin, both alone and in synergism with other endocrine factors, are dealt with elsewhere in the present book (see Chapters 3 and 4) and will not be discussed here, save to mention that the techniques of intraduct injection in the mammary gland of the rabbit and the cultured mammary gland of the mouse have been used to investigate the mammary action of prolactin from different classes of vertebrates.

Following this brief outline of some of the actions exerted by

The physiology of lactation

prolactin, the distribution of these activities among the various classes of vertebrates must be considered (Fig. 2.6). Osmoregulation

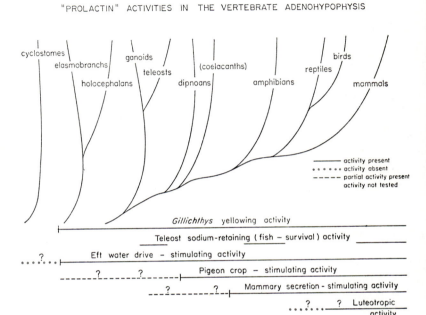

"PROLACTIN" ACTIVITIES IN THE VERTEBRATE ADENOHYPOPHYSIS

FIG. 2.6. Distribution of several of the activities of prolactin among the vertebrates (modified from Bern, H. A., 1967, *Science* **158**, 455–461. Copyright 1967 by the American Association for the Advancement of Science.)

in euryhaline teleosts appears to be a property of all mammalian prolactins so far tested, and of some teleost prolactins (Pickford, Robertson & Sawyer, 1965). While tadpole growth activity makes its appearance in the Amphibia, amphibian water-drive activity is associated with the pituitary of all vertebrates tested so far, with the possible exception of the cyclostomes. Bern & Nicoll (1968) concluded that 'this reflects a more primitive portion of the protein, an active site retained throughout vertebrate phylogeny, despite changes in the molecule that have conferred additional physiological properties'. The prolactins of cyclostomes, chondrichthyeans and teleosts are essentially devoid of pigeon crop-sac stimulating (PCS) activity, while the prolactins of lung-fish and of all classes of tetrapods are fully active in this respect. PCS activity, therefore, appears to have emerged later in vertebrate evolution than either eft water drive or freshwater survival activity. The distribution of mammary gland stimulating activity parallels that of PCS activity very closely, and occurs in all classes of tetrapods. However, unlike PCS activity it does not occur in the lungfish (see Bern & Nicoll, 1968). The latter authors pointed out that three of the actions of prolactin, eft water drive, crop-sac stimulation and mammary stimulation, emerged as properties of the prolactin molecule before the appearance of their target structures and of the animals in which these target structures are to be found. The fact that eft water drive and freshwater survival activity appeared much earlier on the evolutionary scale than the crop-sac or mammary stimulating actions certainly suggests that different portions of the prolactin molecule are responsible for these two pairs of activities. Indeed, the different degrees of response elicited by primate growth hormone in the pigeon crop and rabbit mammary gland bioassays (see p. 66) suggest that even the sites on the prolactin molecule responsible for the two latter activities are not identical.

In summarizing the diverse actions of prolactin, Bern & Nicoll (1968) drew attention to the fact that the common denominator of prolactin action among the vertebrates is its involvement in reproduction, although not, perhaps, in the strictest sense of the word, since prolactin does not appear to play any direct role in the production of gametes. Nevertheless, it is deeply involved on the one hand with movement of the individual to an environment suitable for reproduction, as in the ascent of euryhaline fish from saltwater to freshwater, the return of adult amphibians to water, and even in the premigratory restlessness of birds (Meier, Farner & King, 1965), and on the other hand in parental care of the young in the birds and mammals. In view of its phylogenetic history and the multiplicity of its actions prolactin can well be described as being the least specialized and the most intriguing adenohypophysial hormone.

3

MAMMARY GROWTH

BEFORE discussing the phases of growth of the mammary gland it is convenient to review the problems involved, and the methods used, in assessing mammary growth and differentiation.

METHODS OF STUDYING AND ASSESSING MAMMARY GROWTH

The mammary parenchyma is embedded in adipose and connective tissues and in the non-lactating animal, moreover, the amount of parenchyma relative to stroma is small so that the external size of the mammary gland (i.e. parenchyma and stroma) may give no reliable indication of the amount of secretory tissue embedded within. Cooper (1840) well appreciated the problems of assessing the development of the parenchyma and its functional potential; he writes: 'Nor is the size of the gland a certain criterion of the extent of its secretion, as the very large is often more solid than secretory' . . . 'Although the mammary glands are of simple construction when developed, yet to dissect and prepare their constituent parts and intimate structure for a clear demonstration is a very difficult task.' The methods of study used by Cooper included the injection of the ducts with mercury or preferably with a coloured wax—'by which at once each duct is distinctly shown, and even the cells will be displayed' (it may be noted that the term 'cells' is here equivalent to 'alveoli'). 'To ascertain the quantity of glandulous matter, at different periods of life, it is requisite that the breast be put for a short time in boiling water, when the skin and fat become detached, and the gland, like other albuminous compositions, is left extremely hardened, and perfectly insulated and separated from the surrounding parts. This process furnishes an opportunity of giving an estimate of the quantity of the gland, at puberty, in the adult, and in old age; as will be seen in one of my plates'—and remarkably fine specimens appeared to have been obtained by Cooper by this method. 'To unravel the milk ducts, and to demonstrate the fibrous tissue of the gland, it is to be macerated in warm water, and dissected from day to day; and its ducts and glandules will be separated and shown.'

More recent procedures have been reviewed by Mayer & Klein (1961) and by Munford (1964). We shall first consider the methods available for displaying and visualizing the mammary parenchyma.

Displaying the parenchyma

Whole mounts

In some species (e.g. rat, rabbit, monkey) the mammary gland in the non-pregnant state and in the early stages of pregnancy is a relatively flat sheet of tissue which can be dissected from the body, freed of most of its associated muscular tissue, and which can then be fixed, stained, and cleared so that the epithelial tissues are clearly displayed. This procedure gives excellent visualization of the duct system and the early stages of lobulo-alveolar development. In the later stages of pregnancy the increasing thickness of the gland precludes the use of this method.

Thick sections

In species in which the mammary glands are too thick to examine by the whole mount procedure, and in all species during late pregnancy, the gland after fixation and embedding can be cut in thick sections (80 µm to 5 mm) and these may then be treated as whole mounts. This procedure has been used extensively in the study of the human mammary gland (Dabelow, 1941, 1957; Marcum & Wellings, 1969; Tanaka & Oota, 1970) and for the goat mammary gland (Richardson, 1949).

Thin sections

The classical histological procedures for studying tissues are relevant to all stages of growth of the mammary gland and are the only satisfactory method for studying the lactating mammary gland. In the last decade ultra-thin sections for electron-microscope studies have provided much new information on the mechanisms of milk secretion. For all techniques involving sectioning of the lactating gland it is advisable, indeed essential in any critical study, to fix the whole gland by intravascular perfusion before any attempt is made to remove tissue samples since sampling before fixation will result in much distortion of the tissue and cellular damage (see p. 11). Living mammary cells, moreover, are highly susceptible to mechanical damage and the occurrence of collections of 'light' alveolar cells has been traced to injury during the sampling procedure (Pitelka, Kerkof, Gagné, Smith & Abraham, 1969).

Assessing the growth of the parenchyma

Various methods of assessing the amount of secretory tissue within the mammary gland have been described, some can be used clinically in the living animal, others require that the mammary gland be removed surgically or at autopsy.

Clinical procedures

Volume of gland. In late pregnancy and during lactation measurements of the external volume of the mammae may be a useful index of parenchymal development. Such measurements have been made in lactating women (Hytten, 1954), goats (Linzell, 1966*b*) and cows (Kjaersgaard, 1968*a*). The volumes are obtained by displacement of water from a container (Hytten, 1954; Linzell, 1966*b*) or by producing casts of the udder (Linzell, 1966*b*; Kjaersgaard, 1968*a*). Correlations between gland volumes and milk yield have been demonstrated in these investigations. Such methods, unfortunately, have little value in studying mammary development in the non-pregnant animal or even during early gestation when the volume of stroma in the mammary gland greatly exceeds that of parenchyma (see below).

Radiographic techniques. The use of radiographic techniques in the determination of the normal and abnormal structure of the human breast have been discussed by Ingleby & Gershon-Cohen (1960), Witten (1969) and Gershon-Cohen, Hermel & Birsner (1970). Studies on radiographic techniques combined with the intra-mammary injection of radio-opaque material have been reported by Lombardo (1955) in the goat and similar studies in sheep by Jakovac & Rapić (1963).

Ultrasonograms. An immersion scanner for two-dimensional ultrasonic examination of the human breast has been described by Wells & Evans (1968) who have reviewed earlier studies carried out by ultrasonic techniques; these were mainly concerned in the diagnosis of breast abnormalities. Sonograms or echo-traces have also been used by Caruolo & Mochrie (1967) for locating and identifying structures within the udder of the lactating cow. By this technique changes in the relative positions of suspensory ligaments, milk ducts and lymph nodes can be detected.

Palpation of glandular tissue. Swett and his colleagues (see review by Munford, 1964) introduced a simple palpation procedure, using the thumb and forefinger as calipers to measure the parenchyma within the udder of calves.

Biopsy techniques. Finally, in the living animal, biopsy specimens may be obtained from the mammary gland and evaluated by one of the suitable histological or histometric methods listed below. Numerous instruments have been described for obtaining biopsy samples from the udder of ruminants (e.g. Marx & Caruolo, 1963). The technique has an inherent drawback; it is difficult to be certain that the sample obtained is a representative one; although increasing the size or numbers of samples will reduce the sampling error it increases the trauma to the gland and in the fully secreting gland serious haemorrhage can occur; in short, in mammary biopsy techniques a precarious balance between unsatisfactory sampling and undue damage to the gland must be struck.

Procedures for mammary glands removed at surgery or at autopsy

In many species the removal of a whole mammary gland may well be the more satisfactory research procedure; adequate fixation and sampling can readily be achieved and the growth or functional capacities of the remaining gland (or glands) can be studied. We have used this procedure extensively in studies on mammogenesis in the goat (e.g. Cowie, Folley, Malpress & Richardson, 1952). It should be noted, however, that removal of a mammary gland may eventually induce compensatory hypertrophy in the remaining gland(s) (Linzell, 1963; Kuosaïte, 1965) but in our experience in the goat such hypertrophy is not evident at least for some months after the mastectomy (see Cowie, Cox, Folley, Hosking, Naito & Tindal, 1965).

Several methods are available for assessing mammary growth and development in whole glands obtained by mastectomy under anaesthesia or at autopsy.

Weight of mammary parenchyma. We have already observed that the external volume of the mammary gland as an index of mammary parenchymal growth is of little value in the undeveloped gland but its usefulness increases as the gland develops; similarly the gross weight gives no reliable indication of the amount of parenchyma in the undeveloped gland. In some species, however (e.g. in the goat), when the gland has been fixed by intravascular perfusion and cut into slices much of the adipose and connective tissues surrounding the parenchyma can be trimmed away and the weight of the trimmed gland can be a simple and useful objective measure of mammary development (see review by Cowie, 1971).

Area covered by duct system. In species from which whole mounts of the mammary gland can be prepared, the area covered by the duct system can be measured, preferably by planimeter, giving a useful index of duct growth (provided a sufficient number of glands are studied) which can be readily related to body growth (i.e. relative growth) (see p. 106). Such studies have been reported in the monkey (Folley, Guthkelch & Zuckerman, 1939), in rats (Cowie, 1949; Silver, 1953*a*, *b*) in mice (Flux, 1954*a*, *b*; Nagai & Yamada, 1957). A further refinement of this technique is the determination of the degree of arborescence of the duct systems (see Munford, 1964).

Volume of mammary parenchyma. Fairly accurate determinations of the volume of the mammary parenchyma in the mammary gland of small animals can be made by projecting serial sections of the glands and measuring the areas of parenchyma in the sections. If the thickness of the sections is known then the volume of parenchyma can be readily calculated (see Benson, Cowie, Cox & Goldzveig, 1957). The main drawback of the procedure is that it is time-consuming.

Surface area of secretory epithelium. This ingenious method, based on a technique evolved by Short (1950) to measure the surface area of the alveoli in the lung, was applied to the mammary gland by Richardson (1953). The gland is fixed when full of milk by intravascular perfusion, is then cut into thick slices and numerous blocks (to ensure adequate sampling) are taken from the slices and histological sections prepared. Microscopic fields of the mammary gland are superimposed on grid lines of known length (l) and intersections of the grid with alveolar epithelium (n) are counted. The volume (v) is obtained from the trimmed weight and density of the fixed tissue, then when 'l' is corrected for magnification, the surface area (s) of the alveoli is given by the formula $s = 2nv/l$. It is important that the mammary glands being studied should all be fixed in a similar state of distension. Unfortunately the procedure as described is tedious but if the work of counting the intersections could be carried out by some automatic scanning device then it would become the method of choice in many studies. Very recently an image-processing device for scanning histological sections of lung tissue has been described by Levine, Reisch & Thurlbeck (1970) which may be well suited for mammary epithelium.

Proportion of parenchyma to stroma. By outlining the boundaries of sections of mammary tissue and of the parenchyma within the boundaries and measuring the areas with a planimeter the area of secretory tissue can be expressed as a proportion of the total sectional area (see Benson & Folley, 1957). This ratio is very useful in studies on gland structure but it must be kept in mind that this is a ratio and by itself gives no indication of the total amount of secretory tissue present in the gland, i.e. the ratio may well be the same in a well-differentiated *small* gland and a well-differentiated *large* gland. If, however, the ratio be combined with an estimate of total volume of mammary tissue then an index of total parenchyma can be obtained (e.g. Munford, 1963*a*).

Other indices employed in studies of mammogenesis are (a) number and size of alveoli per unit area, (b) number of cells per alveolar section and (c) the frequency of mitosis (see review by Munford, 1964).

Scoring procedures. In addition to the above objective quantitative

D

procedures for assessing mammary growth subjective scoring methods have frequently been used to assess the degree of lobulo-alveolar growth (e.g. Cowie & Folley, 1947*a*; Jacobsohn, 1948; Benson, Cowie, Cox & Goldzveig, 1957; Khazan, Primo, Danon, Assael, Sulman & Winnik, 1962; Ben-David, 1968). In these the degree of development of a gland is scored against a set of reference slides by several observers. The procedure is relatively quick and if properly conducted (e.g. observers should not know the identity of the slides being scored) useful results are obtained.

Biochemical indices of mammary growth. Histometric methods of assessing mammary growth are generally both time-consuming and tedious and considerable effort has been expended on the development of biochemical indices for assessing the number of cells in the mammary gland and the stromal content of the gland. The most commonly used procedure is the determination of the deoxyribonucleic acid (DNA) content of the gland. This procedure is based on the belief that the amount of DNA per cell nucleus is constant for somatic tissues of a given species. Just as the gross weight of the gland may be of little value as an index of the amount of parenchyma because of the considerable content of stromal tissue in the gland, so the DNA values may be invalidated by the contribution from cell nuclei of non-secretory tissues, e.g. in virgin mice the lymph nodes in the mammary gland may constitute 65% of the total mammary DNA (Nicoll & Tucker, 1965). The assumption that the amount of DNA per nucleus is constant may also be untrue. Sod-Moriah & Schmidt (1968) in studies on mammary gland in rabbits have reported that nuclei of alveolar cells differ in their DNA content, significant differences occurring between individual animals, between different glands of the same animal and between different areas within the same gland.

To counter some of the errors arising from the use of DNA as an index of the amount of secretory tissue in the mammary gland its measurement has been combined with determinations of the content of fat, of hydroxyproline—a measure of collagen, and of hexosamine—a measure of ground substance (Paape & Tucker, 1969*a*).

In short, the total DNA of a gland is at best a measure of the cell population within the gland—all cells, not cells of any specific type—and DNA measurements do not necessarily reveal the character of the parenchymal development (see Sud, Tucker & Meites, 1968). As Munford (1964) has cautioned, the indices of mammary structure derived from histological studies and measures of biochemical change should not be regarded as alternatives but rather as complementary methods of assessing the state of the mammary gland in developmental studies.

Other biochemical methods of assessing mammary growth which have been suggested include (a) determination of the iron content of the gland (Rawlinson & Pierce, 1950), (b) whole mount autoradiographs using ^{32}P (Lundahl, Meites & Wolterink, 1950) and (c) determination of alkaline phosphatase in the mammary gland (Huggins & Mainzer, 1958; Munford, 1963b). Cell proliferation can be studied by the technique of autoradiography using tritiated thymidine which permits the direct visualization of cells synthesizing DNA before mitotic division (Traurig, 1967a, b).

MAMMARY GROWTH IN THE FOETUS

The origin and evolution of the mammary glands have been fertile subjects for discussion. They have been variously derived from anlage of sweat glands, sebaceous glands, or hair follicles or from avian incubation patches. We do not propose to discuss these problems which are dealt with more fully in the reviews by Long (1969) and Raynaud (1969).

Sub-class Prototheria, order Monotremata

In the echidna the primordia of the mammary glands appear as small ectodermal thickenings, one on each flank of the embryo (5 mm crown-rump length), which grow and form elevated lenticular areas. About the time of hatching these two areas extend but diminish in thickness and become difficult to recognize. When the embryo is 2–3 cm long the primordia appear as oval areas devoid of hair. In these areas many epidermal buds are formed (embryo 4–5 cm long) which penetrate the underlying dermis. These primary buds give rise to secondary buds which elongate to become the mammary cords. The primary buds eventually give rise to the mammary hairs and their associated glands (for references see Griffiths, 1968; Raynaud, 1969).

Sub-class Metatheria

In marsupials the mammary primordia also appear as two areas of thickened ectoderm, one on either flank of the embryo during intra-uterine life. Just before birth these areas fragment into small lenticular nodules which grow into epithelial buds. These buds remain for a time in a resting phase during which pause the marsupium is formed. Each primary bud eventually gives rise to a secondary bud which in turn gives rise to a pair of tertiary buds. From the primary buds develop mammary hairs, from the secondary buds the mammary cords and from the tertiary buds the sebaceous glands associated with the hairs. In most marsupials, however, the mammary hairs and their sebaceous glands are transient structures.

Formation of the nipple or teat varies according to the species. In some, the dermis underlying the mammary bud proliferates and gradually pushes the mammary rudiment upwards to form a projection above skin level; in others the mammary bud sinks into the mesenchyme forming a neck which, by a process of cornification, becomes a hollow, termed a nipple pocket, with the mammary cord attached to its deep face. The bottom of the pocket gradually pushes upwards thus everting its walls and eventually forming a projecting nipple bearing the orifices of the ducts.

The unpaired mammary gland which occurs in the Didelphidae is believed to arise by fusion of a pair of adjacent mammary glands.

For further details and references the reader is referred to the review by Raynaud (1969).

Sub-class Eutheria

The various stages in the embryonic and foetal growth of the mammary gland in a number of species of eutherian mammals have been the subject of extensive reviews by Raynaud (1961, 1969, 1971) and we shall briefly describe only the salient features common to most species. The first recognizable structure which may be concerned with development of the mammary gland is a raised band of ectoderm which appears on either side of the midline of the very young embryo and which has been designated the *mammary band*; the significance of this structure for the growth of the mammary gland has, however, been questioned. Along the mammary band there then appears a narrower ridge of ectoderm—

the *milk line* or *milk crest*. The mammary band gradually disappears and the milk line diminishes in length, becomes interrupted to form a series of thickenings or nodules of ectodermal cells, the number and the position of the nodules depending on the species. These nodules sink into the dermis and become *mammary buds*—the primordia of the future mammary glands. The bud, at first lenticular in shape, becomes globular and later conical. A pause then occurs in its development, after which the bud elongates, the base being attached to the epidermis and the distal part penetrates further into the mesenchyme so that a cord-shaped structure is formed—the *primary mammary cord*. In some species the distal end of the cord bifurcates, in others it produces a number of secondary buds which in turn elongate and then branch. These branched cords develop a lumen and become ducts with walls composed of two layers of cuboidal cells. In this manner the duct system of the mammary gland is laid down before term.

During the growth of the mammary bud the mesoderm differentiates into four distinct layers—next to the mammary bud there is a dense zone of mesenchyme which ultimately forms the smooth muscle of the nipple and a second zone from which is derived the stroma of the nipple. As the mammary bud grows it passes through these first two zones; mesenchymal cells from the third zone of loose mesenchyme surround the branching extremities of the ducts to form eventually the connective tissue of the lobules while the fourth zone gives rise to the interlobular septa.

In man the mammary band is discernible in the foetus of 4 mm length; Hughes (1950), however, considers this band of epidermal differentiation to be associated with the growth of the body and its appendages as a whole and that the term mammary band is a misnomer. The mammary crest appears in the human embryo, of 7 mm length. The crest diminishes in length while its cranial end proliferates (embryos of 13–15 mm length) to form the mammary bud which sinks into the differentiating mesenchyme. In the embryo of 20–30 mm length the bud has assumed a spherical shape and lies below the surface of the surrounding epidermis. From the 3rd–4th month of foetal life (20–150 mm length) there is a pause in development while proliferation of the mesenchyme tends to push the mammary bud upwards so producing a slight elevation of the epidermis—the primordium of the nipple. During the 5th month (foetal length 120–170 mm) the surface of the bud spreads out and a depression forms in its centre, at the same time the deeper layer of the bud proliferates and produces 15–25 secondary buds which gradually lengthen and form solid cellular cords which expand at their extremities and become surrounded with concentric layers of mesenchyme. In embryos of 180–200 mm the cellular cords begin to bifurcate, develop a lumen and become ducts; meanwhile the superficial ectoderm of the bud desquamates and keratinizes to leave an inverted nipple area. The ducts continue to grow and, in the 300-mm foetus, have several terminal branches which become separated from each other by septa derived from the 4th layer of mesenchyme. At term (foetal length 330 mm) canalization of the cords is mostly complete, the nipple depression becomes flattened and then somewhat everted as the underlying dermis thickens so that the ducts now open to the exterior at a level which, in the new-born, corresponds to the surface of the skin. Further information about the growth of the mammary glands in the human foetus will be found in the reviews by Geschickter (1945); Dickson & Hewer (1950); Hughes (1950) and Dabelow (1957).

Details of the morphogenesis of the mammary gland have been studied in a number of species including most of the domestic animals and references to these studies will be found in the reviews by Turner (1939, 1952) and Raynaud (1961, 1969, 1971). More recent publications include studies on foetal mammogenesis in the sheep and cow (Wallace, 1953; Biborski, 1961; Martinet, 1962), in the pig (Soloveǐ & Éktov, 1961) and in the monkey (Speert, 1948). There have also been studies on the development of the blood capillary system in the bovine foetus (2–5 months) by Chumakov (1961) and on the formation of the stroma in the bovine foetus by Gorbunov (1963).

Relative growth rates of foetal mammary gland

The technique of relative growth analysis as developed by Huxley (1932) (see also Huxley & Teissier, 1936), in which the rate of growth of an organ is related to that of the body as a whole, has been used in several species to study the growth patterns of the mammary gland during foetal and postnatal life. Balinsky (1950) studied the growth rates of the mammary gland of the foetal mouse by measuring the volume of the mammary rudiments (determined from area measurement of serial sections) and relating them to body size as a whole. He distinguishes three phases in the growth of the gland in the foetal mouse. First there is the formation of the mammary buds during which stage the growth rate of the rudiment decreases far below the high level intrinsic for the epidermis from which it was derived; secondly there is a phase of very slow growth with no progressive differentiation except that the mammary bud changes in shape from lenticular to spherical. This pause in mammary growth lasts from days 11 to 15 and over this period the weight of the foetus increases ten-fold while the volume of the mammary rudiment increases only 4·5 times (i.e. negative allometry). The third phase is the period of sprouting when the primary cord and then the branching duct system are formed; during this period the growth rate of the mammary gland rises above that of the foetus as a whole (i.e. positive allometry). Martinet (1962) has made similar volumetric studies of the mammary glands of foetal sheep of both sexes from the 44th to the 150th day of gestation. Over this period the mammary gland of the male foetus grew 2·8 times as fast as the body as a whole. In the female foetus the mammary buds grew 5 times faster than the body from day 44 until about day 70 when the rate declined to 1·7 times that of the body. Martinet (1962) considers that there may be a connexion between the period of rapid mammary growth (days 44–70) in the female foetus and the occurrence of an increase in mitotic activity in the foetal ovary between days 52–70. In the sheep foetus the second phase or pause in the growth occurs between days 35–48 (Martinet, 1962). Balinsky (1950) considers that the second phase of arrested development occurs in the embryonic development of the mammary gland in most mammals.

Mechanisms controlling the growth of the mammary gland in the foetus
Hormonal factors. Only in the mouse and rat have we any information on hormonal factors regulating the growth of the foetal mammary gland (see reviews by Raynaud, 1961, 1969, 1971). In the mouse the growth and formation of the mammary primordia and of the mammary bud appear to be independent of the influence of any hormones from the foetal gonads and the mammary growth patterns in both male and female foetuses up to the 14th day are the same. After this stage, however, sex differences in mammogenesis occur. In the female foetus on day 15 the mammary

bud sinks into the mesenchyme but remains connected to the epidermis by a neck of ectodermal cells, the bud then elongates into a cord which near term begins to branch at the distal end (Fig. 3.1*a, d*). As the mammary cord grows a circular invagination of the epidermis occurs around the attachment of the cord representing the beginning of the formation of the nipple. In the male mouse foetus the mammary bud also sinks into the mesenchyme but a condensation of mesenchyme forms round the neck of the stalk, the latter disappears leaving the bud isolated in the mesenchyme without any connexion with the epidermis (Fig. 3.1*b, e*). The bud elongates into a cord which becomes slightly branched. In the male mouse foetus there is no nipple formation. Because of these events in the male foetus the mammary gland in the adult male mouse has no connexion to the skin, nor are there nipples. A similar pattern of events occurs in the development of the mammary gland in the male rat save that the mammary bud retains its connexion with the skin although again no nipple is formed (Delost, Jean & Jean, 1962). Studies by Raynaud and his colleagues (see review by Raynaud, 1961), involving destruction of the gonads in the foetal mouse by local X-ray irradiation a few days before the sex differences in the mammary growth pattern appear, have revealed that whereas destruction of the ovaries of the female foetus has no influence on the subsequent development of the mammary gland which continues to grow just as in the intact female foetus, destruction of the testes in the male foetus causes the mammary primordia to develop as in the female, i.e. the buds remain connected to the epidermis and nipples are formed. It was further shown that injection of androgens into the mother or into the foetus before day 14 causes the mammary primordia of the female foetus to follow the male pattern of growth, i.e. the connexion of the primary cord to the skin is broken and nipples fail to develop. Injection of oestrogen, on the other hand, causes a partial or total arrest of the growth of the mammary buds while accelerating the formation of the nipple primordia (see Raynaud, 1961; Jean & Delost, 1965). If injections of hormones are given after day 15, i.e. after sex differentiation has started, then the frequency of mammary malformations are greatly reduced (see review by Raynaud, 1961; also Hoshino, 1965).

The effects of progestogens on the mammary glands of the foetal mouse are very variable. Not only do the different progesto-

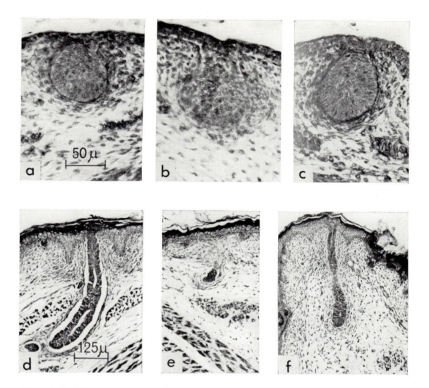

FIG. 3.1. The pattern of development of the mammary anlagen in the foetal mouse.

(a). Mammary bud of normal 14-day-old female foetus.

(b). Mammary bud of normal 14-day-old male foetus; note that the outline of the bud in the male is less clearly defined because of the condensation of the mesenchyme which occurs before rupture of the connexion between the bud and the epidermis.

(c). Mammary bud of the 14-day-old male foetus whose mother has been treated with an anti-androgen (cyproterone acetate, 3 mg/day) from day 12 of pregnancy; note the similarity to the normal female.

(d). Mammary cord of the normal 18-day-old female foetus; the cord is attached to the epidermis and around the base of the cord there is an invagination of the epidermis representing the anlagen of the nipple.

(e). Mammary rudiment of normal 18-day-old male foetus; there is no longer any connexion with the epidermis and the invagination of the epidermis has almost disappeared.

(f). Mammary cord of 18-day-old male foetus whose mother has been treated with cyproterone acetate, 3 mg/day, from day 12 of pregnancy; note the similarity to the normal female (d), the mammary cord is attached to the epidermis and there is evidence of nipple formation.

(From Cowie, A. T. & Folley, S. J., 1970, in *Scientific Foundations of Obstetrics and Gynaecology*, edited by Philipp, E. E., Barnes, J. & Newton, M., pp. 423–432. London: Heinemann Medical Books. Photograph by courtesy of Dr. F. Neumann.)

gens differ somewhat in their action but the same progestogen may exhibit both virilizing and feminizing effects (Cupceancu, Neumann & Ulloa, 1969).

In the pregnant rat androgens administered on day 14 also evoke the male pattern of development in the mammary glands of the female foetus but in an exaggerated fashion, since not only are the nipples not formed but the primary cord loses its connexion with the skin—this connexion is normally retained in the male rat—and two pairs of inguinal mammary glands may disappear—normally only one pair disappears in the male (Jean & Jean, 1969).

Oestrogens administered to the rat on day 14 of gestation result in foetal mammary malformations, the severity of which depends on the dose of oestrogen, ranging from mere hypertrophy of the nipple to complete disappearance of the mammary gland (Delost, Jean & Jean, 1962; Jean & Delost, 1965; Jean, 1968a).

Confirmation of the influence of androgens on foetal mammogenesis has recently been provided by studies on the effect on mammary morphogenesis of an androgen antagonist—cyproterone acetate (1,2a-methylene-6-chloro-$\Delta^{4,6}$-pregnadiene-17a-ol-3,20-dione-17a-acetate) when administered from the 12th day of pregnancy in rats and mice (see Fig. 3.1). This substance induces the female pattern of mammary growth in the male foetus together with feminization of the sexual characters (Neumann & Elger, 1966; Elger & Neumann, 1966). Cyproterone has no oestrogenic activity and its effects are most likely to be related to the blocking of the androgen receptors in the mammary gland primordium.

In the mouse, ox growth hormone (GH) injected on day 14 of gestation either into the mother or directly into the foetuses stimulates the growth of the mammary buds and cords in both male and female foetuses and maintains the attachment of the primary cord to the epidermis in the male foetus. GH, secreted either from the foetal or maternal pituitary, may thus be concerned in the regulation of foetal mammary growth in the mouse (Jean, 1968b). Studies on mammary rudiments from 10–15-day-old foetal mice cultured *in vitro* have also indicated a role for GH in promoting foetal mammogenesis (Lasfargues & Murray, 1959). In the rat, however, recent studies of explants of mammary anlagen from 17-day-old foetuses by Ceriani (1970a, b) gave no indication that growth hormone stimulated mammary growth; the presence of insulin, however, induced growth of the ducts and their pene-

tration into the mesenchyme—an effect enhanced by sheep prolactin; the addition of aldosterone caused branching of the ducts
and some secretory activity. The best growth and secretory
responses were obtained with a combination of insulin + prolactin
+ aldosterone + progesterone. A casein-like material was present
in the secretion. Testosterone inhibited the effects of these hormones on the explants.

Study of the postnatal growth of the mammary glands of mice
which have been subjected to the effects of oestrogens *in utero*
reveals that the atrophy of the mammary glands so induced is
not an irreversible condition since the rudimentary glands grow
rapidly at the onset of puberty and attain normal development,
indeed in the male the degree of growth may exceed that which
normally occurs (Jean, 1969).

The mammary gland of the male rat treated prematurely with
cyproterone grows in the postnatal period as in the normal female
rat, the glands opening to the exterior through normal nipples,
and if such rats are castrated when adult and given injections of
oestrogen, progesterone, cortisol and sheep prolactin then lobulo-
alveolar growth and milk secretion are initiated just as in nulliparous female control rats given identical hormone treatment
(Neumann, Elger & von Berswordt-Wallrabe, 1966; Neumann &
Elger, 1967).

From the studies reviewed it may be deduced that in the foetal
mouse and rat the male pattern of growth is a specialized type
arising from an inhibition or diversion of the neutral (female)
pattern of mammary growth by hormones from the foetal testis.
There is no evidence that oestrogens play any important role in
foetal mammogenesis in these two species. On the other hand,
growth hormone may be concerned and it is possible that some of
the effects of androgens and oestrogens may be mediated by
inhibiting the normal secretion or actions of growth hormone
(see Jean, 1969, and Jean & Jean, 1969).

Whether specialized patterns of foetal mammary growth induced by androgens or other hormones are of common occurrence
in other species awaits further research. The question, moreover,
may not be entirely academic. Raynaud (1961) has discussed the
possible clinical importance and observed that some of the so-
called 'spontaneous' malformations of the mammary gland in man
and animals may possibly be associated with the action on the

mammary rudiments in the embryo or foetus of hormones or other drugs administered to the mother during early pregnancy; in particular he stresses that the administration of oestrogens to gravid females in medical or veterinary treatments should not be lightly undertaken.

Mesenchymal factors. The important role played by the mesenchyme in inducing the differentiation of mammary primordia has been revealed by *in vitro* organ culture studies. Propper & Gomot (1967) observed that explants of mammary-band mesenchyme from 12-day-old rabbit foetuses (i.e. one day before the mammary band appears) when cultured with epidermis taken from other sites in the foetus induced the epidermis to differentiate and to form primary mammary buds. They also noted that epidermis from the mammary band region would differentiate on mesenchyme taken from other regions only if the epidermis was from foetuses 13 days of age or older. These studies suggested that the mesenchyme could induce a specific morphogenesis in a 'neutral' epidermis but that once initiated differentiation could continue on indifferent mesenchyme. Recent organ-culture studies by Kratochwil (1969) with explants from foetal mice have confirmed the essential role of the mesenchyme in mammary differentiation. Explants of mammary primordia from 12–14 day foetuses differentiated normally in culture eventually forming a branching duct system and nipple, but such explants no longer differentiated when their underlying mesenchyme was first removed by treatment with trypsin; growth could be restored, however, to such stripped primordia by adding to them mesenchyme from the mammary region. Mammary rudiments while growing in culture exhibited the characteristic resting phase indicating that this pause in growth is determined not by hormonal but by factors intrinsic to the rudiment. When 16-day-old mammary rudiments were cultured on their own mesenchyme they failed to grow but did so when their own mesenchyme was replaced with 12-day mesenchyme suggesting that during the resting phase some change occurred in the morphogenetic capacity of the mesenchyme—possibly it had now become dependent on hormones. The specificity of the mesenchymal induction suggested by the studies of Propper & Gomot (1967) was further explored by Kratochwil (1969) who demonstrated that when epidermis from the mammary band region of the 12-day foetal mouse (i.e. undifferentiated epidermis) or the mammary rudiments of the 16-day foetus (i.e. differentiated tissue) were deprived of their subjacent mesenchyme and then cultured on mesenchyme from the submandibular salivary gland of the 13-day foetal mouse the subsequent differentiation of the epidermis and rudiments followed the pattern of a salivary gland. Evidence is thus accumulating that the mesenchyme exerts an instructive function on the epidermis through organ-specific factors and, in the case of the salivary mesenchyme these factors are apparently able to override the morphogenetic programme of a mammary rudiment (16-day foetus) in which differentiation has already been induced.

Further organ culture studies are clearly necessary to ascertain to what extent hormonal effects on foetal mammogenesis are mediated by way of the mesenchyme.

POSTNATAL GROWTH

Sub-class Prototheria, Order Monotremata

Little is known of the postnatal phases of growth of the mammary gland of the echidna. A phase of active growth apparently sets in about the onset of the breeding season; glandular differentiation and even milk secretion can occur without the intervention of pregnancy. The stimulus of pregnancy and incubation of an egg, however, is generally, but not invariably, necessary for development of alveoli. The changes in the mammary gland during regression resemble those in eutherian mammals. Further information on the mammary glands of the echidna and on the composition of their milk will be found in the review by Griffiths (1968) (see also Griffiths, McIntosh & Coles, 1969).

Sub-class Metatheria

In marsupials gestation usually falls within the span of the oestrous cycle and it does not interrupt the cyclic recurrence of oestrus provided the new-born young are prevented from reaching the teat. The hormone-induced changes which occur in the reproductive organs, moreover, are identical in both pregnant and non-mated females; thus equivalent post-ovulatory mammary growth occurs in both. In both, the mammary glands can become functional at the equivalent post-oestrous stage and, if a new-born foster young is attached to the teat of a virgin female at this stage the neonate will obtain milk and will grow normally. Thus in the marsupial it appears that all the hormones required for lobulo-alveolar growth of the mammary gland are present in the non-pregnant female after ovulation.

Milk secretion is initiated by the suckling stimulus. At first the milk contains very little fat but in the later stages of lactation the fat content may reach 20%. In the pigmy possum (*Cercartetus concinnus*) only a day or two elapses between the weaning of one litter and the commencement of nursing the next. In this short time the mammary secretion changes from milk to the clear fluid of initial suckling and the enlarged teats regress to a size small enough to be grasped by the jaws of a neonate (Clark, 1967). Some marsupials, notably kangaroos, can be nursing two genera-tions of young at one time; that is there is one young on foot which is suckling one of the four teats while another within the pouch, which is some 200 days younger, is attached to another teat. The two milks being secreted concurrently differ widely in composition. There is some evidence in marsupials that the rate of regression in one mammary gland is slowed down if another gland continues to be suckled. (For further information see Sharman, 1962, 1970.)

Sub-class Eutheria

There is much species variation in the phases of postnatal mammary growth in the female eutherian mammal and even considerable individual differences occur within a species so that any description must inevitably be general rather than detailed.

Several distinct phases, however, can be recognized in the post-natal development of the mammary gland. First there is a quies-cent phase from birth to about the time when ovarian cycles begin when the growth of the ducts just keeps pace with general body growth or in some species may even fail to do so. Secondly, there is a phase of accelerated duct growth associated with the onset of puberty, the nature of this growth process depending on the type of sex cycle and ranging from a rapid extension and growth of the duct system to the development of a lobulo-alveolar system comparable to that occurring in late pregnancy. The third stage is the completion of growth of the mammary gland during pregnancy and early lactation when the lobulo-alveolar tissues become fully developed and functional. Lastly after lactation there is a phase of regression when the gland may lose much of its lobulo-alveolar structure and return to a state similar to that before pregnancy.

Birth to puberty

Although this is the quiescent phase when mammary growth is minimal, occasionally in some species and in both sexes at birth or a few days thereafter there may occur a transient burst of mammary activity believed to be associated with hormonal changes in the foetus at the end of gestation. Most commonly observed in man, this transient activity has also been described in the guinea-pig, rabbit, cat and horse (see reviews by Courrier, 1945; Mayer & Klein, 1961). In man there is a hypertrophy of the primary ducts, there may be a proliferation of buds on the walls of the milk sinuses and the terminal ducts may divide and expand into alveolar-like vesicles (Dabelow, 1957; Dosset, 1960). The epithelium of the ducts and vesicles secretes a colostrum-like fluid—'witch's milk'. (The origin of this term with its implications of superstition and sorcery has been discussed by Forbes, 1950.) This mammary activity may last for about three weeks. The gland then returns to a state of rest, the end vesicles and ducts regress and their epithelium becomes double layered.

During the rest of the quiescent phase, according to the species, the mammary ducts may remain short and confined to the nipple area or may grow and branch dichotomously so that their extension keeps in step with the growth of the body surface (see reviews by Folley, 1952; Mayer & Klein, 1961).

Puberty

Upon the onset, or just before the onset, of regular ovarian cycles there is a marked acceleration in the growth processes in the mammary gland. The extent and nature of these changes reflects the type of sex cycle exhibited by the species in question (see review by Turner, 1939). In species in which the duration of the cycle is short (e.g. rat, mouse) the growth is limited to a rapid extension and branching of the duct system. A striking feature of these rapidly growing glands is the presence of club-shaped terminal end buds around their periphery (Fig. 3.2.*a*). Cyclic changes in mammary growth have been described in some species,

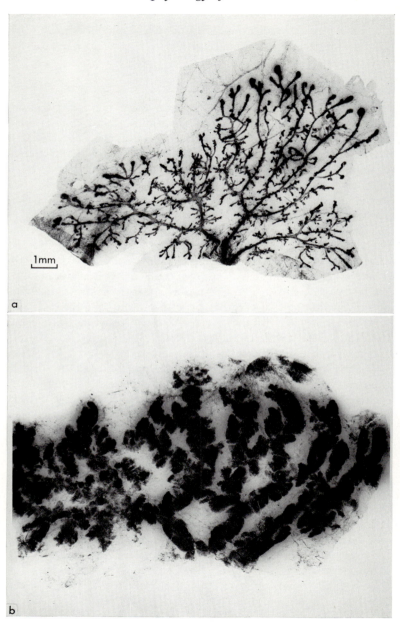

1mm

a

b

Fig. 3.2.

there being a more active phase of duct growth in early oestrus followed by some regression towards dioestrus (see review by Folley, 1952). In general in the species with short cycles the growth is limited to the duct system but in some strains of mice the formation of rudimentary alveoli at about the 75th day of age has been observed (Nandi, 1959; Nagai, 1962). In the young female goat the occurrence of precocious udder growth associated with hypertrophy of the udder cistern is not uncommon and small regions of alveolar tissue may be present (Cowie, 1971).

In species such as man and monkeys in which the luteal phase of the cycle is more prolonged, as the duct system extends and branches, the foundations of the lobules are laid down. Collections of epithelial buds appear clustered about the terminal portions of the ducts. These buds elongate, become canalized to form ductules, and are surrounded by a loose and delicate stroma thus forming the rudimentary lobules. These ductules have been termed alveoli but as both Dawson (1935) and Richardson (1947) have stressed it is difficult in the mammary gland to distinguish alveolar cells from the epithelium of the fine ducts. In histological sections, both alveoli and intralobular ducts are lined by a single layer of epithelium and all of it is capable of secretion. In man it is generally agreed that true alveoli are not usually present until the 3rd month of pregnancy (see Dawson, 1935; Dabelow, 1957). Cyclic proliferation changes have been described in the human mammary gland during the menstrual cycle. Active growth of duct tissue is said to occur before ovulation, reaching a maximum in the premenstruum and then showing some regression.

Speert (1948) examining biopsy specimens of the mammary gland from rhesus monkeys throughout the sex cycle considered that the most consistent change was an increase in the size of the lobules during the premenstruum followed by some regression in the post-menstrual period. From studies by Folley *et al.* (1939) and

---

FIG. 3.2. (*a*) Whole mount of second thoracic mammary gland from a normal female rat, 30 days of age. Note the presence of club-shaped end buds. The nipple has been removed during preparation of the whole mount.
(*b*) Whole mount of second thoracic mammary gland from a normal male rat, 100 days of age. The duct system is covered with dense clusters of alveoli.
Both figures are at the same magnification, see scale on (*a*).

Speert (1948) it appears that true lobulo-alveolar growth may occur in the adolescent female rhesus monkey.

In species in which pseudopregnancy occurs (e.g. dog, fox, opossum) lobulo-alveolar growth continues to a degree similar to that observed in late pregnancy (see reviews by Richardson, 1947; Folley, 1952). Similarly in species such as the rabbit, rat and mouse in which a short phase of pseudopregnancy can be induced by a sterile mating the mammary gland will develop to a stage comparable to early pregnancy. In mice, moreover, the occurrence of alveolar formation may be associated with the long oestrous cycles that occur when mice are kept in groups rather than singly— the Whitten effect (Nagai, 1962; Kobayashi, Nagai & Naito, 1963).

The use of the technique of relative growth analysis in studying foetal mammary growth has already been noted (see p. 94). The earliest attempt to correlate postnatal mammary growth with the growth rate of a reference organ was by Aberle (1934) who compared the increase in area of the mammary glands of the rhesus monkey with the rate of weight increase of the kidney over a period from birth to maturity; the kidney showed a constant growth rate whereas the mammary gland showed a variable rate which was highest at puberty. The first detailed study of mammary growth using relative growth analysis proper was that by Folley *et al.* (1939) on the rhesus monkey in which it was shown that over the body weight range 3·4 to 6·1 kg the rate of increase in area of the mammary gland was some 2·7 times that of the body surface as a whole indicating that the mammary gland was being influenced by some specific growth stimulus. Subsequently relative growth studies (see Cowie, 1949; Silver, 1953*a*, *b*; Flux, 1954*a*; Sinha & Tucker, 1966; Nagasawa, Iwahashi, Kanzawa, Fujimoto & Kuretani, 1967) revealed that the acceleration of the mammary growth rate began in the rat some 12 days, and in the mouse about 4 days before the onset of oestrous cycles; during the quiescent phase the rate of growth in both species was similar to that of the body as a whole (i.e. isometric growth) but at the times indicated above the rate of growth of the mammary gland of the rat became 3 times and of the mouse 5–8 times faster than body growth (i.e. allometric growth). The maximum mammary duct extension is reached in the rat and mouse at an approximate age of 100 days.

Recent studies by Sinha & Tucker (1969) in which mammary growth, based on determinations of DNA, RNA, collagen and lipid, was studied in heifers from birth to 1 year of age have shown that mammary DNA increases 1·6 times faster than body weight between birth and 2 months, then a phase of greatly accelerated mammary growth sets in when the DNA increases some 3·5 times faster than body weight. This phase of allometric growth continues to about 9 months of age when the rate falls to 1·5 times the increase in body weight. Although in rats there is some discrepancy between estimates of mammary growth rate derived from area measurements and from DNA measurements (Sinha & Tucker, 1966) it is probable that the above observations do indicate the onset of a phase of rapid allometric growth of the mammary gland in the heifer some months before the first oestrous cycle (about 6–7 months). Sinha & Tucker (1969) also studied the same biochemical constituents in the udder of 16-month-old heifers throughout the oestrous cycle (mean length 20·6 ± 0·2 days) and observed that all constituents increased sharply at the onset of oestrus but declined during the progestational phase. It thus appears that at oestrus there is a proliferation of mammary cells but that some of this tissue regresses during the progestational phase.

Pregnancy

During pregnancy further extension and branching of the duct system may occur according to the species, alveoli are developed and the lobulo-alveolar system progressively takes over most of the space occupied by stroma so that the gland becomes a compact mass of lobules of alveoli separated from each other by septa of connective tissue. Some years ago it was widely held that most of the growth of the parenchyma arising from cell division was completed during the first two thirds of gestation and that subsequent increases in mammary size were due to hypertrophy of the cells and the filling up of the alveoli with secretion. There is, however, now clear evidence that cell division occurs throughout pregnancy and also during the early stages of lactation (see reviews by Munford, 1964; Denamur, 1965a). In the rat and mouse during pregnancy the histometric and biochemical changes in the mammary glands have been studied in detail by Munford (1963a, b, c) who showed that there is an increase in the total

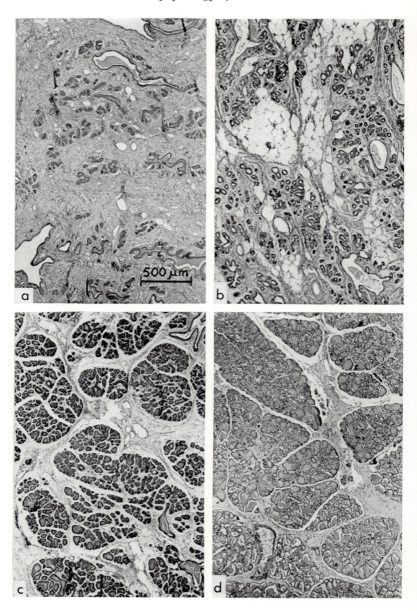

Fig. 3.3.

number of alveolar cells in late pregnancy and early lactation. More recent studies on epithelial cell proliferation in the mammary glands of pregnant and lactating mice by Traurig (1967*a*, *b*) with an autoradiographic technique, using tritiated thymidine, revealed that the rate of mammary gland cell proliferation during pregnancy followed a bimodal distribution, the highest rate of cell proliferation being recorded on day 4 while a second peak in activity occurred on day 12. A third wave of proliferation occurred on the second day of lactation, and thereafter mitotic activity fell to near zero by day 7 of lactation. In the rabbit Denamur (1963) observed in the mammary parenchyma a phase of rapid mitosis starting with day 20–23 of pregnancy and continuing to day 5 of lactation; on the basis of DNA studies Denamur (1963) considered that on days 14 and 30 of pregnancy the development of the mammary gland in the rabbit was 15% and 75% respectively of the development on the 5th day of lactation. Studies on the rabbit by Sod-Moriah & Schmidt (1968), however, indicated that proliferative activity of the mammary parenchyma was most intense during the first half of pregnancy, diminished during the second half of gestation, but showed a sharp rise at the time of parturition followed by a sharp drop in intensity during lactation. Further studies are necessary to resolve these discrepancies although some of the problem may lie in the difficulty of interpreting the biochemical and autoradiographic results.

The growth of the human mammary gland during pregnancy has been discussed by Dawson (1935), Geschickter (1945) and Dabelow (1957). In the first trimester there is an extension and branching of the duct system and by the tenth week the formation of immature lobules is evident. Alveolar formation is said to

---

FIG. 3.3. Structure of the mammary gland of the goat during pregnancy (gestation = 145–150 days).

(*a*) day 35   (*b*) day 72

In the first half of pregnancy the gland consists of collections of ducts within the stroma.

(*c*) day 82   (*d*) day 120

By day 82 the lobulo-alveolar formation is now distinct, secretion is present in many of the alveoli. By day 120 the lobulo-alveolar growth is complete, the alveoli are distended with secretion containing numerous fat globules (from Cowie, A. T. 1971, in *Lactation*, edited by Falconer, I. R., pp. 123–140. London: Butterworths).

occur early in the second trimester and later during this period secretion appears in the alveolar lumina, fat droplets being present both in the alveolar cells and in the secretion. By the last third of pregnancy the growing lobules have taken over much of the space previously occupied by connective and fatty tissues.

The growth of the mammary gland in the rhesus monkey during pregnancy (165 days) has been described by Speert (1948). During the first 2 months there is a high degree of individual variation; by the third month lobulo-alveolar development is extensive and secretory activity becomes evident by the beginning of the fourth month.

The growth of the lobulo-alveolar tissue in the udder of the goat during pregnancy has been briefly described by Cowie (1971); not until early in the second half of gestation, 70–100 days, is there a distinct and rapid formation of lobulo-alveolar tissue (Fig. 3.3).

The ultrastructure of the mammary gland during pregnancy has been studied in the rat by Murad (1970). The epithelium of the ductules shows an increase in the numbers of cytoplasmic ribosomes and polysomes from day 2 of gestation; on day 6 lipid droplets appear throughout the cytoplasm and become more plentiful as pregnancy proceeds. Two types of protein particles appear in the cytoplasm on day 7; formed in the region of the rough endoplasmic reticulum these migrate towards the apex of the cell and are totally excreted into the lumen before parturition. Murad (1970) considers that these particles are related to antibody formation in the colostrum and that, unlike the protein particles formed in late pregnancy and lactation, the Golgi apparatus plays no role in their formation. In the first half of gestation swelling of the mitochondria occurred but most mitochondria returned to the resting form by day 14. These cellular changes were observed only in the epithelium of the ductules and alveoli, not in the epithelium of the large ducts.

Ultrastructural changes in the mammary gland in late pregnancy associated with the initiation of milk secretion are discussed in Chapter 4.

Lactation and regression

The phases of functional activity and regression of the mammary parenchyma will be considered in the next chapter.

Stroma

So far we have discussed the growth of the mammary paren-chyma. The stroma, however, also undergoes important changes during the growth of the gland. The nature of the stroma varies with the species; in the ruminant, mouse and rat it is composed mainly of adipose tissue with some connective tissue, whereas in man it is mostly connective tissue (see Mayer & Klein, 1961). There is evidence that the disposition of the stroma predetermines the ramifications of the duct system and of the lobulo-alveolar growth of the gland (see Turner, 1939; Dabelow, 1957; Mayer & Klein, 1961). Studies involving the transplantation of mammary glands have thrown some light on these local mechanisms regu-lating parenchymal growth. In 3-week-old female mice Faulkin & DeOme (1960) transplanted a piece of homologous primary mam-mary duct into the 4th mammary fat pad from which the host mammary gland had been removed, while into the contralateral fat pad in which the host mammary gland was still intact two similar transplants were made. Two months later the single transplant filled $72 \pm 17\%$ of the fat pad whereas on the contra-lateral side the host gland occupied $32 \pm 19\%$ of the fat pad, and the two transplants $22 \pm 10\%$ and $44 \pm 22\%$. This indicates that there is a growth regulating system determining the spacing and extent of the growth of the mammary parenchyma, and which affects not only the transplanted gland but also the host gland. In such studies the ductal elements of the opposing edges of two or more outgrowths in a single fat pad do not interdigitate and a distinct duct-free zone exists at the border of the gland. The failure of advancing ducts to occupy these areas of pad is not due to a loss of growth potential since in many instances ducts have turned away from these zones and grown into unoccupied areas of pad; moreover, if portions of these ducts are transplanted to a cleared fat pad they will grow and fill it. Faulkin & DeOme (1960) point out that this growth-restricting force provides a mechanism whereby the general architecture of the adult mammary gland can be explained. Although the mammary ducts appear to fill the fat pad only a small portion of the total fat pad volume is actually occupied; ducts do not touch one another except at the point of origin and it would seem that around each duct there is a cylinder of fat about 0·25 mm diameter into which adjacent ducts do not enter. In short the spacing of the gland growth appears to be determined by a growth inhibiting system imparted to the surrounding fat pad by existing ducts, and the extent of the gland appears in some way to be associated with the border of the fat pad. While these forces regulating ductal growth within the individual fat pad are local phenomena the growth and development of the mammary gland in the mouse is under systemic hormonal control and the hormones involved have been determined (see p. 116). Faulkin & DeOme (1960) consider that the systemic hormones are the 'go' stimulus and must be present before growth can occur but the 'go' signal can be superseded by the local duct-inhibiting 'stop' signal. During pregnancy ductules and alveoli develop from the terminal buds and occupy previously unoccupied interductal spaces and begin to replace the fatty stroma which virtually disappears by the end of pregnancy. This invasion of the interductal spaces by the developing lobules implies some modification of the regulating mechanism. Faulkin & DeOme (1960) suggest that either (a) the terminal ducts are less sensitive to the inhibiting mechanism and the alveoli still less sensitive so that the alveoli grow in contact with one another; or (b) the mammogenic hormones responsible for lobulo-alveolar development alter the local growth inhibiting mechanism; or (c) the 'stop' signal may be specific and may regulate only duct growth.

Not only is the growth of the duct system controlled by mechanisms within the fat pad but, in mice at least, some property of adipose tissue is essential for mammary growth since transplants of mammary parenchyma will grow in a variety of intra-abdominal and subcutaneous deposits of fat (Hoshino, 1964, 1967) but will not grow in a variety of other sites (see also Nicoll, 1965a). The fat pad, moreover, may be considered to be a protected and privileged transplantation site in that the immunological responses evoked by the tissue implanted into it are limited.

Nicoll (1965a) has demonstrated in a series of experiments that removal of 84% of the mammary duct system from three-week-old female mice did not influence the rate of growth of the remaining 16% nor did injections of extracts of mammary tissue influence the growth from which he concluded that there was no evidence for the existence of a systemically operative humoral autoregulatory mechanism of mammary origin for the control of mammary duct growth which, as already noted, is subject to local regulators within the fat pad and to a variety of hormones. The possible relevance of these observations to neoplastic transformations of mammary cells is discussed by Nicoll (1965*a*). Normal mammary gland eventually ages and its growth rate declines on serial transplantation whereas preneoplastic gland appears to have an unlimited ability to proliferate in serial passage (Daniel, DeOme, Young, Blair & Faulkin, 1968).

Mammary growth in the male

In many species the mammary gland in the male consists of a restricted duct system hardly extending beyond the base of the rudimentary teat and in some species (e.g. rat, mouse) teats are absent in the male, the excretory ducts ending in the subcutaneous tissue or in the skin. In the rat and mouse the male gland keeps pace with the growth of the body as a whole (isometric growth), i.e. there is no period of accelerated growth such as occurs in the female. Between days 40–60, however, alveoli begin to form on the limited duct system of the male rat, these clusters of alveoli becoming dense (Fig. 3.2*b*). At first the epithelium of the alveoli consists of a single layer of cells but after some weeks the walls become several layers thick and some alveoli may eventually become solid clumps of proliferated epithelial cells (see Cowie, 1949; Ahrén & Etienne, 1957).

In boys there is usually no marked proliferation of the mammary gland at puberty, branched ducts are present but there is no true lobular formation. Occasionally duct proliferation may be sufficiently extensive to be regarded as gynaecomastia (see Jull & Dosset, 1964).

Detailed references to studies on the male gland in man will be found in the review by Dabelow (1957). Gynaecomastia has been dealt with in a book by Hall (1959) and the ultrastructural changes occurring in this condition have been recently described by Bässler & Schäfer (1969*b*).

In the male rhesus monkey Speert (1948) has observed a wide variation in the extent of development of the mammary glands ranging from tiny glands with unbranched ducts which did not extend beyond the base of the nipple to glands with extensive branching of the ducts and even with lobules of alveoli.

HORMONAL CONTROL OF MAMMARY GROWTH

Sub-classes Prototheria and Metatheria

We are not aware of any studies on the hormonal control of mammary growth in either Prototheria or Metatheria.

Sub-class Eutheria

In 1910 Marshall wrote, 'It was formerly supposed that the connection between the growth of the mammary glands and that of the embryo in the uterus was a nervous one—that is to say, that the hypertrophy of the glands was determined reflexly through the central nervous system. There is now, however, abundant evidence that such is not the case.' Marshall, after reviewing the relevant literature on the control of mammary growth (about a dozen references), concluded that 'the stimulus to mammary growth, which arises originally in the ovary, is afterwards derived from the developing embryo' and 'the inference is that the relation between the growth of the mammary glands and the development of the foetus in the uterus is chemical in nature'. At the time when Marshall wrote, the phenomenon of pseudopregnancy in bitches and rabbits (although it had been described and rediscovered on several occasions in the bitch since the late 18th century) was not generally recognized and the growth of the mammary gland in the non-pregnant bitch and rabbit was a source of some confusion in a number of early studies (see Frank & Unger, 1911). When, however, the classical studies of Ancel & Bouin (see review by Mayer & Klein, 1961) revealed the role of the corpus luteum in mammary growth in the pseudopregnant rabbit the interpretation of subsequent studies was greatly facilitated. Lyons (1958) has reviewed the major steps of the subsequent story which indeed forms a substantial part of the history of endocrinology. As the ovarian steroids became available in the 1930s it became possible to analyse the mammary responses observed earlier in response to crude ovarian extracts and the mammary-growth stimulating potency of the oestrogens and progesterone was clearly demonstrated in a variety of experimental animals. In rats and mice oestrogen alone stimulated growth of the duct system while lobulo-alveolar formation appeared to require the presence of both oestrogen and progesterone (see review by Folley, 1952). The studies of Stricker & Grueter (1928, 1929) on the involvement of the anterior pituitary in mammary function (see p. 144) stimulated research on the possible role of the pituitary in mammary growth and evidence soon accumulated which clearly indicated that the integrity of the anterior pituitary was essential for the ovarian hormones to manifest their mammogenic actions. Turner and his group in Columbia, Missouri, proposed the existence of two specific pituitary hormones concerned in the growth of the mammary gland: Mammogen I secreted from the anterior pituitary under the influence of oestrogens was considered to be responsible for duct growth, while Mammogen II released in response to oestrogen + progesterone caused lobulo-alveolar growth (see review by Cowie, 1966). Although the concept of *specific* mammogens of pituitary origin was never widely accepted (see reviews by Folley & Malpress, 1948*a*; Folley, 1952; Cowie, 1966) the 'Mammogen' theory rightly centred attention on the role of the anterior pituitary in mammogenesis and stimulated much research in the field. The early studies on the mammogenic effects of anterior pituitary extracts in hypophysectomized animals have been reviewed in detail by Folley & Malpress (1948*a*) and Folley (1952).

Studies on mammary growth in hypophysectomized animals

Major elucidation of the roles of the ovarian and pituitary hormones in mammogenesis came from a series of studies by Lyons and his colleagues who worked on the hypothesis that the ovarian hormones synergized with the hypophysial hormones to induce the two main phases of mammary growth, namely ductal and lobulo-alveolar mammogenesis; their problem was to identify the synergizing hypophysial substances, which they believed to be some of the already known anterior pituitary hormones rather than specific 'Mammogens', the preparation, in the late 1930s and early 1940s, of relatively pure prolactin, GH and ACTH having now made such studies possible. The procedure used by Lyons and his colleagues was that of replacement therapy, i.e. they studied the effects of various combinations of ovarian and hypophysial hormones on mammary growth in young rats from which the pituitary or pituitary and ovaries (double operation) or pituitary, ovaries and adrenals (triple operation) had previously been removed. Thus at the start of the hormonal treatments the mammary glands consisted of atrophied duct systems; the removal of the pituitary and other endocrine glands, moreover, eliminated the possibility of endogenous mammogenic hormones participating in the responses with the exogenous hormones and so complicating the interpretation. These extensive studies have been well reviewed by Lyons (1958), Lyons, Li & Johnson (1958) and Lyons & Dixon (1966) and we shall limit comment on them to a summary of the main conclusions. In the triply-operated rat the ovarian and adrenal steroids are only mammogenic in the presence of anterior pituitary hormones, the minimal hormonal requirements for duct growth being oestrogen, adrenal steroids and ox growth hormone, lobulo-alveolar growth being subsequently induced by adding progesterone and sheep prolactin to the above three hormones. By the local application of prolactin and GH it was demonstrated that both acted directly on the mammary parenchyma. To what extent are these findings applicable to other species? As Lyons & Dixon (1966) have stated: 'It should be emphasized that conclusions regarding these activities have been drawn from experiments done with endocrinectomized Long-Evans rats; and to a lesser extent with hooded-Norway rats. . . . No suggestion should be inferred, therefore, that our findings on mammogensis necessarily apply to other forms. . . .' Only in one other species, the mouse, have similar detailed studies been carried out on endocrinectomized animals. Several hormonal combinations have been associated with duct growth after hypophysectomy in the mouse and some of the variations in response may be associated with differences in strain. Oestrogen + progesterone + sheep prolactin, or oestrogen + progesterone + ox GH, induced vigorous duct growth in Strong A2G strain hypophysectomized mice (Hadfield & Young, 1958). Extensive studies by Nandi (1959) on triply-operated mice (C3H/He Crgl strain) indicated that oestrogen + ox GH, or oestrogen + corticoid + ox GH, stimulated duct growth although from his studies Nandi concluded that oestrogen + GH + corticoid were the hormones normally concerned in duct growth in the mouse. The hormonal requirements for ductal mammogensis in the mouse and rat are therefore similar. For lobulo-alveolar development in triply-operated mice a number of hormonal combinations were reported by Nandi to be effective but a very efficient one was oestrogen + sheep prolactin + progesterone + ox GH + corticoid which is again in conformity with Lyons's observations in the rat. Nandi, however, observed that a combination of oestrogen + progesterone + ox GH stimulated lobulo-alveolar development to a greater degree than did oestrogen + progesterone + sheep prolactin, i.e. either prolactin or GH in combination with the ovarian hormones evoked lobulo-alveolar growth. Subsequent studies by Nandi & Bern (1961) revealed that the combination of ovarian hormones and ox GH was effective in inducing lobulo-alveolar growth only in some strains of mice. Despite small variations in mammogenic responses it is clear that in both the rat and mouse full mammary growth can be induced by the anterior-pituitary hormones—prolactin + GH—acting in combination with ovarian and adrenal steroids. While these studies do not exclude the possible existence of specific pituitary mammogens, they do rather diminish the necessity to postulate their existence. In 1960 Clifton & Furth noted that lobulo-alveolar mammary growth was induced in ovariectomized-adrenalectomized rats grafted with pieces of rat pituitary tumours which secreted both prolactin and GH. This observation which suggested that hypophysial hormones alone in sufficient doses were mammogenic in the absence of ovarian hormones was followed up by Talwalker & Meites (1961, 1964) who demonstrated that lobulo-alveolar development could be induced in triply-operated rats given frequent doses of prolactin + GH. Talwalker & Meites emphasize that this observation should not be interpreted to mean that ovarian and adrenocortical hormones are not concerned in normal mammogenesis in the rat. However, since the hypophysial hormones given by themselves in frequent and large doses can stimulate lobulo-alveolar growth they must therefore be regarded as being of major importance in mammogenesis in the rat.

Only in the rat and mouse have such detailed analyses of the hormones concerned in mammogenesis been made. In a small study on goats in which an attempt was made to build up the mammary gland by suitable replacement therapy Cowie, Tindal & Yokoyama (1966) concluded that in this species in the absence of the pituitary, oestrogen (hexoestrol) alone or in combination with progesterone exerted no significant mammogenic effect nor did the ovarian hormones prevent the regression after hypophysectomy of an already developed gland. In the hypophysectomized-ovariectomized goat significant lobulo-alveolar growth was induced by the combination of hexoestrol, progesterone, prolactin, GH and ACTH (Fig. 3.4). In this study there was no indication

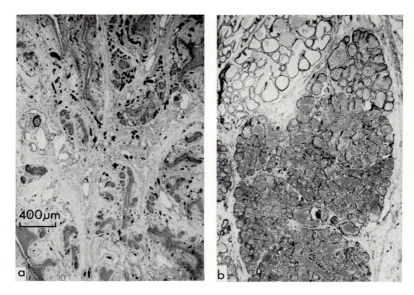

FIG. 3.4. Induction of mammary growth in the hypophysectomized goat. (*a*). Section of mammary gland from a hypophysectomized goat which had been injected daily for 40 days with hexoestrol (0·5 mg) and ACTH (20 i.u.). The parenchyma is quite undeveloped, consisting of scattered groups of ducts. (This gland was not fixed by intravascular perfusion and the capillaries contain darkly staining red blood cells.)

(*b*). Section of the mammary gland from a hypophysectomized goat injected daily for 40 days with hexoestrol and ACTH (as (*a*) above), for a further 40 days with these hormones plus bovine GH (12·5 mg) and then for a further 20-day period with these three hormones plus progesterone (70 mg) + sheep prolactin (225 i.u.). Observe the moderately developed lobulo-alveolar tissue and the presence of secretion in the alveoli.

Both figures are at the same magnification (from Cowie, A. T., Tindal, J. S. & Yokoyama, A., 1966, *J. Endocr.* **34**, 185–195).

of a combination of hormones that stimulated duct growth alone. The degree of lobulo-alveolar development achieved in the hypophysectomized-ovariectomized goat was, moreover, far from complete being equivalent to that observed soon after mid-pregnancy. Whether the poor response was due to inadequate hormone dosage, to an incomplete hormone combination or both is not known. It is of interest, however, that subsequently evidence was obtained that hypophysial hormones will induce mammogenesis in the goat in the absence of ovarian hormones indicating their prime importance in this species as in the rat (see p. 126).

Although there are extensive studies on experimental mammogenesis in the rabbit from which it appears that after hypophysectomy the mammary gland is still partially responsive to ovarian hormones (see p. 120) there is, at present, little information on its responses to the hypophysial hormones. Norgren (1968), however, in preliminary studies reported that GH alone, or in combination with oestrone or oestrone and progesterone, did not stimulate mammary growth in hypophysectomized rabbits.

While such studies as those of Lyons and his colleagues and of Nandi have delineated the minimal hormone requirements for mammary growth in the rat and mouse under experimental conditions it is most likely that for normal mammogenesis during pregnancy hormones from the placenta, possibly steroid, and certainly protein play important roles in mammary growth. There is evidence for the existence of a rat chorionic mammotrophin which imitates its hypophysial counterpart—prolactin—by being both directly mammogenic and indirectly so by activation of the corpus luteum (see review by Lyons, 1958; Matthies, 1967). Studies by Desjardins, Paape & Tucker (1968) on the effects of the surgical removal of the foetuses and placentae from pregnant rats on the nucleic acid content of the mammary glands suggest that placental hormones play a major role in mammary development in the second half of pregnancy. The presence in the primate placenta of chorionic somato-mammotrophin (see Chapter 2) which is both mammogenic and lactogenic in test animals suggests a physiological role for this hormone in the development of the mammary glands in primates.

As already noted, experimental studies in the rat, mouse and goat have shown that the presence of a functional anterior pituitary is essential for the mammary gland to respond to steroid hormones, whereas mammary growth can occur in response to hypophysial hormones by themselves suggesting that the hypophysial hormones are the essential factors in mammogenesis. Hypophysectomy, however, by removing all the hypophysial hormones causes a vast upset to a variety of essential metabolic processes either directly, or indirectly through the endocrine target organs; the question must therefore be asked as to what extent such metabolic deficiencies influence the ability of the mammary gland to respond to ovarian hormones. Hypophysectomy, for example, depresses appetite and various attempts have been made to assess the significance of this factor (see review by Jacobsohn, 1958). Using the observation by Salter & Best (1953) that alterations in the intermediary metabolism of rats after hypophysectomy can be partially remedied by giving daily injections of long-acting insulin combined with a carbohydrate-rich diet (see review by Jacobsohn, 1958), Jacobsohn noted that the mammary glands of rats so treated did show some growth response to ovarian hormones although the benefits of insulin did not appear to be associated with increased food intake. She further observed that the beneficial effects of insulin were enhanced by thyroxine but counteracted by cortisone. While the partial restoration of the metabolic deficiencies in the hypophysectomized rat can facilitate the growth response of the mammary gland to ovarian hormones the responses so obtained are nevertheless small in comparison with those observed in the rat with intact pituitary thereby confirming the essential and specific roles of the hypophysial hormones in mammogenesis in this species.

In the rabbit, hypophysectomy appears to have a less inhibitory effect on mammogenesis than in the rat, mouse and goat. Norgren (1968), after a series of studies, reached the following conclusions: (a) extensive mammary duct growth occurred in the completely hypophysectomized rabbit injected with oestrogen alone or in combination with progesterone but responses were submaximal and alveoli did not form; (b) the responsiveness of the mammary glands to ovarian hormones could be modified by other hormones— thyroxine markedly increased duct growth and alveolar development, cortisone tended to depress duct growth, while insulin with or without thyroxine caused a slight increase in duct growth. Cortisone, thyroxine and insulin in various combinations in the absence of ovarian hormones did not stimulate mammary growth in the hypophysectomized rabbit. The mammary development obtained with ovarian hormones in hypophysectomized rabbits treated with cortisone, thyroxine and insulin was not so extensive as that obtained in rabbits with intact pituitary; (c) in rabbits with intact pituitary, duct growth was depressed by cortisone and by thyroidectomy. It is thus clear that in rabbits the metabolic effects of hypophysectomy are such that they still permit the mammary gland to respond partially to doses of oestrogen and progesterone —a situation somewhat different from the rat although the presence of the anterior pituitary appears to be essential for full growth.

Organ culture studies

Studies of mammary gland tissue from the mouse and the rat explanted and cultured *in vitro* in media containing hormone supplements have in general confirmed the observations made *in vivo* on the hormonal requirements for mammary growth and have also implied that much of the synergism between the hormones lies at the target tissue level (see Rivera, 1964*a*, *b*; Gadkari, Chapekar & Ranadive, 1968).

It is possible to induce some degree of lobulo-alveolar growth in mammary transplants from virgin mice cultured in medium containing insulin, ovarian and adrenal steroids, prolactin and growth hormone but to obtain extensive lobulo-alveolar proliferation it is necessary to pretreat the mice with ovarian steroids, prolactin and growth hormone (Ichinose & Nandi, 1966). In culture such explants require the presence of insulin in the culture medium irrespective of other hormone supplements if regression of the parenchyma is to be prevented. Culture media must contain anterior-pituitary and steroid hormones for lobule formation to occur in mouse mammary gland (Ichinose & Nandi, 1966).

Mammary explants from young female rats behave somewhat differently in culture in that pretreatment of the rat is not a necessary prerequisite for obtaining extensive lobulo-alveolar growth. Indeed some lobulo-alveolar proliferation of the rat mammary gland can be obtained in medium containing only insulin and prolactin although the degree of proliferation can be much enhanced by adding oestrogen, progesterone and adrenal steroids (Dilley & Nandi, 1968).

Organ culture studies relevant to alveolar cell differentiation previous to secretory activity are discussed in the next chapter. A comprehensive review by Forsyth (1971) of organ culture techniques and studies on the mammary gland has recently been published.

E

Studies in animals with intact pituitary

So far, this chapter has dealt almost exclusively with studies specifically designed to determine the role of the various hormones in mammogenesis and the simplest hormonal combinations required for duct and lobulo-alveolar growth using animals from which the pituitary, ovaries and frequently the adrenals had been removed in order to eliminate the participation of endogenous hormones. There is, however, a vast literature on the mammogenic potencies of ovarian steroids in various species of normal animals which provides information on the most effective dose levels of the ovarian hormones required for stimulating extensive duct and lobulo-alveolar growth. In all such studies the essential role of the anterior pituitary must be stressed since much of the apparent mammogenic activity of the ovarian hormones may be exerted by way of the anterior pituitary hormones whose release they effect. There is, of course, clear evidence that in the intact animal oestrogens can act directly on the mammary parenchyma and stimulate its growth as shown by the local application of oestrogens (see review by Lyons, 1958); moreover, the accumulation of tritiated oestrogen in the mammary tissue of the rat may well be associated with its direct mammogenic activities (Sander, 1968; Puca & Bresciani, 1969). Nevertheless such direct mammogenic effects involve the co-operation of anterior pituitary hormones.

Folley (1952, 1956) extensively reviewed and discussed the earlier studies of this nature and the general conclusion which emerged, and which is still valid, is that both oestrogen and pro-gesterone are necessary for stimulating extensive normal lobulo-alveolar growth, i.e. comparable to that developed in the course of pregnancy. Mammogenic responses to the ovarian hormones vary, however, with the species both in the qualitative and quanti-tative nature of the growth response and, with regard to the response to oestrogen, three main categories may be recognized among laboratory and farm animals. First there are those species such as the rat, mouse, cat and rabbit in which oestrogen in physiological doses evokes growth of the ducts alone, alveoli only appear if the dose of oestrogen is high or its administration prolonged. Secondly, in species such as the guinea-pig, goat and cow, oestrogen at physiological dose levels induces lobulo-alveolar growth. Lastly there are some species such as the bitch and ferret in which oestrogen alone evokes little or no mammary growth (see reviews by Folley, 1952, 1956).

The phase of allometric duct growth which occurs in the adolescent female rat and mouse has already been discussed (see p. 106). That this phase of accelerated mammary growth is evoked by the ovary was demonstrated by the fact that ovariectomy prevented the onset of allometric growth, the ducts continuing to grow isometrically (Cowie, 1949; Silver, 1953*a*, *b*; Flux, 1954*a*, *b*). Replacement therapy studies have indicated that oestrogen alone appears to be responsible for the phase of allometric duct growth in both rats and mice. Silver (1953*a*) could best reproduce the normal duct growth in young ovariectomized rats by injecting 0·1 µg oestradiol dipropionate every other day from day 21 of age and increasing the dose stepwise with body weight; in the ovariectomized mouse 0·055 µg oestrone/day restored duct growth to normal (Flux, 1954*a*).

Some of the early studies on the role of the ovarian hormones in mammogenesis were concerned with the possible existence of an optimal progesterone : oestrogen ratio and a good deal of confusion arose because it was not fully realized that the various oestrogens differed widely in their biological activities not only between species but within the same species and for a comparison of ratios to be meaningful the oestrogen must be the same in all ratios being compared. Detailed studies of the responses of the mammary gland to various doses of oestrone and progesterone, singly or in combination, have been reported in the guinea-pig (Benson, Cowie, Cox & Goldzveig, 1957) and in the gonadectomized rabbit (Norgren, 1966). It was confirmed that oestrone alone in the guinea-pig induced considerable lobulo-alveolar growth; more extensive growth was obtained when progesterone was also administered, the best responses being obtained with daily doses of 1 mg progesterone in combination with 10–50 µg oestrone. Progesterone alone evoked lobulo-alveolar growth if the dose was sufficiently large (2·4 mg/day). Optimal dose levels were somewhat similar in the rabbit—1·2 or 5 mg progesterone in combination with 5, 10 or 20 µg oestrone. In both the guinea-pig and rabbit the absolute quantities of the hormones were the important factors in determining the mammogenic response, the progesterone : oestrone ratio *per se* being unimportant since altering the dose levels while maintaining the ratio gave quite different results. Similar conclusions were reached by Sud, Tucker & Meites (1968) using progesterone and oestradiol-17β to induce maximum lobulo-alveolar growth in heifers.

In the late 1930s when synthetic oestrogens became available in quantity, studies began on the feasibility of using these substances—diethylstilboestrol, hexoestrol, dienoestrol—to induce udder growth and lactation in cows and goats. Extensive investigations on the artificial induction of lactation in sterile heifers and cows were conducted during the second world war and were fully reported in the *Journal of Endocrinology* (vol. 4, no. 1, 1944); they have moreover been discussed at some length by Folley & Malpress (1948*b*) while subsequent studies have been reviewed by Folley (1956) and Meites (1961). In these studies on cows oestrogen only was administered, synthetic progesterone being not then available, and although extensive and detailed morphological studies of the mammary tissue were not performed the occurrence of extensive lobulo-alveolar growth was evidenced from the preliminary studies of the mammary tissue and from the considerable milk yields obtained. A striking feature was the marked variation in response between individual animals to the oestrogen therapy, varying from little growth of the udder and virtually no milk to marked udder growth and maximum daily yields of over 13 kg of milk. Only in about 50% of the treated animals were economic yields of milk attained (considered at the time to be about 7 kg/day). Subsequently when synthetic progesterone became available, further small-scale studies suggested that better mammary growth responses and higher milk yields could be attained by combined oestrogen + progesterone therapy (see Folley, 1956; Meites, 1961). A series of experiments were conducted in this laboratory on goats to determine the effects of various doses of oestrogen (hexoestrol) alone or in combination with progesterone on mammary structure and function. To avoid interference from endogenous ovarian hormone the goats (young virgin goatlings) were ovariectomized before the treatments were started. The structure of the lobulo-alveolar tissue was evaluated by new histometric procedures devised by Richardson (see p. 89) which permitted the surface area of the secretory epithelium to be calculated. From these studies it emerged that while hexoestrol alone could induce very considerable lobulo-alveolar growth several abnormalities in structure were generally present; first, the alveoli tended to be excessively large or cystic resulting in an overall deficiency of secretory epithelial surface area per unit volume of tissue in comparison with the mammary tissue of normally lactating goats; secondly, immature lobules of alveoli were frequently present, and thirdly the alveolar walls sometimes showed the presence of papillomatous outgrowths. The addition of progesterone to the treatment greatly reduced the incidence of such abnormalities in udder structure and usually increased milk yields (see review by Folley, 1956). Satisfactory dose levels of hexoestrol and progesterone were 0·5 mg/day and 70 mg/day respectively and when these were given over a period equivalent to that of normal gestation in the goat (140–150 days) the lobulo-alveolar structure of the udder at the peak of lactation was virtually normal although milk yields were only two thirds of the expected yield had the goats come into lactation after a normal pregnancy (Benson, Cowie, Cox, Folley & Hosking, 1965). A further study (Cowie, Cox, Folley, Hosking, Naito & Tindal, 1965) using the same daily dose levels of hexoestrol and progesterone explored the effects, in ovariectomized goats, of the duration of the treat-ment period on mammary growth and function. Histological studies were carried out on half-udders removed at the end of the treatment period (35, 70 or 140 days), that is just before milking was started, while the contralateral halves were studied after 25–40 weeks of lactation. In general the longer the treatment period the sooner were peak milk yields attained after the start of milking, the interval from the start of injections to attainment of peak yield being 32 to 41 weeks. The best milk yields over a 24-week period (4·97 l./wk per goat and 3·24 l./wk per goat, respectively) were obtained with hexoestrol and progesterone given for 140 or 70 days (these yields are from one mammary gland only, the other having been removed before milking started). With hexoestrol alone the duration of treatment did not affect the milk yields, the mean yields after 35-day treatment being 2·06 l./wk per goat and after 140 days 2·10 l./wk per goat. The lowest yield (0·34 l./wk per goat) occurred in the goats receiving hexoestrol and progesterone for 35 days. These observations indicate that for the practical induction of lactation a combination of oestrogen and progesterone over prolonged periods will result in the higher milk yields but that therapy with oestrogen alone may be the better procedure if treatments can only be given for short periods. Comparison of the glands at the end of the hormone treatments with the contralateral glands removed at the peak of lactation showed, rather surprisingly, that most of the lobulo-alveolar growth and maturation occurred during lactation, i.e. after hormone injections had been stopped. While it was possible that the growth during milking might have resulted, in part, from residual hormone depots after injections had ended it seemed more probable that the mammary growth was due to the release of mammogenic hormones from the anterior pituitary in response to the milking stimulus; moreover, since the goats had been ovariectomized any indirect pituitary effects mediated by way of the ovarian steroids could be excluded. This latter explanation was confirmed by Cowie, Knaggs, Tindal & Turvey (1968) who showed that the regular application of the milking stimulus to nulliparous ovariectomized goats induced mammary growth and lactation without the necessity of any pre-treatment with ovarian hormones; it was further demonstrated that the mammogenic response was of anterior pituitary origin since surgical transection of the pituitary stalk completely abolished the response. Milk yields were, however, less than would have been expected had pre-treatment with hormones been given and the lobulo-alveolar structure was somewhat abnormal in that there was present an excess of interalveolar connective tissue. These observations indicate that in the goat, as in the rat (see p. 117), the pituitary hormones by themselves are capable of inducing considerable lobulo-alveolar growth and would appear to play the major role in mammogenesis since in the hypophysectomized goat the ovarian hormones have no mammogenic activity (Cowie, Tindal & Yokoyama, 1966). The above observations would also suggest that in the artifical induction of lactation in farm animals the best results are likely to be achieved by reinforcing the mammogenic effects of the administered ovarian hormones by the regular application of the milking stimulus.

Recently Sud, Tucker & Meites (1968) studied the effects of progesterone and oestradiol in various doses on mammary growth in ovariectomized heifers over a period of 20 weeks; the best growth responses occurred with doses of 0·8 mg oestradiol and 200 mg progesterone or 0·4 mg oestradiol and 100 mg progesterone. Histological and biochemical studies of the mammary tissue at the end of the injection period showed that the above dose levels of progesterone and oestradiol induced differentiation of the lobulo-alveolar tissue to a degree qualitatively similar to that in 5-month-pregnant control heifers but quantitatively there was an overall deficiency of lobulo-alveolar tissue in comparison with the pregnant controls.

It would seem that seldom, if ever, has it been possible in farm animals to induce the development of full lobulo-alveolar growth comparable in quality and quantity to that occurring at the end of normal pregnancy with the aid of ovarian hormones alone in the absence of the milking or suckling stimulus. It is likely that in normal pregnancy increased levels of hypophysial mammogenic hormones (prolactin, GH) and, in some species, the presence of placental mammogenic hormones play the prime role while the ovarian hormones have a subsidiary role in mammary growth and that such hormonal conditions cannot be reproduced or even approximated in the non-pregnant animal by the administration merely of oestrogen and progesterone possibly because of their limited ability to increase the output of pituitary hormones and because of the total absence of placental mammogenic hormones.

Oral contraceptives and mammary growth

There have been occasional clinical reports suggesting that oral contraceptives cause enlargement of the breast (see Kahn & Baker, 1964; Pincus, 1965). There is, as would be expected, considerable evidence that the oestrogen-progestogen combinations used can induce mammogenesis in rats and mice (Griffith, Williams & Turner, 1963; Kahn & Baker, 1964, 1969; Kahn, Baker & Zanotti, 1965; Browning, Larke & Talamantes, 1968) but whether these steroid combinations induce proliferation of the parenchyma of the human breast has still to be demonstrated.

Self-licking and mammary growth

Roth & Rosenblatt (1968) observed that in rats as pregnancy advanced self-licking of the nipple lines increased. If this behaviour was prevented by fitting a wide collar round the animal's neck then normal mammary growth was retarded. This observation is discussed in Chapter 6.

Growth of nipple or teat

The growth of the nipple or teat appears to be influenced mainly by oestrogens although studies are relatively few. Most widely investigated has been the guinea-pig in which the growth of the nipple was at one time used as a sensitive indicator of oestrogen activity (Jadassohn, Uehlinger & Margot, 1938; Jadassohn & Fierz-David, 1943; Wheeler, Cawley & Curtis, 1953). In the male guinea-pig the nipple grows isometrically relative to body growth but as castration suppresses teat growth it appears that androgens are required to maintain the isometric growth (Bottomley & Folley, 1938). In female rats also nipple growth can be stimulated by the local application of testosterone propionate and this effect is not dependent on the presence of anterior pituitary hormones (Ahren & Hamberger, 1962). Norethynodrel alone or with mestranol induces pronounced growth of the nipples in virgin female rats (Kahn & Baker, 1964).

In the female goat teat growth is initially isometric but at an early age, even at 6 weeks, allometric growth may set in but may be interrupted during the annual period of oestrous cycles (Folley, Scott Watson & Bottomley, 1941).

The topical application of oestrogen to one nipple in prepubertal male rhesus monkeys causes localized growth of the nipple and areola (Speert, 1948).

Changes in areolar size during adolescence in the human female have been described by Garn (1952).

Levels in the peripheral blood of ovarian, pituitary and placental mammogenic hormones during pregnancy

From our review of the studies on mammogenesis it will have become obvious that our knowledge of the role of hormones in mammary growth has been derived principally by studying the effects on the mammary glands of the addition or subtraction of the hormones under experimental conditions. In most experiments the doses of the hormones administered were chosen empirically because of the complete lack of information about the normal levels of hormones in the blood during the various phases of mammary growth. Over the last decade, however, assay methods of sufficient sensitivity and specificity have been developed, with the result that information on hormone levels in blood is now accumulating, certainly regarding the steroid hormones, and to a lesser extent for the mammogenic protein hormones of the pituitary and placenta.

Oestrogens. The methods of assay and levels of oestrogens present in the blood of women have been reviewed by O'Donnell & Preedy (1967) while their metabolism in the foetal, placental and maternal compartments has been discussed by Diczfalusy (1969) and Diczfalusy & Mancuso (1969). Approximate levels of the three classic oestrogens in peripheral blood during the menstrual cycle and gestation are set out in Table 3.1 (for recent studies on oestriol, see also Fischer-Rasmussen, 1970). The levels of all three oestrogens increase markedly in the peripheral blood during pregnancy.

Table 3.1. Approximate levels (ng/ml.) of oestrone, oestradiol-17β and oestriol in the peripheral blood or plasma of women (derived from review by O'Donnell & Preedy, 1967)

Reproductive state	Blood or plasma	Oestrone	Oestradiol-17β	Oestriol
Menstrual cycle				
(a) proliferative phase	blood	0·2	0·1	0·2
(b) ovulatory peak	plasma	0·6	0·3	0·2
(c) secretory phase	plasma	< 0·6–2·2	< 0·7	< 1·5–3·0
Pregnancy				
6th week	blood	1·4	0·5	0·9
12th week	blood	3·9	0·9	2·0
last 5 weeks	plasma	26–260	12–30	40–240

Studies of oestrogen levels in bovine blood have been reviewed by Mellin & Erb (1965) who concluded that, while no endogenous oestrogen had been specifically identified in the peripheral blood of ruminants, oestrogen activity in the second half of pregnancy had been detected by several investigators, the values ranging from 0·1 to 3·7 ng oestradiol equivalent/ml. blood. Pope, Jones & Waynforth (1965) also reported oestrogenic activity in the peripheral blood of cows in oestrus equivalent to 1–10 pg/ml., while at the 5th–6th months of pregnancy activities were equivalent to 1 ng/ml. rising to 7 ng/ml. in cows 7–9 months pregnant; it was moreover, shown that in late pregnancy the activity was mainly due to the presence of oestrone in a water-soluble form.

In the rat information on oestrogenic hormones in blood is limited to studies on the ovarian venous blood. Whether such

The physiology of lactation

studies will accurately reflect changes in the peripheral blood will depend *inter alia* on the possible secretion of oestrogen from other sites, e.g. placenta. According to Yoshinaga, Hawkins & Stocker (1969) in non-pregnant rats the highest activity in ovarian plasma occurred at pro-oestrus when the concentration was 4·5 ng oestradiol equivalent/ml. plasma or 9·0 ng oestradiol equivalent/ ovary per hour; during pregnancy there was a transient peak of activity on day 4 (1·1 ng oestradiol equivalent/ml. or 2·3 ng equivalent/ovary per hour), thereafter values remained low until day 13 when for seven days the concentration was about 0·5 ng oestradiol equivalent/ ml.; on day 20 the activity increased rapidly to 1·1 ng equivalent/ml. reaching a peak on day 23, i.e. day of parturition, when the concentration was 3 ng equivalent/ml. or 14·6 ng equivalent/ovary per hour; the day after parturition oestrogenic activity in the plasma could not be detected.

Pope & Waynforth (1970) have recently assayed levels of oestrone and oestradiol-17β in the ovarian venous blood of pregnant rats; oestrone levels were always very low but on day 2 oestradiol levels were about 100 pg/ovary per hour rising to 500 pg/ovary per hour on day 3; this level was maintained until day 16 but by day 21 levels of 2–4 ng/ovary per hour were reached; similar high values occurred at pro-oestrus.

Progesterone. The various methods of assaying progesterone in blood and studies on the levels present in the blood of women have been reviewed by van der Molen & Aakvaag (1969) while its placental synthesis and metabolism have been discussed by Hellig, Lefebvre, Gattereau & Bolté (1969) and Younglai & Solomon (1969) respectively. In the follicular phase of the menstrual cycle mean levels of progesterone in the peripheral plasma during the first and second weeks are about 0·49 and 1·3 ng/ml. plasma respectively; in the luteal phase the highest level in the blood (15·2 ng/ml. plasma) occurs about day 24 falling to 7·1 ng/ml. in the last week. During the first trimester of gestation the progesterone level is 20–70 ng/ml. plasma, the level increasing slightly in the second trimester and then more steeply in the last trimester when levels of 40 to 360 ng/ml. occur.

Earlier studies on progesterone levels in the blood of cows and other farm animals have been reviewed by Gomes & Erb (1965); levels of progesterone in the peripheral plasma from days 60 to

260 were in the region of 10 ng/ml. and after day 260 there was a rapid fall. Subsequent studies in non-pregnant and pregnant cows have indicated rather high concentrations of progesterone in peripheral blood, 10 ng/ml. and 26 ng/ml. plasma at oestrus and mid-cycle respectively with levels varying between 30–40 ng/ml. over the greater part of gestation (Plotka, Erb, Callahan & Gomes, 1967; Erb, Estergreen, Jr., Gomes, Plotka & Frost, 1968). These higher values have not, however, been confirmed in two recent studies. Pope, Gupta & Munro (1969) report mid-cycle values for the cow of 9·0 ng progesterone/ml. plasma with levels in the last month of gestation mostly between 2·5 and 7·5 ng/ml., there being a significant decline during the last month. Progesterone levels of 0·5 ng/ml. plasma at oestrus, increasing to 7 ng/ml. at peak luteal phase, have been found by Stabenfeldt, Ewing & MacDonald (1969) while studies by the same group in pregnant cows from day 140 to parturition indicated progesterone levels of about 5 ng/ml. plasma increasing to 7 ng/ml. by day 250; levels then declined to 4 ng/ml. 10 days before calving followed by an abrupt fall to less than 1 ng/ml. 24 hr before parturition (Stabenfeldt, Osburn & Ewing, 1970). Possible technical reasons for disagreements regarding levels of progesterone in the peripheral blood of cows as found by various teams have been discussed by Hunter, Erb, Randel, Garverick, Callahan & Harrington (1970) who also showed that levels of progesterone in peripheral blood in the last week of gestation are apparently associated with the length of the gestation period of the individual animal.

In the pregnant goat progesterone levels of about 10 ng/ml. peripheral plasma were attained in the first two weeks reaching a maximum of about 15 ng/ml. in about five weeks, then declining near parturition (Heap & Linzell, 1966). In the pregnant goat, the ovary appears to be the main source of progesterone, some 10 mg progesterone being produced by the ovaries per day and about 2 mg of this are taken up by the mammary glands (Heap & Linzell, 1966; Heap, Linzell & Slotin, 1969). The significance of this uptake so far as mammary growth is concerned is unknown and the problem is perhaps further complicated by the apparent ability of the mammary gland to synthesize progesterone from pregnenolone (Slotin, Heap, Christiansen & Linzell, 1970). The mammary gland of the rabbit also takes up quantities of progesterone from the blood (Chatterton, Jr., Chatterton & Hellman, 1969).

In the sow in early pregnancy (days 20–28) a level of 20 ng progesterone/ml. plasma has been observed which is slightly lower than the peak level (24 ng/ml.) during the oestrous cycle (days 10–12) (Tillson, Erb & Niswender, 1970).

In the pregnant rat high levels of progesterone are present in peripheral plasma, about 260 ng/ml. plasma at day 10 falling to 200 ng by day 18, and to 114 ng by day 21; there is then an abrupt fall on day 22 to 10 ng/ml. rising within 6 hr post partum to 43 ng/ml. (Grota & Eik-Nes, 1967). Kuhn (1969a) has reported values of 65 ng/ml. 5 days before parturition declining to less than 10 ng/ml. before parturition.

Prolactin. The problem of the existence of human prolactin has been discussed in Chapter 2. If it exists its assay in the blood during pregnancy will have to depend on a specific assay since bioassays normally measuring mammotrophic activities (i.e. mammogenic and/or lactogenic responses) will respond to the large quantities of chorionic somato-mammotrophin (HCS) present in the blood during gestation.

Attempts to measure pigeon crop-stimulating activity in the blood of women during pregnancy have been reviewed by Forsyth (1967, 1969). The unsatisfactory nature of the extraction procedure (see p. 70) and the doubtful appropriateness of the pigeon as a test animal for mammotrophic activity throws grave doubts on the value or significance of any results so obtained either in women or other mammals. Recently a promising bioassay, based on a lactogenic response in explants of rabbit mammary gland, has been used to detect lactogenic activity in the plasma of goats during pregnancy and parturition, when considerable activities have been found (Brumby & Forsyth, 1969; Forsyth, personal communication). This technique is also applicable to human blood (Forsyth, 1969) (see also Fig. 2.4). As already noted, this assay will not normally differentiate between hormones of pituitary and placental origin but the addition of a suitable immune serum to the system thereby inhibiting the biological effects of either prolactin or HCS may introduce a high degree of specificity to the bioassay (Forsyth, personal communication). Information about blood levels of prolactin during pregnancy in several species is now being gathered by new radioimmunoassay procedures. In the goat in late pregnancy levels of 720 ng prolactin/ml. plasma rising to 3000 ng/ml. after delivery have been reported by Bryant, Greenwood & Linzell (1968). In the sheep several studies have indicated the presence of prolactin in the blood during pregnancy but the levels and trends differ widely in the several reports and further studies are essential before drawing any conclusions about trends in concentration (Saji, 1967; Arai & Lee, 1967; McNeilly, 1971). In the cow levels of 50–70 ng prolactin/ml. serum in the last week of pregnancy rising to over 800 ng/ml. just before parturition have been reported (Schams & Karg, 1969, 1970).

In an extensive study on prolactin levels in the peripheral blood of rats in various phases of reproduction Amenomori, Chen & Meites (1970) found that in pregnancy the greatest concentrations (19–30 ng/ml. serum) occurred during the first three days whereas during the next eighteen days the values were low (8–11 ng/ml.); on day 22, i.e. just before parturition the level rose to 29 ng/ml. The highest levels of prolactin in the peripheral blood of the rat occurred outside pregnancy—68 ng/ml. at oestrus, 65 ng/ml. on the first day post partum and 130 ng/ml. after nursing when the litter had been previously separated from the mother for 12 hr.

Human growth hormone (HGH). The problem of the interference of chorionic somato-mammotrophin (HCS) in radioimmuno-assays for human growth hormone (HGH) in blood during pregnancy has been discussed by Greenwood (1967a). It would appear that HGH levels in the blood during pregnancy are low and this has been confirmed in a recent study by Spellacy & Buhi (1969) who used a radioimmunoassay system, in which interference from HCS was considered to be slight, to study levels of HGH in the last month of pregnancy both during fasting and after injection of insulin. Katz, Grumbach & Kaplan (1969) postulate that HCS may inhibit the release of HGH in late pregnancy and that the suppression may persist into the early post-partum period.

Chorionic somato-mammotrophin (HCS). Studies on the peripheral blood levels of human chorionic somato-mammotrophin (HCS) have been reviewed by Forsyth (1967). HCS can be detected in blood in the 6th week after the last menstrual period, levels of about 0·1 μg/ml. plasma being recorded. The level rises steeply to reach a peak in the third trimester with values of 2–9 μg/ml.

plasma, with term values of about 3 µg/ml. Somewhat higher values, about 10 µg/ml., during the last month have been reported by Spellacy & Buhi (1969). It is of interest to note the different pattern of secretion of HCS compared with human chorionic gonadotrophin which reaches peak values in the first trimester.

In view of the known mammotrophic activities of HCS in animals and man (see Lyons, Li, Ahmad & Rice-Wray, 1968) it seems highly probable that it plays an important role in mammary growth during pregnancy.

Studies on the possible existence of placental mammotrophin in non-primate mammals are now overdue (see p. 63), particularly as it seems that in some species levels of prolactin may be low in pregnancy.

From the above brief review of hormone levels during pregnancy it will be noted that only in some instances are levels greatly increased over values occurring in certain phases of the sex cycle in the non-pregnant female. It is thus likely that the maintenance of raised levels of the hormones over considerable periods of time may be an important factor in mammogenesis.

Hormonal control of mammary growth in the male

Androgens may stimulate duct and alveolar growth in the mammary glands of laboratory animals although there are some species variations, e.g. mainly alveolar growth occurs in the rat, duct growth in the guinea-pig (see review by Folley, 1952).

Castration of male rats before puberty does not affect duct growth but does largely inhibit the growth of alveoli which normally sets in between days 40–60 (Cowie, 1949; Ahrén & Etienne, 1957). This alveolar growth can be restored in castrated rats by injections of testosterone but not when the rats are hypophysectomized as well as castrated (Ahrén & Etienne, 1959) unless growth hormone is given with the androgen (Ahrén, 1959). In the castrated rabbit testosterone is only effective in inducing mammary growth when combined with oestrogen (Bengtsson & Norgren, 1961) and in the rat evidence has been obtained that the mammogenic action of testosterone may be dependent on the concomitant action of oestrogen and adrenal steroids (Jacobsohn, 1962; Jacobsohn & Norgren, 1965). Hamberger & Ahrén (1964), while confirming that adrenal steroids play a role in the action of testosterone in the rat reaffirm the essential role of growth hormone but doubt whether oestrogen plays any essential part. The action of testosterone appears to be at least partly a direct action on the mammary parenchyma as evidenced by a local response after topical application to a mammary gland (Ahrén & Hamberger, 1962).

In the male rhesus monkey administration of testosterone resulted in stunted duct growth and alveolar formation (Folley, Guthkelch & Zuckerman, 1939; Speert, 1948).

4

MILK SECRETION

Reference has already been made to the limited information about milk secretion in prototherian and metatherian mammals (see p. 101) and this chapter will deal exclusively with the phenomenon in eutherian mammals.

TERMINOLOGY

It is customary and convenient to regard milk secretion as comprising two main phases, (a) the synthesis of milk by the cells of the alveolar epithelium and (b) the passage of milk from the cytoplasm of the alveolar epithelium into the alveolar lumen (see Folley, 1947; Cowie, Folley, Cross, Harris, Jacobsohn & Richardson, 1951).*

It is usual, moreover, to differentiate between the initiation of milk secretion (lactogenesis) and the maintenance of an established milk secretion, but the precise features characteristic of these two phases have never been clearly defined. Folley (1969a) observed that lactogenesis can be studied at many levels and from a number of different viewpoints. The enzymologist, for example, may equate lactogenesis with dramatic increases in the amounts of certain enzymes within the alveolar cells; the biochemist with the appearance of some or all of the constituents peculiar to milk, e.g. lactose, casein; the cytologist with an increase in the granular endoplasmic reticulum; the histologist with the sudden distension of the alveoli with milk-like secretion; and the clinician with the surge of

* Milk as ultimately removed from the mammary gland by the act of milking or suckling may not precisely correspond in chemical composition to that excreted by the alveolar cells since fluctuations in the osmotic pressure of the blood may cause an exchange of water and water-soluble constituents between the blood and milk in the alveoli and fine ducts (see review by Rook & Wheelock, 1967; also Linzell, 1967).

secretory activity which occurs just before (e.g. in the cow) or after (e.g. in women) parturition when there is change-over from the secretion of colostrum to the secretion of increasing amounts of milk of normal composition. It is therefore necessary in discussing mechanisms controlling lactogenesis to note in what sense the term is being used. There has been a tendency of late to equate hormonal mechanisms controlling the synthesis of one milk constituent with those controlling the phenomenon as a whole but until more evidence is available to establish that the same hormonal complex is concerned it would be preferable to discuss the initiation of the synthesis of lactose, casein etc. as such and not in general terms of the initiation of milk secretion.

The term galactopoiesis was originally applied to the enhancement of an established milk secretion such as occurs in the lactating cow in response to bovine growth hormone or thyroid hormone (see Bergman & Turner, 1940; Folley & Young, 1940); the term is, however, frequently used synonymously with 'maintenance of lactation' which is unfortunate since a hormone that by itself may be galactopoietic, e.g. thyroxine in the cow, will not by itself maintain milk secretion.

MEASUREMENT OF MILK YIELD

Measuring milk yields in the large domestic animals (e.g. cows, goats, sheep) which can be milked either by machine or by hand presents no great problem provided a quiet regular routine is followed at milking times to ensure proper functioning of the milk-ejection reflex. Milking is usually carried out twice daily (although somewhat higher yields will be obtained on a three- or four-times a day schedule (see Linnerud, Caruolo, Miller, Marx & Donker, 1966; Wheelock & Dodd, 1969). Milk samples for chemical analysis should be composite samples from morning and evening milkings.

In the smaller laboratory animals assessment of milk yields may be made directly on the basis of weight increases in the litter after suckling, or indirectly from the growth rate of the litter as a whole. The direct method is particularly suited to those species that normally only nurse their litter once (e.g. rabbit) or twice daily. In this procedure it is necessary to separate the litter and the mother except during the nursing period. The litter is weighed, the mother may be injected with oxytocin to ensure milk ejection, and the litter allowed to suckle; when suckling is completed the litter is again weighed. Samples for analysis can be hand milked from a gland immediately after the injection of oxytocin (Cowie, Hartmann & Turvey, 1969; Cowie, 1969*a*). It is, of course, necessary to have sufficient young in the litter to ensure complete milking out; in the rabbit this requires litters of 6–8 young. Milk yields may be under-estimated by this procedure if the young urinate while suckling (see Cowie, 1969*a*; Fuchs, 1969). A modified direct method may also be used under experimental conditions in which the milk-ejection reflex of the mother has been destroyed (e.g. in hypophysectomized rats on replacement therapy). The litter can be left with the mother and milk yields obtained by allowing the weighed litter to suckle after injecting the mother with oxytocin (see Cowie, 1957). Otherwise in species which nurse their young frequently throughout the 24 hr it may be necessary to base estimates of milk yield on the growth rate of the litter. The rat nurses its young almost at hourly intervals and apart from the impracticability of weighing the litter so frequently separation upsets the mother and tends to depress lactation (Cowie, unpublished observations). Cowie & Folley (1947*b*) proposed for use in rats the 'litter growth index' (LGI), defined as the mean daily increase in total litter weight over the 5-day period from the 6th to 11th days of lactation, the size of the litter being standardized at 8 pups (not 6 as later stated by Reddy & Donker, 1964); this particular period was chosen because the daily increase in total litter weight was approximately constant and at a maximum during this stage of lactation. The index was used extensively in studies on the effects of adrenalectomy and replacement therapy in lactating rats. Subsequently in studies on the possible galactopoietic effects of growth hormone in rats it was observed that litters of 8 young might be too small to detect galactopoietic responses since the LGI could be increased by increasing the number of pups in the litter, indicating that the mothers were capable of producing more milk than was required by 8 pups for their normal growth. Because, with 16 pups the individual pup growth was markedly depressed it was considered that 12 pups might be the most suitable number (Cowie & Tindal, 1957). The problem of litter size and milk yield, moreover, is not one solely relating to the suckling capacity of the young for there occurs an accommodation of lactation to variable numbers of young and to their demand which seems to be effected by an alteration of the involution rate of the mammary gland which is at least in part dependent on the intensity of the milking stimulus (see Blaxter, 1961). Subsequent studies (Reddy & Donker, 1964; Edwardson & Eayrs, 1967; Kumaresan, Anderson & Turner, 1967; Ôta & Yokoyama, 1967; Moon, 1969) have extended the above observations and shown that in the rat, litter weight gains during lactation increase steadily as the numbers of pups in the litter increase from 2 to 12, thereafter the litter gain remains steady; on the other hand gain in weight of individual pups is inversely related to litter size although the differences between the individual pup gains between litters of 2, 3, 4 and 6 are small indicating the pups in these litters are getting all the milk they can consume although the mothers are not lactating to their full capacity. Clearly with litters of 6 pups or less one cannot expect to detect galactopoietic responses.

Turner and his colleagues (Grosvenor & Turner, 1959c; Kumaresan & Turner, 1966) considered that litter weight gains were unsatisfactory for assessing galactopoietic responses and since they used only 6 pups per litter their conclusions were clearly valid in the circumstances. As an alternative they assessed milk yield from the intake of milk by the litter over a 30 min suckling period following a 10-hr interval when mother and litter were separated; 1 i.u. oxytocin was injected into the mother at the beginning of the suckling period and a further 1 i.u. some 15 min later. This procedure was carried out once or at more frequent intervals during lactation. Since litters of only 6 were used the reliability of this procedure must also be questioned; indeed Moon (1969) using an isolation period of 16 hr on day 13 of lactation, anaesthetizing the mother and then giving oxytocin and allowing suckling for 20–30 min, found that milk intakes were significantly higher with litters of 12 than with litters of 6. Because differences between milk intakes were more highly significant than difference in total litter weight gains, Moon reached the not very convincing conclusion that a single determination of milk yield is a more precise measure of lactational performance than litter weight gain. It seems more likely that gains in the weight of the litter over a considerable period of lactation using litters of 12 will provide a better index of milk yield than will the isolated determination of actual milk intake recorded under rather artificial conditions of nursing.

In the guinea-pig Nagasawa, Tôzaki, Shôda & Naito (1960) recommend that yields be measured every other day by separating the young from the mother and allowing them to suckle for 4 periods of 30 min, the pups being weighed before and after each suckling period; during intervening days the young suckle normally.

Devices have been described for milking small laboratory animals (e.g. Cox Jr. & Mueller, 1937; Temple & Kon, 1937; Mueller, 1939; Kahler, 1942; Nelson, Kaye, Moore, Williams & Herrington, 1951; McBurney, Meier & Hoag, 1964; Feller & Boretos, 1967; Gupta, Conner & Langham, 1970) and for milking the baboon (Buss & Kriewaldt, 1968).

Lactation curves

Information and references about the daily milk production throughout lactation in several species will be found in the following papers:

guinea-pig	Nagasawa, Tôzaki, Shôda & Naito (1960).
rabbit	Cowie (1969*a*).
mouse	Hanrahan & Eisen (1970).
sheep	Coombe, Wardrop & Tribe (1960).
	Robinson, Foster & Forbes (1969).
pig	Barber, Braude & Mitchell (1955).
cow	Dodd (1957); Wood (1969).

Composition of milk

It is outside the scope of this review to discuss the chemical composition of the milk of various species. References to the composition of the milks of a wide variety of species will be found, however, in the reviews by Evans, (1959), Macy & Kelly (1961), Ling, Kon & Porter (1961) and Glass, Troolin & Jenness (1967). Some recent studies are listed in Table 4.1.

CYTOLOGY OF LACTOGENESIS

The major light-microscope studies of cytological changes in the mammary gland associated with the onset of milk secretion

Table 4.1. Chemistry of Milks

Species	References
Echidna	Griffiths (1968), Griffiths, McIntosh & Coles (1969), Jordan & Morgan (1969)
Kangaroo (red)	Lemon & Bailey (1966)
Kangaroo (grey)	Lemon & Poole (1969)
Baboon	Buss (1968)
Bear (polar and grizzly)	Cook, Lentfer, Pearson & Baker (1970)
Elephant	McCullagh & Widdowson (1970)
Moose	Cook, Rausch & Baker (1970)
Rabbit	Cowie (1969a)
Reindeer	Aschaffenburg, Gregory, Kon, Rowland & Thompson (1962)
Seal	Cook & Baker (1969)
Whale	Lauer & Baker (1969)

were reviewed at some length by Mayer & Klein (1961) who commented that 'there can be few glands whose histophysiological mechanism of excretion has been the subject of more controversies than that of the mammary gland' (see also Chapter 1). Histometric studies of the morphological changes occurring in the lobulo-alveolar tissue in late pregnancy and early lactation have been the subject of a review by Munford (1964).

Electron-microscope studies, which have given us much new information, have been discussed by Bargmann & Welsch (1969), Hollmann (1969) & Wellings (1969) and the description that follows is based mainly on their reviews.

Although in mice (Fig. 4.1) evidence of secretory activity has been noted in the alveolar cells as early as day 10 of pregnancy (Girardie, 1968; Hollmann, 1969), it is not until late gestation that marked changes occur. The alveolar cell in late gestation (18–19 days) is characterized by small amounts of rough endoplasmic reticulum, the Golgi apparatus is small and inconspicuous, the mitochondria are few and are scattered throughout the cytoplasm, apical cytoplasm may show the presence of one or two large fat droplets, and a few microvilli may be present on the apical surface. Shortly before parturition the rough endoplasmic reticulum hypertrophies forming large groups of flattened parallel sacs, mitochondria increase in number, the Golgi apparatus enlarges, numerous milk protein granules appear within the Golgi vacuoles and the vacuoles progress towards the cell apex where their

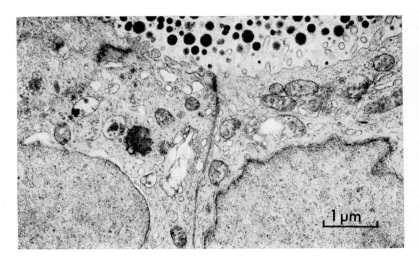

FIG. 4.1. Apical portion of alveolar cells of the mammary gland of a 10-day pregnant mouse. Protein granules are present in the lumen; the cytoplasm is more abundant than in the resting state and contains mitochondria and Golgi elements (from Hollmann, K. H., 1969, in *Lactogenesis: the Initiation of Milk Secretion at Parturition*, edited by Reynolds, M. & Folley, S. J., pp. 27–41. Philadelphia: University of Pennsylvania Press).

granules and other fine material are released into the lumen. The number of fat globules in the cytoplasm increases and on reaching the cell apex the fat droplets are released into the lumen by a process of "pinching off", a portion of the apical membrane enveloping them and forming their outermost envelope as described in Chapter 1. The microvilli greatly increase in number.

From morphometric studies of the mouse mammary gland by Hollmann (1969) see also Hollmann & Verley, 1970) it is clear that the cytoplasmic organelles in the alveolar cell develop independently (Fig. 4.2); the mitochondria increase early in pregnancy and attain their definitive volume some days before parturition while the rough endoplasmic reticulum, Golgi membranes and vacuoles develop progressively with parturition and then more rapidly during the first days of lactation. Thus while the alveolar cell can secrete before parturition it cannot be considered as fully differentiated until several days of lactation have elapsed.

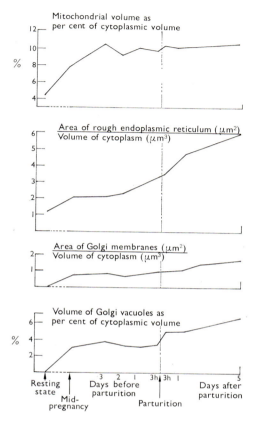

Fɪɢ. 4.2. Graphical representation of the development of the organelles in the alveolar cells of the mammary gland of the mouse during pregnancy and lactation. There is a progressive increase in the volume of the mitochondria, the surface area of the rough endoplasmic reticulum and of the Golgi elements (volume of vacuole and area of membranes) during pregnancy. Two days before parturition the definitive mitochondrial volume is reached but the rough endoplasmic reticulum and the Golgi components continue to develop during the early stage of lactation (from Hollmann, K. H., 1969, in *Lactogenesis: The Initiation of Milk Secretion at Parturition*, edited by Reynolds, M. & Folley, S. J., pp. 27–41. Philadelphia: University of Pennsylvania Press.

In the rabbit, fat droplets and other granules can be detected in the alveolar lumen from days 21–22 (i.e. at the beginning of the last third of pregnancy); also at this stage milk protein granules appear within the Golgi apparatus and lactose can be detected (see Girardie, 1968; Bousquet, Fléchon & Denamur, 1969). In the rat secretory changes may be observed in the alveolar cells only a little later than in the mouse whereas in the guinea-pig pregnancy is well advanced before such changes are obvious (Girardie, 1968).

HORMONES AND MILK SECRETION

Anterior pituitary

The first conclusive demonstration that a hormone (or hormones) from the anterior pituitary played an active role in lactogenesis was in 1928 when Stricker and Grueter, while studying the gonado- trophic activities of anterior pituitary extracts, observed the onset of copious milk secretion in pseudopregnant rabbits injected with the extracts (see Stricker, 1951). The subsequent identification by Riddle and his colleagues of this lactogenic principle—pro- lactin—with the anterior pituitary factor which stimulates the crop-gland of the pigeon provided a useful means of assay which greatly aided the purification of the hormone (see Chapter 2). Early studies with purified prolactin in species other than the rabbit soon revealed differences in the responses obtained with purified prolactin and with anterior pituitary extracts. For example, in the hypophysectomized guinea-pig prolactin was not lacto- genic unless combined with adrenocorticotrophin (ACTH); in the cow in declining lactation anterior pituitary extracts would readily increase milk yield (galactopoietic response) whereas prolactin was inactive. Because of such discrepancies in the actions of purified prolactin and crude anterior pituitary extracts Folley & Young (1938, 1941) queried the contemporary concept of regarding prolactin as the lactogenic hormone and suggested it would be more realistic to consider lactogenesis as a response of the suitably developed mammary gland to a lactogenic hormone complex (see reviews by Folley & Malpress, 1948b; Folley, 1952; Cowie, 1966). Subsequent studies on galactopoiesis indicated that growth hormone and thyrotrophin (TSH) were likely to be components of a complex of hormones concerned in the maintenance of milk secretion in cows, while ACTH appeared to be a component of the complex in the guinea-pig (see review by Folley 1956).

Hypophysectomy and hormone replacement studies

In the species so far studied hypophysectomy during lactation causes a rapid decline in milk yield even when adequate exogenous oxytocin is given to ensure milk ejection (removal of the posterior pituitary abolishes the milk-ejection reflex at least for a time— see Chapter 5). The interval between hypophysectomy and virtual cessation of milk secretion varies. In the rat milk secretion is completely suppressed within 1–3 days (Cowie, 1957), whereas in the lactating goat the effects of hypophysectomy are less rapid for although there is an immediate precipitous drop in milk yield, a low level of secretion may continue for a month or more. The severity of the decline in milk yield immediately after hypophysectomy is in part due to surgical stress and trauma and the nature of the decline is better revealed by observing the effects of withdrawing replacement therapy when the yield has been restored. Under these circumstances the milk yield of the goat takes 4–6 weeks to fall to negligible quantities, and moreover the immediate fall is much less precipitate. Similarly in the lactating rabbit milk yields are reduced to trace amounts in 3 to 7 days after hypophysectomy whereas after the cessation of successful replacement therapy the decline in milk yield is somewhat slower, taking 5–10 days. Whether the slow tailing-off of milk secretion after removal of the anterior pituitary indicates that the alveolar cells can continue for a time to carry out their synthetic activities in the complete absence of the anterior pituitary hormones or that there is a small hormonal output from that part of the pars tuberalis which usually remains on the pituitary stalk after hypophysectomy, is not known. Whatever the explanation, it seems that there are species variations in the length of the period during which the alveolar cells can continue their synthetic activities in the absence of anterior pituitary hormones.

The first detailed study of the components of the lactogenic complex was carried out in rats by Lyons and his colleagues (Lyons, Li & Johnson, 1958) using triply-operated (i.e. hypophysectomized-ovariectomized-adrenalectomized) animals in which lobulo-alveolar growth had been developed to a stage comparable to that occurring in late pregnancy by suitable injection of oestro-gen, progesterone, adrenal steroids, ox growth hormone (GH) and sheep prolactin (see Chapter 3). If the injections of GH, oestrogen and progesterone were stopped while those of prolactin and adrenal steroids were continued then lactogenesis occurred. In similar studies on triply-operated mice Nandi (1959) (see also Nandi & Bern, 1961; Wellings, 1969) found that lactogenesis occurred when the ovarian steroids were withdrawn while con-tinuing to inject prolactin and adrenal steroids. However, in some strains of mice bovine GH + adrenal steroids were lactogenic, and indeed the effect of prolactin + GH appeared to be additive so that the best lactogenic responses were obtained with prolactin + GH + adrenal steroids. These studies, in addition to providing information on the essential components of the lactogenic complex,

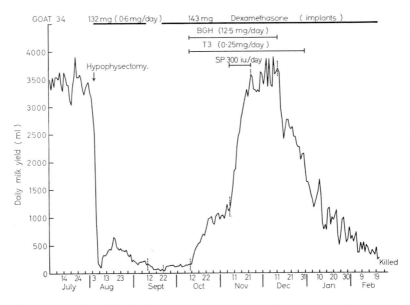

FIG. 4.3. Daily milk yields of a goat before and after complete hypophy-sectomy and during replacement therapy. BGH = bovine growth hormone, T3 = tri-iodothyronine, SP = sheep prolactin. Horizontal lines indicate periods over which the hormones were administered (from Cowie, A. T., 1969*b*, in *Lactogenesis: The Initiation of Milk Secretion at Parturition*, edited by Reynolds, M. & Folley, S. J., pp. 157–169. Philadelphia: University of Pennsylvania Press.

also suggested that the ovarian hormones prevented the anterior pituitary hormones from eliciting their lactogenic response in the mammary gland while co-operating in their mammogenic action. That a similar hormonal complex was required to maintain lactation in rats was demonstrated by hormone replacement studies in rats hypophysectomized during lactation (Cowie, 1957; Bintarningsih, Lyons, Johnson & Li, 1958; Cowie & Tindal, 1961*a*) when a substantial restoration of milk yield was obtained with prolactin + ACTH, or prolactin + adrenal steroids. In sum there is much evidence to indicate that in the rat and mouse the hypophysial hormones prolactin and ACTH are both essential for the induction and maintenance of milk secretion with the proviso that in some strains of mice GH may play a role as important as prolactin.

Studies on the hormonal requirements for milk secretion have also been conducted on goats and rabbits. In the goat the maintenance of lactation has been studied after surgical hypophysectomy and after destruction of the pituitary by proton irradiation (for references see review by Cowie, 1969*b*). In the hypophysectomized goat restoration of milk yield to pre-hypophysectomy levels can be achieved by administering sheep prolactin + bovine GH + tri-iodothyronine + adrenal steroids (Fig. 4.3); low levels of milk secretion will occur when prolactin + GH + adrenal steroids, GH + adrenal steroids or prolactin + adrenal steroids are administered. The important role of GH in the maintenance of milk secretion in the goat is not unexpected in view of the marked galactopoietic effects of GH in the cow in declining lactation (see p. 162).

Frederikson (1939) first reported that prolactin was lactogenic in rabbits hypophysectomized during pseudopregnancy or in late pregnancy and that it would reinitiate lactation in rabbits hypophysectomized during lactation. Frederikson's observations remained unconfirmed until Kilpatrick, Armstrong & Greep (1962, 1964) noted, during studies in the rabbit on the maintenance of the corpus luteum after hypophysectomy, that while prolactin alone failed to maintain the corpus luteum it induced copious milk secretion. This response to prolactin is apparently not dependent on the presence of endogenous adrenal steroids since prolactin will induce milk secretion in the pseudopregnant adrenalectomized or adrenalectomized-ovariectomized rabbit

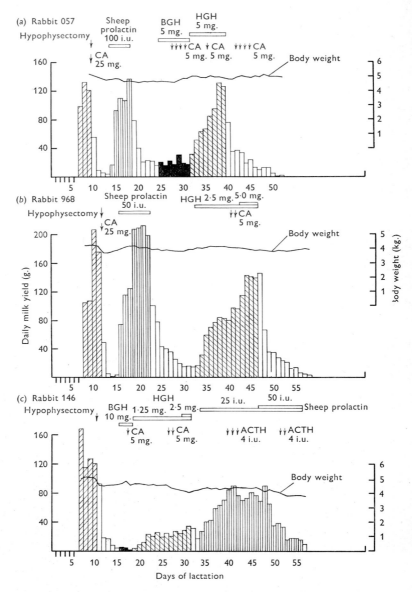

FIG. 4.4. Daily milk yields of three rabbits after surgical hypophysectomy and during replacement therapy with purified anterior pituitary hormones and cortisol acetate. Dose level of hormones = dose/day; ACTH = adrenocorticotrophin; BGH = bovine growth hormone; CA = cortisol acetate; HGH = human growth hormone (from Cowie, A. T., Hartmann, P. E. & Turvey, A., 1969, *J. Endocr.* **43**, 651–662).

(Cowie & Watson, 1966) or hypophysectomized-adrenalectomized-ovariectomized rabbit (Denamur, 1969). Further studies by Cowie, Hartmann & Turvey (1969) on the restoration of lactation in rabbits hypophysectomized during lactation confirmed that sheep prolactin alone was capable of restoring milk secretion to pre-hypophysectomy levels; no significant beneficial effects were noted when either ACTH or adrenal steroids were administered in addition to the prolactin (Fig. 4.4). Bovine GH had little restorative effect on the milk yield although it delayed the regression of the gland which occurs after hypophysectomy (see also Hartmann, Cowie & Hosking, 1970). Human growth hormone, on the other hand, was just as effective as sheep prolactin in restoring milk secretion in the rabbit in accord with the known lactogenic properties of this hormone (see Chapter 2). It was observed in the rabbit that after restoration of the milk yields with sheep prolactin, or human GH, the yields began to decline despite continued injections of the hormone; this decline could be stopped and yields would again increase if one hormone was replaced by the other; some evidence was obtained that the decline in effectiveness of the hormone was due to the development of an immune response (Cowie, Hartmann & Turvey, 1969). The question of species specificity of anterior pituitary hormones is one of considerable importance and it requires that some caution should be exercised in the interpretation of experiments in which heterologous prolactins are used (see also Chapter 2).

The rabbit thus appears to be a species in which the hormonal complexes required for the initiation and the maintenance of milk secretion are in the simplest form—a single hormone, prolactin. The considerable diversity in the components of the hormonal complexes for initiating and maintaining milk secretion already revealed in the few species so far studied make an extension of these studies to a wider variety of species highly desirable. Further discussion on these problems will be found in the reviews by Denamur, 1969, 1971).

The cytomorphology of hormonally induced lactogenesis in triply-operated mice (see p. 146) has been studied by Wellings (1969) who concluded that the ultrastructure of the artificially stimulated tissue closely paralleled that of normal cells in all the accepted changes associated with normal lactogenesis. Similarly in the pseudopregnant rabbit (Bousquet, Fléchon & Denamur,

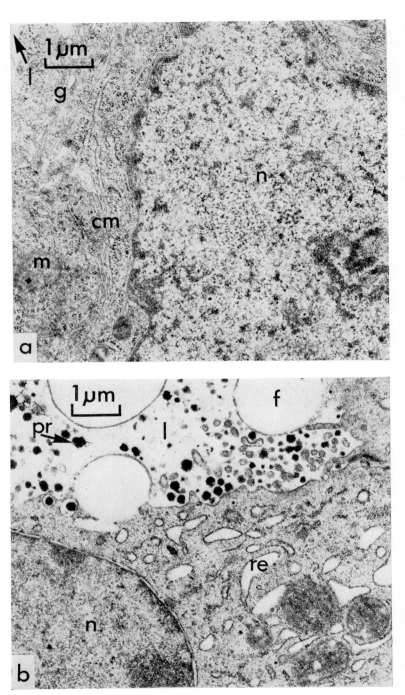

Fig. 4.5.

1969) injection of prolactin resulted within 12 hr in the appearance of fat droplets in the cytoplasm and protein granules in the Golgi vacuoles; after 48 hr the rough endoplasmic reticulum was vesicular and dilated, the Golgi vacuoles distended with granules and there were abundant fat globules and protein granules in the alveolar lumen (Fig. 4.5).

Information concerning the hormonal requirements for lactation in primates is as yet limited. The question of the existence of a primate prolactin has been discussed in Chapter 2 where reference has also been made to the interesting prolactin-like properties which primate growth hormone exhibits. Studies bearing on the hormonal requirements for milk secretion in primates have recently been discussed by Forsyth (1969). Clinical observation on the effects of hypophysectomy during pregnancy and on postparturient pituitary necrosis (Sheehan's syndrome) suggest that while placental hormones can, in the absence of the pituitary, induce mammary growth and milk secretion it is likely that pituitary growth hormone and chorionic somato-mammotrophin both have roles in the initiation of lactation. For the maintenance of lactation the presence of a pituitary hormone, or hormones, is necessary and in view of the galactopoietic effects of human growth hormone in women (see p. 162) this hormone may well have a role.

Initiation of milk secretion

Hormonal control

The time when secretion can first be detected in the mammary alveoli during pregnancy differs widely in different species (see

FIG. 4.5. (opposite) Ultrastructural changes in the mammary gland of the pseudopregnant rabbit which occur when lactogenesis is induced with prolactin.
(a) Portion of epithelial cell of mammary gland of rabbit on day 14 of pseudopregnancy. The nucleus (n) is large and the surrounding cytoplasm is narrow. m = mitochondrion; g = Golgi apparatus; cm = cytoplasmic membranes; l = lumen.
(b) Portion of epithelial cell of mammary gland of pseudopregnant rabbit 48 hr after injections of prolactin (4 × 50 i.u. every 12th hr) beginning on day 14 of pseudopregnancy. The lumen contains free protein granules (pr) and fat droplets (f). There are large vesicles in the rough endoplasmic reticulum (re) (from Bousquet, M., Fléchon, J. E. & Denamur, R., 1969, *Z. Zellforsch. Mikrosk. Anat.* **96**, 418–436).

p. 141 and review by Denamur, 1971). In the rat in which parturition normally occurs during day 22 evidence of marked secretory activity occurs only some 1–2 days earlier (see review by
Turner, 1939); similarly in the sow alveolar secretion is minimal
until 2 days before parturition (Cross, Goodwin & Silver, 1958).
In ruminants secretory activity of the alveolar epithelium is
marked during the second half of pregnancy, indeed very considerable quantities of milk may be produced before parturition
and the pre-partum milking of cows was at one time recommended
as a routine procedure in dairy husbandry (see Dodd, 1957).
In the rhesus monkey colostrum is usually present in the alveoli
by the beginning of the 4th month of pregnancy (gestation =
$5\frac{1}{2}$ months) although copious milk secretion does not occur until
a day or two after parturition (Speert, 1948). Similarly in man the
alveoli become distended with colostrum in the last third of
pregnancy although copious secretion does not appear until
3–4 days after childbirth (Geschickter, 1945). However, irrespective of the stage of gestation at which the early stages of secretory
activity may first be detected in the mammary gland there occurs
in most species, even in the cow milked pre-partum, a marked
increase in the secretory activity of the mammary gland at the
time of parturition.

There have been numerous theories derived from observations
in a variety of species concerning possible endocrine mechanisms
involved in the initiation of lactation (for references see Cowie,
1969*b*). Probably the most popular concept is that the secretory
activity of the alveolar epithelium during pregnancy is kept in
check by the ovarian and placental steroids in the blood exerting
an inhibitory effect either directly on the mammary epithelium
rendering it less responsive to the lactogenic hormones of the
anterior pituitary or placenta, or both; or indirectly by depressing
the release of lactogenic complex from the anterior pituitary;
or by a combination of these mechanisms. At parturition a fall in
the concentration of the steroids in the blood permits the mammary
epithelium to respond to the lactogenic complex, while the lowered
levels of oestrogen may even increase the output of lactogenic
hormones from the anterior pituitary. Secondly, it has been
postulated that the onset of copious milk secretion is associated
with increases in the level of physiologically active adrenal steroids
in the blood at the time of parturition. Thirdly, it has been con-

tended that the commencement of suckling may stimulate the release of prolactin and probably other anterior pituitary hormones concerned in milk secretion (see Chapter 6). Fourthly, the secretion of oxytocin in response to the suckling stimulus may release lactogenic hormones from the anterior pituitary as suggested by Benson & Folley (1956), or in some other manner stimulate milk secretion.

The relevance of such mechanisms will certainly vary according to the species. At present only in the rat do we have much detailed information on the precise mechanisms involved. The early studies concerned with the inhibitory effects of the ovarian hormones on lactation in the rat have been reviewed in detail by Mayer & Klein (1949) and Cowie (1961). It was generally believed (see Mayer & Klein, 1949, also Desclin, 1952) that the ovarian hormones acted by inhibiting the release of hormones from the anterior pituitary, but there was also evidence of a direct effect on the mammary epithelium. Further, in the rat with suitably developed mammary glands whether or not exogenous prolactin exerted a lactogenic response depended on its effects on the ovary; if a luteotrophic effect occurred then there was no lactogenic response. Thus, in the pregnant rat it was possible to have prolactin in the circulation without the occurrence of milk secretion. Desclin (1952) noted that the inhibitory effects of the ovarian steroids were not absolute and could be overcome by higher levels of prolactin, hence the ability in some species to lactate *while pregnant.* Mayer & Klein (1949) discussed various theories as to how, in the rat, the luteotrophic effect of prolactin could change to a lactogenic effect at the end of pregnancy; they suggested a possible competition between ovary and mammary gland for prolactin but no very satisfactory explanation emerged. Confirmatory evidence of these observations came from the studies by Lyons and his colleagues (see p. 116) who noted that in triply-operated rats the mammogenic hormone combination of prolactin + GH + adrenal steroids + oestrogen + progesterone became a lactogenic combination when oestrogen and progesterone were omitted.

Further confirmatory and additional information accrued from the studies of Yokoyama and his colleagues (see review by Yokoyama, Shinde & Ôta, 1969) who used the appearance of lactose in the mammary gland as an indicator of the early stage of lactogenesis. In rats, removal of the ovaries in late pregnancy (18th or

F

19th day) permitted a sharp increase in the lactose content of the mammary gland within 1–2 days and this increase could be prevented by daily injection of large doses (5 mg) of progesterone. In addition, from studies of rats hypophysectomized on day 19 it was shown that the placenta could inhibit lactose synthesis by a luteotrophic effect on the ovary, removal of the ovaries allowing the placental hormones to exert a lactogenic effect. Removal of both placenta and pituitary abolished any stimulatory effect on lactose synthesis, indicating an essential need in lactose synthesis for lactogen derived either from the anterior pituitary or placenta. Yokoyama concluded that the loss of the placenta might contribute to the initiation of lactation, but since lactose could be detected in the mammary gland two days before parturition clearly other mechanisms were initially involved. Kuhn (1969*a*, *b*), also using lactose synthesis as an indicator of the early stages of lacto-genesis, concluded that the physiological lactogenic signal in the rat could be expected to occur 30 hr before parturition and he showed that at this time there occurred a fall in plasma progesterone due to a decreased steroidogenic activity of the ovaries and in particular to an abrupt redirection of the metabolism of pregneno-lone away from progesterone and towards 20α-hydroxypregn-4-en-3-one (Kuhn & Briley, 1970). He, therefore, suggested that lactogenesis in the rat resulted from a fall in the plasma concentra-tion of progesterone which occurred about 30 hr before parturition and that this change acted directly on the mammary gland. Kuhn considered that prolactin, adrenal steroids and perhaps other hormones might participate in lactogenesis in a supporting capacity but that change in their concentrations in the plasma either did not occur or did not constitute the lactogenic signal. Kuhn (1971) later postulated that the alteration in the steroidogenic capacity of the ovaries might be associated with a fall in prolactin levels in the blood. Studies by Amenomori, Chen & Meites (1970) indicate, however, that levels of pituitary prolactin in the blood are low in the pregnant rat from days 4 to 21 and that a rise occurs just before parturition. Nothing is known, however, about the levels of rat placental lactogen in pregnancy and it might be that a decrease in placental hormone rather than in pituitary prolactin is concerned in changes in ovarian activity.

    While there is strong evidence for the assumption that lacto-genesis in the rat is triggered off by the removal of a progesterone block on the secretory activity of the mammary alveolar cells, there is also ample evidence from both *in vivo* and *in vitro* studies that the lactogenic complex of hormones plays an essential role in lactogenesis, and that lactogenesis does not occur if both pituitary and placental lactogenic hormones are absent (Yokoyama, Shinde & Ôta, 1969). Recent biochemical studies also indicate an essential role for prolactin in the synthesis of lactose. The final step in the pathway of lactose synthesis is one in which the enzyme lactose synthetase transfers galactose from UDP-galactose to glucose. Lactose synthetase is composed of two protein subunits, A and B, both of which are required for lactose synthesis; protein A is now known to be a galactosyl transferase while protein B is the well-characterized constituent of milk—α-lactalbumin (see review by Jones, 1969). In mice, organ culture studies by Turkington & Hill (1969) have indicated that prolactin in the presence of insulin and cortisol induces the synthesis of both A and B proteins in the mammary gland, but that progesterone selectively inhibits the formation of α-lactalbumin. It thus seems evident that the fall in the level of circulating progesterone at the end of pregnancy permits the stimulation of α-lactalbumin synthesis by prolactin thereby completing the lactose synthetase unit and so the catalysis of the final step in lactose synthesis. There is evidence that α-lactalbumin is the rate-limiting subunit of lactose synthesis at all stages of pregnancy and lactation and it is also likely that the rate of lactose synthesis may be linked to the rate of milk protein synthesis (Brew, 1969; Palmiter, 1969a).

Koch (1969) observed an almost 3-fold increase in plasma corticosterone in the rat between days 18 and 21 of gestation and considered that the high levels reached by unbound adrenal steroids played an important role in lactogenesis. Kuhn (1969a) was unable to confirm the occurrence of significant changes in the concentration of plasma corticosterone at the time of lactogenesis and parturition and excluded corticosterone as a lactogenic trigger mechanism. Davis & Liu (1969) while confirming Kuhn's contention that changes in adrenal steroid levels in the blood do not initiate lactation in the rat, consider that the presence of glucocorticoids are essential for lactogenesis. Clearly more research is required even in the rat and mouse to unravel the complex interplay between pituitary, ovarian, adrenal and placental hormones occurring at the initiation of milk secretion.

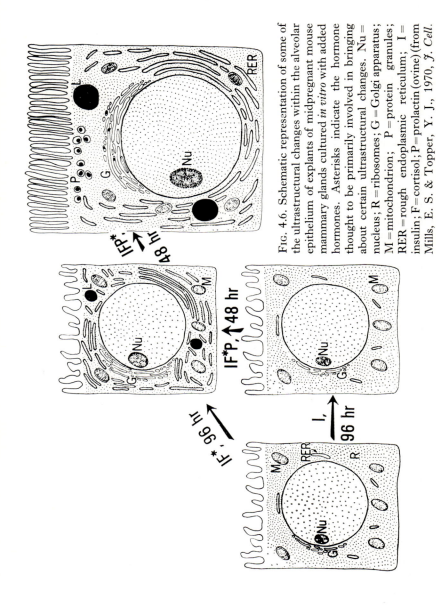

Fig. 4.6. Schematic representation of some of the ultrastructural changes within the alveolar epithelium of explants of midpregnant mouse mammary glands cultured *in vitro* with added hormones. Asterisks indicate the hormone thought to be primarily involved in bringing about certain ultrastructural changes. Nu = nucleus; R = ribosomes; G = Golgi apparatus; M = mitochondrion; P = protein granules; RER = rough endoplasmic reticulum; I = insulin; F = cortisol; P = prolactin (ovine) (from Mills, E. S. & Topper, Y. J., 1970, *J. Cell. Biol.* **44**, 310–328).

insulin, cortisol and prolactin, casein synthesis by the insulin–cortisol explants could be detected within 12 hr but not by the insulin explants, even at 48 hr. Study of the ultrastructure of the alveolar cells of explants during the second incubation in insulin–cortisol–prolactin medium (48 hr) revealed marked differences between the insulin and insulin–cortisol explants. The alveolar cells of the explants first cultured in insulin–cortisol medium resembled those seen in late pregnant mice: the nuclei and nucleoli were large, the bulk of the rough endoplasmic reticulum was basal, the Golgi apparatus was supranuclear and large and many Golgi vacuoles contained protein granules, the apical cytoplasm was filled with membrane-bounded protein granules, lipid droplets of various sizes were plentiful, and the microvilli were long, regular and abundant. In contrast the insulin explants incubated for 48 hr in insulin–cortisol–prolactin medium varied greatly in appearance, about a third of the alveoli were unchanged and the rest had cells which resembled those seen in the alveoli in the insulin–cortisol explants at the end of the first incubation period. When the second incubation was extended to 96 hr, however, the cells of the insulin explants now resembled those of the insulin–cortisol explants at 48 hr. Mills & Topper (1970) consider that cortisol is concerned in the formation and maintenance of the rough endoplasmic reticulum and the Golgi apparatus, and that the presence of these organelles enables the cells to respond rapidly to prolactin in terms of milk protein synthesis. (It may be noted, however, that the absence or minimal development of these organelles need have no deleterious effect on the capacity of the cells to synthesize intracellular, i.e. non-milk, proteins.) While earlier studies had indicated that cortisol did not act post-mitotically the above study suggests that it may do so since the insulin explants with their peak of proliferation over did eventually respond when incubated in insulin–cortisol–prolactin medium for 96 hr. The above studies show that there is an excellent correlation between the ultrastructure of the alveolar cells and their capacity to synthesize milk proteins.

Whether or not the role played by insulin in these explant studies is a physiological one is still uncertain for the minimal effective concentration of insulin which induces DNA synthesis *in vitro* is some 100 times greater than the levels obtaining *in vivo* (Turkington, 1968). Palmiter (1969*b*) has suggested that insulin

may play a permissive role in that it is necessary for the maintenance of normal cellular metabolism in the mammary gland and
that the addition of insulin to the culture medium may merely
restore the tissue to its predissection rates of metabolic function.

While such studies have provided much information on the
functional differentiation of the alveolar cells of the mouse mammary gland under conditions of organ culture, the pattern obtained
clearly does not represent the precise picture of the *in vivo*
changes leading to lactogenesis during the latter part of gestation.
The cell population *in vivo* appears to be less synchronized than
in vitro and there is a steady growth of alveolar tissue in the mouse
from mid-pregnancy to about day 10 of lactation (see Munford,
1964). *In vivo* other hormones such as oestrogen and progesterone
affect cell differentiation (see Bresciani, 1964); the role of progesterone in inhibiting the induction of α-lactalbumin and hence
the completion of the enzyme lactose synthetase has been noted
(see p. 155). However, despite limitations, such organ culture
studies are providing useful information for the analysis of the
complex interplay of hormones on the growth of the mammary
gland and on the cytological and functional development of its
epithelial cells (see also review by Forsyth, 1971).

Hormone–enzyme relationships

In recent reviews on enzymic and metabolic changes in the
mammary gland associated with lactogenesis Baldwin (1969*a*, *b*)
lists three crucial events which are highly interrelated, regulated
by the same hormones and often occur almost simultaneously.

The first of these events is the formation of functionally
differentiated secretory cells. As already discussed, *in vitro* studies
have shown that the alveolar cells of mouse mammary gland
explanted at mid-pregnancy must divide in the presence of certain
hormones before the cells can synthesize milk proteins (see p. 156).
Comparable *in vivo* studies are lacking but Baldwin (1969*a*, *b*),
after reviewing the evidence, considers that in rodents alveolar
cell proliferation and differentiation must occur *in vivo* for the
initiation of milk secretion but that the situation in other species
is far from clear.

The second event listed by Baldwin is the development of a
characteristic enzyme complement and the ability to synthesize
milk proteins by the differentiated secretory cells. In rodents there

is evidence that after differentiation secretory activity is in part an inherent property of the alveolar cells requiring only a hormonal environment consistent with the maintenance of the cells; for example, studies on the effects of hypophysectomy and replacement therapy in lactating rats have shown that the activities of a number of enzymes, i.e. activities per cell, are not regulated by pituitary hormones. On the other hand there is evidence that hormones may regulate the activities of certain key enzymes and affect patterns of RNA and protein synthesis within the alveolar cells (see Baldwin, 1969*a*, *b*; Denamur, 1969). The role of the hormonal environment in the maintenance of the alveolar cells would also appear to be a factor of some importance on which further information is required; a recent study on the effects of hypophysectomy and replacement therapy in the lactating rabbit suggests that the rate of milk synthesis depends upon the degree of maintenance of secretory cells rather than on a block in the synthetic pathways within the cells (Hartmann, Cowie & Hosking, 1970).

The third event involves the regulation of the expression of the capacity for milk synthesis resulting from the occurrence of the first two events. Baldwin (1969*a*, *b*) comments that while little is still known concerning the intracellular metabolic regulatory mechanisms it seems that such mechanisms may play important roles in the initiation of copious milk secretion, particularly in ruminants in which alveolar cell proliferation and differentiation occur and high enzyme activities are present in the mammary gland some time before the initiation of lactation (see also Baldwin & Chang, 1969).

Further information on the biochemistry of lactogenesis will be found in the review by Jones (1969). Much research is still required into the cellular and enzymic changes in the alveolar epithelium during pregnancy and lactation and into the regulation of secretory cell development and function before the mechanisms controlling the initiation of lactation are fully understood.

Effect of hormones on established lactation—galactopoiesis

Anterior pituitary

As with lactogenesis the effects of hormones on established lactation differs from species to species.

Primates. Significant increases in milk yield have been observed in lactating women by Lyons and his colleagues in response to daily injections, over 7–8 days, of a human growth hormone preparation (Lyons, Gutiérrez, Cervantes & Rice-Wray, 1968; Lyons, Li, Ahmad & Rice-Wray, 1968).

So far as we are aware no similar studies have been made in monkeys although human growth hormone will initiate milk secretion in rhesus monkeys (Lyons, 1962).

Rat. Galactopoiesis in rats after treatment with sheep prolactin, alone, or in combination with bovine GH, and with thyroid hormones has been reported (see von Berswordt-Wallrabe, Moon & Turner, 1960) but Talwalker, Meites & Nicoll (1960) failed to detect any response of milk yield to prolactin (see also Thatcher & Tucker, 1970). Increases in milk yield in response to treatment with bovine GH have been reported by Grosvenor & Turner (1959a) and Moon (1965) but others have not confirmed this (see review by Cowie, 1961; also Thatcher & Tucker, 1970). Most of these studies on rats were carried out with too few young per litter to ensure efficient milking (see p. 139) and the significance of the results is in some doubt.

Guinea-pig. Neither sheep prolactin nor bovine growth hormone are galactopoietic in the guinea-pig (Nagasawa & Naito, 1962, 1963).

Rabbit. In the rabbit sheep prolactin is galactopoietic in declining lactation increasing both the yield and the lactose content of the milk (Gachev, 1963, 1968b; Cowie, 1969a)

Cow and Goat. Apart from one report of increases in milk yield in response to injections of sheep prolactin in cows recovering from foot-and-mouth disease, studies with purified prolactin in cows have provided no evidence of galactopoietic responses (see review by Cowie, 1966).

In the cow and goat there is clear evidence that GH will cause marked increases in milk yield during declining lactation (see review by Cowie, 1966). There is some evidence that part of the galactopoietic activity of GH preparations in ruminants may be due to TSH contamination as Bullis, Bush & Barto (1965) have reported that highly purified bovine GH is less active than commercial GH. Nevertheless there is good evidence that the two hormones exert galactopoietic effects independently of each other (see review by Cowie, 1966).

[Research workers and veterinarians should note that, in the United Kingdom, extracts of the anterior pituitary and purified anterior pituitary hormones of animal origin intended for use in farm animals come within the provisions of the Foot-and-Mouth Disease (Sera and Glandular Products) Order of 1939 and permission to inject such extracts or hormones into farm animals must first be obtained from the Ministry of Agriculture.]

The other trophic hormones of the anterior pituitary exert their activity by way of their target organs and it is convenient to discuss these with hormones of the target gland.

Adrenal Cortex

Removal of the adrenal glands from lactating animals impairs lactation and replacement studies in the rat and goat indicate that both mineralo- and glucocorticoids are concerned in the maintenance of lactation (see review by Cowie, 1961). Thatcher & Tucker (1970) also found that glucocorticoids may be rate limiting in milk synthesis during prolonged lactation in the rat. The biochemical effects of adrenalectomy on the mammary gland of the lactating rat have been studied by Greenbaum & Darby (1964) who observed decreased activity in both the Embden–Meyerhof and the pentose phosphate pathways of glucose degradation, the latter being particularly affected. Glucocorticoids effectively restore the levels of hexosemonophosphate shunt enzymes in the mammary gland and liver to normal in lactating adrenalectomized rats (Willmer & Foster, 1965).

The administration of adrenal steroids to intact lactating rats and mice have given somewhat conflicting results. Adrenal steroids may be inhibitory in high doses but galactopoietic in smaller doses (see review by Cowie, 1961; also Talwalker, Meites & Nicoll, 1960; Hahn & Turner, 1966). In the rabbit cortisol may give increases in milk yield and lactose content (Gachev, 1966). ACTH and adrenal steroids will induce lactogenesis in several species when injected during pregnancy, e.g. cow, sheep and rabbit (see review by Cowie, 1969*b*). In the lactating cow

ACTH and the adrenal steroids tend to depress milk yield (see Cowie, 1961; also Campbell, Davey, McDowall, Wilson & Munford, 1964).

Thyroids

The effects of thyroidectomy on lactation are conflicting and in some species (e.g. rat) confused by the concomitant loss of the parathyroids. The evidence in general suggests that the intensity and duration of lactation is reduced in the absence of the thyroid (see review by Cowie, 1961). Grosvenor (1961) has noted that in the rat the level of lactation is correlated with the intensity of thyroid hormone output. Histological and cytological studies have also indicated that thyroid activity is increased during lactation in the cat (Racadot, 1957) and in the golden hamster (Curé, 1965). The effects of thyroidectomy on the pathways of glucose metabolism in lactating rat mammary glands have been studied by Walters & McLean (1967); a number of biochemical parameters were depressed but unlike adrenalectomy there was no marked differential effect on the relative activities of the two alternative pathways of glucose metabolism.

There is evidence that thyroid hormones are galactopoietic when administered to lactating rats in physiological doses (Desclin, 1949; Grosvenor & Turner, 1959*b*; von Berswordt-Wallrabe, Moon & Turner, 1960); in large doses milk yield is depressed in rats (Schmidt & Moger, 1967) and both yield and lactose content depressed in rabbits (Gachev, 1967). In cows and goats the galactopoietic effect of thyroid hormones and TSH is well established (see reviews by Meites, 1961; Cowie, 1966). In man, also, beneficial effects of thyroid hormones on lactation have been reported (Robinson, 1947; Lelong, Giraud, Roche, Liardet & Coignet, 1950).

Thyrocalcitonin, secreted by the mammalian thyroid, will be referred to when dealing with parathyroid hormone (see below).

Parathyroids

Removal of the parathyroids from lactating animals depresses lactation (see review by Cowie, 1961; von Berswordt-Wallrabe & Turner, 1960; Payne & Chamings, 1964). In the rat total milk solids tend to increase while the effect on milk Ca is variable (Neuenschwander & Talmage, 1963). Successful replacement therapy has been reported in this species by von Berswordt-Wallrabe & Turner (1960).

In the cow the parathyroid gland increases in size due to increase in secretory tissue just before parturition and then decreases during early lactation. Despite the large amounts of Ca secreted in the milk the activity of the gland appears to be depressed at the height of lactation (Stott & Smith, 1964).

There is little information about the effects of thyrocalcitonin (the hypocalcaemic polypeptide hormone secreted by the thyroid) on lactation but Capen & Young (1967) on the basis of ultra-structural studies and assays of the thyrocalcitonin content of the thyroid in cows have noted that milk fever (parturient paresis) is associated with an abrupt release of thyrocalcitonin from the 'C' cells of the thyroid gland (see also review by Hirsch & Munson, 1969).

Endocrine Pancreas

Early studies showed that insulin was necessary for the proper functioning of the mammary gland (see Cowie, 1961). It has since proved an essential constituent of the medium for successful organ culture of the mammary gland (see p. 156). Daily injections of insulin are said to increase milk yield in lactating rats; milk yields fall somewhat in rats made diabetic with alloxan but are restored when insulin is given (Kumaresan & Turner, 1965*a*, *b*). Injections of insulin depress milk yield in goats and cows, the milk lactose content falls while fat and protein concentrations increase and these increases cannot be explained entirely by a decrease in the milk volume (see Cowie, 1961; also Kronfeld, Mayer, Robertson & Raggi, 1963; Rook, Storry & Wheelock, 1965; Schmidt, 1966; Rook & Hopwood, 1970).

Ovaries

Removal of the ovaries has no detrimental effects on established lactation but the ovarian hormones themselves have important roles in the initiation of milk secretion (see p. 152).

Galactopoietic effects of oestrogen, particularly in farm animals, have been observed but high dosage or a constant infusion of oestrogen depresses milk yield and it has been suggested that the accelerated decline in yield from the 5th month of pregnancy in lactating cows is due to an increasing level of oestrogen (see reviews by Folley & Malpress, 1948*b*; also Hutton, 1958; Ben-David, Roderig, Khazen & Sulman, 1966; Forbes & Rook, 1970).

Oestrogens are much used for the suppression of unwanted lactation in women but since the suckling stimulus is also stopped the precise mode of action of the oestrogen is still a matter of controversy (see Gold & Cohen, 1959; Toaff & Jewelwicz, 1963; Steele, 1968). The possibility that oestrogen suppression of lactation in the puerperium may be associated with puerperal thromboembolism has recently stimulated re-evaluation of this therapy (Daniel, Campbell & Turnbull, 1967; Stewart, Kerridge & Dennis, 1969; Hakim, Elder & Hawkins, 1969) and interest in alternative synthetic oestrogens (Brown & Snell, 1968; Firth, 1969).

There is much evidence that oestrogen–progestogen combinations depress lactation (see review by Cowie, 1961). Fresh interest in the effects of oestrogen–progestogen combinations on lactation has recently arisen because many oral contraceptives currently available contain oestrogenic and progestogenic substances which could possibly impair lactation in women who are breast feeding. Some inhibition of lactation occurs in the rat with norethynodrel combined with mestranol (Enovid) (Saunders, 1967; Joshi & Rao, 1968) but not in the mouse or rabbit (Joshi & Rao, 1968); since, however, the mice nursed litters of only 6 young, and the rabbits only 3, mild depression of milk yield would hardly have been detected. Pincus (1965) reported that inhibitory effects on lactation in women declined as the dose of norethynodrel + mestranol (Enovid) was reduced from 20 to 2·5 mg/day. Later Kaern (1967) concluded from a controlled study on lactating women using a combination of norethisterone + mestranol (Norinyl-1) that in no case was the initiation of lactation suppressed by the drug but there was evidence indicating a diminution in the quantity of the milk. Significant depression of milk yields, however, was observed in mothers taking ethynodiol diacetate + mestranol (Ovulin) in as short a period of medication as two cycles (Kora, 1969). In view of the present low dosage rates, oral contraceptives are unlikely to have serious detrimental effects on lactation, particularly if their use is postponed until lactation is established (see also Toaff, Ashkenazi, Schwartz & Herzberg, 1969). However, further studies are desirable in view of the vital importance of satisfactory breast feeding in countries where milk substitutes are too costly for many mothers.

The question of contraceptive steroids and their metabolites being excreted in the milk is discussed on p. 184.

Oxytocin

As discussed in Chapter 5 the hormone oxytocin is mainly concerned in the phenomenon of milk ejection which results in the transfer of pre-formed milk from the alveoli into the ducts, sinuses and cisterns of the mammary gland thereby making the milk available to the suckling or milker. There is evidence, however, at least in some species, that oxytocin may also exert a galactopoietic action, that is, it may promote milk secretion. This galactopoietic response has been observed in cows, goats and sheep and has been associated with the routine use of oxytocin to obtain the residual milk from the udder, i.e. the milk which is retained in the udder after normal milking, but the effect was not observed when oxytocin was injected between milkings (for references see Morag, 1968*a*). Exogenous oxytocin may also depress milk yields when injected regularly into lactating ruminants by interfering with the release of endogenous oxytocin resulting in incomplete milking (Donker, Koshi & Petersen, 1954; Morag & Fox, 1966; Morag, 1968*b*). Studies by Morag (1968*a*) have shown that it is this partial inhibition of the milk-ejection reflex which may mask galactopoietic responses to oxytocin. If oxytocin is given both between and immediately before milking, proper evacuation of the udder occurs and the galactopoietic response is evident. Linzell (1967) has demonstrated that for experimental purposes the milking of goats at hourly intervals is a practicable procedure and, provided that low doses (50–400 mu.) of exogenous oxytocin are given, the quantity of milk, fat and lactose obtained each hour for 10–12 hr is equal to or slightly more than the mean hourly yield calculated from the yield on twice daily milking. Large doses of oxytocin are not only unnecessary but may induce changes in milk composition. The influence of repeated injections of oxytocin on the milk of the cow has recently been discussed by Lane, Dill, Armstrong & Switzer (1970).

Galactopoietic effects of exogeneous oxytocin have been described in rats (Kumaresan & Turner, 1966; Morag & Brick, 1969), but if the interval between nursings was extended from 8 to 16 hr oxytocin then depressed milk secretion although there was no evidence that the endogenous release of oxytocin was inhibited as in the cow (Morag & Brick, 1969). In mice oxytocin depresses lactation (Mizuno & Shiiba, 1969; Mizuno & Satoh, 1970).

How oxytocin effects its galactopoietic response is not known although several mechanisms have been suggested; first, it may stimulate the release of hormones from the anterior pituitary as was initially suggested by Benson & Folley (1957); secondly, by moving the milk from the alveoli into the ducts it may prevent the build-up of inhibitory pressures within the alveoli; thirdly it may increase the permeability of membranes thereby increasing supply of nutrients to the alveolar cells (see Morag, 1968*a*).

Oxytocin administered regularly to cows during the dry period reduces their milk yield in the next lactation as when the dry period is of too short a duration (Gorman & Swanson, 1968) see also p. 180.

REGRESSION AND INVOLUTION OF THE MAMMARY GLAND

Types of regression

Regression of the mammary gland may be a rapid or a slow process depending on the pertaining circumstances. In the course of normal lactation both the total volume and the secretory activity of the parenchyma may decline; thus in the lactating mouse the total mammary DNA and the ratio of RNA/DNA decline from day 14 of lactation (Mizuno, 1961) while in the rat the mean alveolar diameter diminishes from the 2nd day of lactation (Bässler & Flörchinger, 1966*a*, *b*). In the cow diminution of lobule volume with corresponding increase in stromal tissue is said to occur in the course of lactation (see Turner, 1952) while in the goat total alveolar surface area decreases in proportion to the milk yield but no increase in stromal tissue was noted (Schmidt, Chatterton & Hansel, 1962). Clearly the intensity of such changes will vary with the species and with the duration of lactation but they will tend to accelerate during the natural self-weaning process as the young acquire other sources of food and, as lactation ends, the mammary gland eventually returns to a state somewhat similar to that before the onset of pregnancy. These gradual changes during lactation may be retarded if a further pregnancy supervenes (Mizuno, 1961; Paape & Tucker, 1969*a*).

A more intense and dramatic regression of mammary tissues

occurs when for experimental reasons or accidental causes the suckling or milking stimulus suddenly ceases, i.e. premature weaning; under these circumstances the rate of regression will depend on whether cessation of suckling or milking has occurred at the height of lactation, at the onset of lactation or towards its natural end. Again these rapid changes may be modified if suckling or milking of some of the mammary glands is continued so that the non-suckled gland continues to be influenced by hypophysial hormones (both adeno- and neurohypophysial) liberated into the blood stream in response to the milking or suckling stimulus.

Yet another type of mammary regression is that occurring at the end of reproductive life and this again may present characteristic features which differentiate it from the other types of regression.

In any investigation of mammary involution it is therefore necessary to indicate the type of involution under study. Mayer & Klein (1961) apply the terms 'post-lactational involution' and 'senile involution' which are more or less self-explanatory save that several varieties may come within the 'post-lactational' category. Hollmann & Verley (1967) apply the term 'regression' to the post-lactational varieties of involution as described above and restrict the term 'involution' to the senile type.

Observations on senile involution of the mammary gland have centred almost exclusively on man and the various studies have been reviewed by Geschickter (1945) and Dabelow (1957); after the age of 35 years the peripheral mammary lobules gradually diminish in size and are replaced by adipose tissue, indeed because of the deposition of fat the breast may enlarge as the parenchyma regresses. With advancing years there is eventually a loss of the lobular structure of the parenchyma and all but the mammary ducts and their major branches disappear; the fibrous stroma becomes increasingly dense and hyalinized, even sclerotic, and some of the smaller ducts become obliterated.

Studies on the various types of post-lactational regression have been reviewed by Turner (1939, 1952), Folley (1952) and Mayer & Klein (1961) and we need only give references to selected papers or those which have appeared in the last decade.

Biochemical studies

Numerous biochemical investigations, some with particular reference to nucleic acids, have been reported on the mammary glands during premature weaning (e.g. Greenbaum & Slater, 1957; Slater, 1962; Levy, 1964; Ôta, 1964; Helminen, Ericsson & Orrenius, 1968; Helminen & Ericsson, 1970). In rats at mid-lactation weaning produces within 24 hr a rapid increase in the weight of the mammary gland, in its total content of protein, phosphoprotein-P and of lactose—the increase of the latter being particularly striking; these parameters then decrease, the lactose very rapidly, so that by the third day their values have fallen below the preweaning levels. The total DNA increases for the first 24–48 hr and then declines whereas the total RNA decreases rapidly from 6 to 12 hr after removal of the litter (Slater, 1962; Ôta, 1964; Tucker & Reece, 1964). When rats were weaned towards the end of lactation (day 21) an increase in total DNA was not observed in the early stages (Tucker & Reece, 1963). The increases in gland weight, protein and phosphoprotein-P and lactose are evidently the result of the increase in the amount of milk retained in the gland during the first 24 hr when more than 70% of the gland weight may represent milk. The rise in DNA in the first 48 hr must result from an increase in cells other than those of the mammary parenchyma, possibly leucocytes (Slater, 1962; Ôta, 1964; Tucker & Reece, 1964). Since lactation can be readily re-established in the rat after premature weaning if suckling is resumed within 24 hr, the changes observed during this period clearly do not represent any irreversible atrophy of the secretory cells; however the marked decreases in gland weight, RNA content and RNA : DNA ratio occurring from days 2 to 5 indicate the disappearance of secretory function although the changes are apparently still reversible up to 110 hr after weaning (Silver, 1956).

Histological studies

Histological studies have revealed the general nature of the tissue changes during mammary regression (see reviews by Turner, 1939, 1952; Folley, 1952; Mayer & Klein, 1961). The pattern appears similar in all species studied save that the duration of the process varies, e.g. 15 days in the mouse (Sekhri, Pitelka & DeOme, 1967a); 36 days in the rat (Oshima & Goto, 1955); about 32 days in the ewe (Lee & Lascelles, 1969a); and 48 days in the goat (Turner, 1952). In the smaller laboratory animals during the first 24–48 hr there is a period of engorgement with milk, the alveoli are distended and the alveolar cells stretched and flattened. The distension may not be uniform throughout the gland for histometric studies have shown that in the rat after ligation of a teat the maximum alveolar distension occurred in the centre of the gland after some 55 hr whereas in the peripheral regions of the parenchyma the maximum distension was reached at 24 hr but the degree of distension was less (Bässler & Flörchinger, 1966*a*, *b*). As resorption of the milk constituents begins the alveolar distension diminishes and by day 5 the alveoli are collapsed and disintegrating and the gland is infiltrated with phagocytic cells. The lobular structure disappears, the stromal tissue becomes predominant and eventually, when the involutionary process is completed, the mammary parenchyma is only slightly better developed than it was before the onset of pregnancy.

The mode of resorption of the lobulo-alveolar tissue has presented some problems. While various types of phagocytic cells have been described in the regressing tissues their numbers, in the absence of infection, were too small to suggest that a significant inflammatory action was active in the process of involution. In a study on the numbers and distribution of stromal macrophages in the mouse mammary gland Mayberry (1964) observed but few macrophages in the lactating gland and these were distributed in the intralobular stroma; after premature weaning on the 8th day post partum the macrophages remained few in numbers till the fifth day of regression when along with lymphocytes and plasma cells their numbers increased in the stroma as it encroached upon and replaced the parenchyma; by the 9th day their numbers had much increased and they were found within and around the disintegrating and shrunken alveoli. Mayberry (1964) considered that the stroma was active in supplying phagocytic cells to aid in the removal of residual secretion and necrotic epithelium in the late stages of regression. In cows and ewes macrophages appear to play a major role in the removal of fat from the regressing mammary gland. Macrophages pass into the milk within the alveoli and ducts, phagocytose fat droplets and then migrate into the tissues to pass by way of the lymphatics to the regional lymph nodes. Presumably lipolysis of the fat occurs within the cytoplasm of the macrophages (Lee, McDowell & Lascelles, 1969).

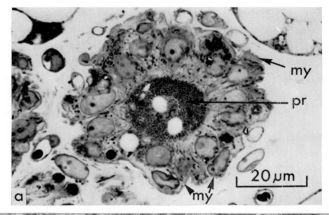

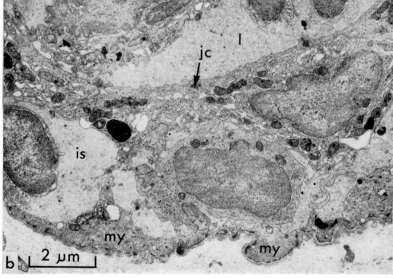

Fig. 4.7.

Ultrastructural studies

In the last decade detailed information has become available about the ultrastructural changes during regression. These studies have been reviewed by Sekhri, Pitelka & DeOme (1967a, b) with particular reference to the mouse and the following description is based on their conclusions. Within 12 hr of the cessation of suckling, colostral corpuscles are present in the lumina of the alveoli and ducts; within 24 hr vacuoles bounded by a single membrane appear in the cytoplasm of the alveolar cells, some of the vacuoles are empty while others contain protein granules; these vacuoles tend to coalesce and their contents undergo lysis. While these changes are occurring microvilli slough off thereby smoothing the luminal surface. The endoplasmic reticulum breaks down into isolated membrane fragments and possibly into microvesicles; mitochondria fuse with one another. On days 3 and 4 after the cessation of suckling the breakdown products of some autophagic vacuoles are demonstrable in the form of residual bodies sometimes termed 'lamellated inclusions', 'vacuolated bodies' or 'myelin figures'. Dense irregular droplets of fat appear in the cytoplasm and there is a depletion in the numbers of mitochondria, ribonucleoprotein particles and other cell constituents. By day 5 there is a disintegration of the architecture of the cell which now consists

---

FIG. 4.7. (*a*) Light micrograph of araldite-embedded 0·5 μm thick section of alveolus of mammary gland of mouse 2 days after premature weaning. The lumen is packed with protein granules; the alveolar cells are tall but the volume of the cytoplasm relative to the size of the nucleus is becoming reduced; fat droplets are no longer present in the cytoplasm; the contour of the alveolus is becoming irregular because the myoepithelial cells are becoming prominent and are projecting into the perialveolar tissue. pr = protein granules; my = myoepithelial cells (from Verley, J. M. & Hollmann, K. H., 1967, *Z. Zellforsch. mikrosk. Anat.* **82,** 212–221). (*b*) Electron micrograph of alveolar cells in mammary gland of a rabbit 8 days after premature weaning showing the disruption of the architecture of the gland which occurs during regression. Note the occurence of large intercellular spaces containing flocculent material similar to that present in the lumen. The junctional complexes adjacent to the lumen are intact and there is also an intact network of myoepithelial processes around the alveolus; pieces of degenerating alveolar cells are present in the lumen. l = lumen; jc = junctional complex; is = intercellular space; my = myoepithelial cell (from Hollmann, K. H. & Verley, J. M., 1967, *Z. Zellforsch. mikrosk. Anat.* **82, 222**–238).

mostly of lipid droplets and residual bodies. The basement membranes generally remain intact until the 8th day although some alveoli seem to rupture in the early stages from extreme intraluminal pressure of milk. By day 10 the mammary gland is composed of necrotic alveoli; residual bodies fill most of the cytoplasm and nuclei may be floating freely in the interstitial spaces. The alveoli are no longer identifiable by the 15th day, and the remaining ducts are lined with epithelial cells resembling the duct cells of resting glands.

Further observations on regression after premature weaning in mice and rabbits have been made by Verley & Hollmann (1967) (also Hollmann & Verley, 1967). In the early stages of involution there is a loss of contact between epithelial cells (Fig. 4.7*b*), the intercellular spaces increase although contact at the junctional complexes remains; milk protein granules pass from the lumen into these intercellular spaces and so into the tissue spaces where

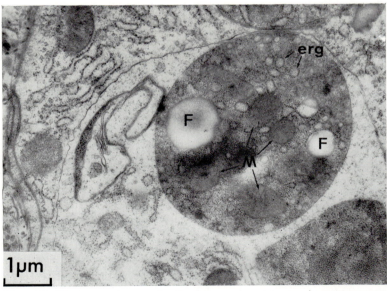

Fig. 4.8. Electron micrograph of a large cytosegrosome in a mammary alveolar cell of a lactating rat after weaning. The cytosegrosome contains mitochondria (M), fat droplets (F) and vesiculated endoplasmic reticulum (erg) (from Helminen, H. J. & Ericsson, J. L. E., 1968*b*, *J. Ultrastruct. Res.* **25**, 214–227).

they are removed by the capillaries. Not all alveolar cells are cytolyzed but some return to the resting state. During the degeneration process the myoepithelial cells seem to play an active role by contracting around the acini as the epithelial cells disappear thereby drawing together those cells which have passed into the resting state and simultaneously aiding the expulsion of cellular debris (Fig. 4.7*a*, *b*). Hollmann & Verley believe that two systems assure the cohesion of the epithelial elements and thereby the integrity of the gland tree throughout regression; first, the junctional complexes which remain secure until the actual death of the cell, and secondly, the myoepithelial cells which form a retaining and contracting network over the epithelial cells.

Studies on the effects of premature weaning on the ultrastructure of the mammary glands of lactating rats have been carried out by Helminen & Ericsson (1968*a*, *b*, *c*) who observed that autophagic vacuoles (cytosegresomes) (see p. 178) were extremely rare in the epithelial cells of normal lactating mammary

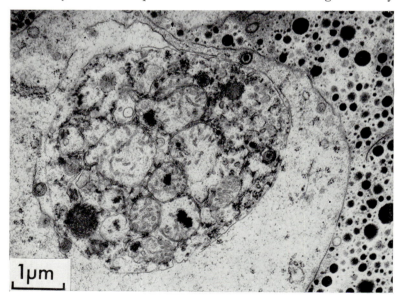

Fig. 4.9. Electron micrograph of a large cytosegrosome in a mammary alveolar cell of a lactating rat three days after weaning. The cytosegrosome contains numerous altered mitochondria (from Helminen H. J. & Ericsson, J. L. E., 1968*b*, *J. Ultrastruct. Res.* **25**, 214–227).

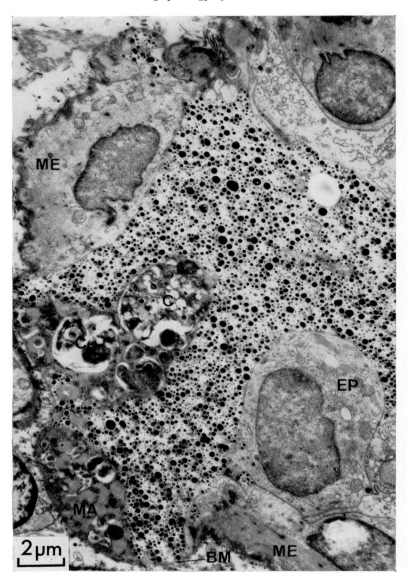

Fig. 4.10

glands but that in the first three days after weaning there was a marked increase in their numbers, several often being present in a cell (Fig. 4.8). By day 3 the cytosegresomes were larger and contained altered mitochondria as well as other cytoplasmic organelles and ground substance (Fig. 4.9). After day 3 the cytosegresomes became fewer and were replaced by large cytosomes (lysosomes). From days 3 to 10 there appeared to be a heterophagocytic uptake of portions of epithelial cells, cytoplasm and milk protein droplets by macrophages present between epithelial cells in the alveoli (Fig. 4.10).

Some divergence from the above general pattern of involutionary changes may occur when the mammary regression is produced by ligature of a teat so that the gland becomes distended with milk while adjacent glands continue to be regularly suckled. In such circumstances the unsuckled gland remains under the influence of anterior and posterior pituitary hormones released in response to the suckling stimulus so that the regression changes are delayed and the gland architecture partially maintained. Electron microscopic studies on such glands are few; in rats, Bässler (1961) noted progressive cytolytic changes often involving rupture of the basement membrane followed by the dispersal of the secretory products and cell debris into the interstitial spaces. Wellings (1961) carried out similar studies in mice but found no ultrastructural changes indicative of cytolysis even on the 4th day. Sekhri, Pitelka & DeOme (1967b) have suggested that the divergence of observations may arise because in the ligated gland while autolytic processes do occur, they occur more slowly than in the absence of the suckling stimulus and that while many lobules are diminished some survive and manage to maintain themselves with the hormones arriving in the residual blood supply although they show no evidence of secretory activity.

FIG. 4.10 Survey electron micrograph of portion of an alveolus of mammary gland of a lactating rat three days after weaning showing macrophage-like cell (MA), myoepithelial cell (ME) and epithelial cell (EP) bordering the lumen. In some areas the basement membrane (BM) is naked. There are numerous protein droplets in the lumen. C = large cytosomes in apparent macrophage (from Helminen, H. J. & Ericsson, J. L. E., 1968c, *J. Ultrastruct. Res.* **25**, 228–239).

Role of lysosomes

In lactating rat mammary tissue particles having properties similar to the lysosomes of rat liver have been demonstrated by Slater, Greenbaum & Wang (1963) who suggested that these particles might be concerned in the cytologic processes occurring in involution. It will be recalled that lysosomes,* first discovered by deDuve and his colleagues—see review by deDuve (1969)—are believed to play a role as an intracellular digestive system—the processes involved being (a) autophagocytosis (i.e. digestion of portions of the cell's own cytoplasm in cytosegresomes); (b) heterophagocytosis, i.e. digestion of whole or disintegrating cells by other cells such as macrophages; and (c) release of lysosomal hydrolytic enzymes from damaged lysosomes. Woessner Jr. (1969) has recently reviewed studies relevant to the role of lysosomes in mammary involution. The resting mammary gland has been little studied but it appears to contain lysosomes and lysosomal enzymes but they are neither prominent nor very active. In the rat during pregnancy lysosomal enzymes in the mammary gland increase and to a greater extent than does the weight of the enlarging glands, β-glucuronidase, cathepsin D, acid phosphatase and acid ribonuclease all following this pattern. The role of lysosomes during this period is not known. Acid phosphatase and cathepsin continue to increase during lactation. On premature weaning there is a gradual increase in the specific activity of acid phosphatase, aryl sulphatase, β-glucuronidase and cathepsin D from the first to the seventh day, while the total activities of these enzymes (i.e. per gland) increase on days 1, 2 and 3; the lysosomal enzymes being the only enzymes which do not decline sharply during mammary regression. There is, moreover, an increased activity of these enzymes in the macrophages, as well as in the epithelial cells

* The terminology relating to lysosomes is somewhat confusing. Many electron microscopists regard the term 'lysosome' as representing a biochemical concept and since there is uncertainty as to the precise relationship it has to the various membrane-limited bodies seen in the cytoplasm they consider it inappropriate to give the term a morphological connotation. It has therefore become customary in electron microscope studies to refer to large inclusion bodies containing vesiculated and dense material of variable appearance within a single membrane as 'cytosomes', and to autophagic vacuoles containing recognizable organelles bordered by a double membrane as 'cytosegresomes' (see Ericsson, Trump & Weibel, 1965; deDuve & Wattiaux, 1966).

(see Helminen, Ericsson & Orrenius, 1968; Zarzycki, Peryt, Klubińska, Zak & Hajac, 1969; Helminen & Ericsson, 1970).

How do these biochemical observations relate to what is occurring at the cellular level? It has already been noted that while the macrophage population increases in the later stages of regression these cells do not appear to play any major role in early tissue breakdown and it is likely that autophagic processes are the main mechanisms involved during this period. This is in accord with the observed occurrence of autophagic vacuoles (cytosegresomes) in the cytoplasm in early regression (see p. 175), and the fact that as cellular damage proceeds there is an increase in the lysosome-like vesicles and eventually most of the cell organelles are transformed into residual bodies (cytosomes). Although autophagocytosis is comparatively pronounced Helminen & Ericsson (1968c) consider it unlikely that the rapid reduction in cytoplasmic organelles, particularly the endoplasmic reticulum, is solely due to digestion within cytosegresomes or that the diffuse cytoplasmic alterations in early involution are associated with the release of lysosomal enzymes since they have not observed breaks in cytosomal membranes or focal degeneration in the neighbourhood of cytosomes. Helminen & Ericsson (1968c, 1970) further believe that the rise in lysosomal enzymes is a symptom not the cause of regression of the glandular tissue and that the primary triggering effect—resulting from increased intra-alveolar pressure, intracellular stasis of milk protein, diminished levels of anterior pituitary hormones, or other factors—is directed towards cytoplasmic structures other than the lysosomes. In the later stages when the degenerating epithelial cells become detached into the alveolar lumen then heterophagocytosis in macrophages appears to play a dominant role. In sum, lysosomes appear to play a role in regression in two ways—in autophagocytic processes which reduce the cytoplasm of the epithelial cells, and in heterophagocytic processes by which macrophages remove the debris of dead cells and secretion. Not all losses of material are accounted for by lysosomes for some substances diffuse into the interstitial spaces and are carried away in the lymph and capillaries.

Concurrent pregnancy and mammary regression

In the rat a new pregnancy during the early stages of postlactational involution retards but does not prevent the regression changes in the mammary gland and the rats enter their second lactation with less nucleic acid, hydroxyproline (a measure of collagen) and hexosamine (a measure of ground substance) in the mammary glands than were present at the time of weaning in their first lactation (Paape & Tucker, 1969*a*).

In the cow histometric and biochemical studies provide little indication that significant regression occurs during the usual dry period of some two months duration (Swanson, Pardue & Longmire, 1967). This short dry period and interval of rest for the mammary gland is of great physiological importance for the next lactation for if the dry period be unduly shortened (e.g. less than 6 weeks) then the milk yields in the subsequent lactation may be reduced by some 70% (Swanson, 1965). It has been said that the beneficial effect of the dry period arises from the better nutrition of the cow when the drain of lactation ends but Swanson's study suggested that the dry period itself, independently of nutritional effects, affected the next lactation. Further proof of this contention was provided by Smith, Wheelock & Dodd (1966) who dried off two quarters of the udder (i.e. two mammary glands) in identical-twin cows while continuing to milk the other two quarters to the end of pregnancy. When the cows calved all four quarters were again milked; during the first three months of their second lactation the experimental quarters which had been milked throughout gave about half the milk yield of the quarters which had been dried off. Since all quarters in the same cow received blood of the same composition and containing the same milk precursor substances and hormones then, as Smith *et al.* (1966) emphasize, the reduced yields of the quarters milked regularly to the second lactation cannot be ascribed to nutritional or hormonal factors but must be due to some change within the mammary gland itself. The continued milking might inhibit the renewal and regeneration of the alveolar cells which may occur in the dry period or early in the next lactation (see also Paape & Tucker, 1969*b*; Wheelock & Dodd, 1969). Subsequently Gorman & Swanson (1968) showed that injecting oxytocin twice daily during the dry period simulated the effects of continued milking up to parturition by depressing the subsequent lactation. It was observed that the oxytocin injections maintained the presence of secretions in the udders thus greatly reducing the resting phase of the alveolar cells. In this connexion it is of interest that injections of oxytocin retard the decline in mammary DNA in late lactation in the rat (Thatcher & Tucker, 1970).

Role of anterior pituitary hormones

In part the regressive changes within the mammary gland after the cessation of the suckling or milking stimulus may be associated with a decline in the levels of prolactin since the administration of prolactin will retard such changes (see review by Folley, 1947; Cross, 1961*b*). In the rat, moreover, injections of oxytocin will also delay some aspects of mammary regression (Benson & Folley, 1957; Richards & Benson, 1969; Thatcher & Tucker, 1970) so that a reduced secretion of both adeno- and neurohypophysial hormones may be involved. In the rat the most effective combination of hormones in retarding mammary regression is said to be prolactin, cortisol and oxytocin (Meites & Hopkins, 1961). The problem of the role of the anterior pituitary hormones is however, a complicated one, since the direct effects of milk accumulation within the alveoli may simulate effects of anterior pituitary hormone deficiency (see p. 182).

Vascular changes

The vascular changes in the rat mammary gland during regression have been studied by Silver (1956). At the end of the first 24 hr after weaning the capillaries are full of blood despite the great distension of the alveoli; between 36 and 48 hr there is a reduction in the number of patent capillaries and the alveoli no longer contract in response to intravenous injections of oxytocin. Attempts to re-establish lactation were successful only if suckling was recommenced within 110 hr of weaning. Cross & Silver (1956) do not consider that the capillary closure is wholly a matter of a passive occlusion due to alveolar distension but is probably associated with the presence of some substance in the retained milk which has a direct constrictor effect on the capillaries.

Milk accumulation

Studies on the effects of varying the interval between milkings in the cow have indicated that for intervals of up to 12 to 18 hr the rate of milk secretion remains unaffected (for references see Wheelock, Rook, Dodd & Griffin, 1966; also Porter, Conrad & Gilmore, 1966; Linnerud, Caruolo, Miller, Marx & Donker,

1966). In the ewe the rate of milk secretion declines after 12 hr of non-milking (Morag, 1969). A recent investigation on the effects of extending the milking interval up to 36 hr in the cow has shown that after 12–18 hr the rates of secretion of milk and its constituents decrease curvilinearly with the duration of the interval but that the degree of curvilinearity differs between the constituents (Wheelock *et al.*, 1966). The inhibitory effect of milk accumulation on the functional activities of the alveolar cells is a complex problem involving physical factors such as pressure on the alveolar cells and on the blood vessels supplying them (for pressure changes in cow udder, see Graf & Lawson, 1968) and the possible presence of factors in the retained milk which may affect alveolar cell function. In this connexion Levy (1964) has postulated the presence of an inhibitor substance in the milk of rats which shuts off the synthesis of fatty acids within 24 hr of weaning by decreasing the activity of the enzyme acetyl-CoA carboxylase.

Also, in the lactating rat, within 24 hr of removal of the litter there is a rapid decline in the activities of a number of enzymes in the mammary parenchyma, changes which, moreover, can be reproduced almost exactly by hypophysectomizing lactating rats (Jones, 1967, 1968). However, in studies involving the ligation of the galactophores of the mammary glands on one side of the lactating rat, thereby preventing the emptying of the ligated glands while permitting suckling and therefore normal hormone levels in the blood, the fall in enzyme activities still occurred in the ligated glands while in the contralateral glands, which would be emptied by the young, levels remained normal (Jones, 1968). Thus despite the similarity to the changes after hypophysectomy the alterations in enzyme activities in response to milk engorgement appear to be a direct effect on the mammary epithelium of milk accumulation. As Jones (1968) points out this direct effect of milk engorgement represents a useful feed-back system for adjusting milk production in response to demand.

EXCRETION OF DRUGS AND HORMONES BY MAMMARY
GLAND

The excretion of drugs in the milk is a subject of increasing importance both in domestic animals and man. In an early review on this subject Burns (1947) discussed the excretion in milk of nicotine (from smoking), sulphonamides, purgatives, sex hormones and insecticide (DDT). More recently Rasmussen (1966) has listed over 400 references to the mammary excretion of drugs and pesticides and discussed the mechanisms of excretion involved; recent reviews include those by Sisodia & Stowe (1964), Knowles (1965) and Smithells & Morgan (1970). While many drugs are excreted in such small quantities as to be pharmacologically inactive in the infant, the levels of laxatives may be sufficient to cause purgation, salicylates and sulphonamides may cause skin rashes while antibiotics in the milk may cause sensitivity symptoms (see Smithells & Morgan, 1970). Excretion studies of two recent fenamate analgesic drugs—mefenamic acid ('Ponstel', Parke, Davis & Co.) and flufenamic acid ('Arlef', Parke, Davis & Co.) indicate that only very small quantities are found in breast milk (Buchanan, Eaton, Koeff & Kinkel, 1968, 1969).

The ability of the thyroid gland to accumulate iodide against a concentration gradient and to maintain a high gland : plasma concentration ratio of iodide is well known, but the mammary gland also has this ability of concentrating iodide and of passing it into the milk (Honour, Myant & Rowlands, 1952; Brown-Grant, 1957). This ability may vary with species, the lactating goat concentrating iodide in the milk to a greater extent than the cow (Lengemann, 1970). This ability of the mammary gland to concentrate iodide should be kept in mind when radio-iodide is administered to lactating women. Recently Bland, Crawford, Docker & Farr (1969) have reported that when routine blood-volume studies using serum albumin labelled with ^{125}I are used in women at the time of delivery a considerable amount of radio-active iodine is transmitted to the infant in the breast milk so that the dose taken up by the infant thyroid may well constitute a health hazard by increasing the risk of subsequent cancer of the thyroid.

Astatine, the only member of the halogen family without a stable isotope, is also accumulated by the mammary gland and is passed into the milk (Asling, Durbin, Johnston & Parrott, 1959).

The problem of sex hormones in milk has been investigated in connexion with the administration of oestrogen to cows for the artificial induction of lactation (see p. 124) but this does not appear to present any serious problems (Lawson, Stroud & Williams, 1944; Melampy, Gurland & Rakes, 1959; Mellin &

Erb, 1965). However, it is well to note that the amount of oestrogen excreted in the milk is a matter of dosage for a single high dose of diethylstilboestrol (1·2–2·5 mg) injected into rats on day 4 of lactation will cause a permanent sterility in the female sucklings (Mayer & Duluc, 1967).

Recently the possibility of oestrogens and progesterone and their metabolites being excreted in the milk of women taking oral contraceptives has aroused interest. The various investigations have been reviewed by van der Molen, Hart & Wijmenga (1969) who studied the presence of labelled mestranol and lynestrol and their metabolites in breast milk (see also Wijmenga & van der Molen, 1969). Small quantities of the steroids or their metabolites certainly entered the milk but the authors reached no conclusions as to whether they could be pharmacologically active. Ethynyloestradiol and its 3-cyclopentyl ether (quinestrol) can also be detected in the milk when administered to lactating rats (Cargill, Meli, Giannina & Steinetz, 1969). Further studies are necessary before any conclusions can be made regarding a possible health hazard to the infant from the excretion of such steroids. In this connexion the fact must not be overlooked that in the first 3 weeks of lactation there is normally a not inconsiderable excretion of endogenous steroids in breast milk. Sas, Viski & Gellén (1969) have assayed various steroids in the milk of ten healthy women over a 25-day period after delivery. The concentration of oestrogens (oestriol, oestrone and oestradiol) reached a peak on day 5 and then declined to negligible quantities after 3 weeks; 5β-pregnene-3α, 20α-diol was present in the milk on days 3, 4 and 5 but 5β-pregnane-3α, 20β-diol was present on day 2 alone; 17-ketosteroids (chlor-dehydroepiandrosterone, androstanedione, androstenedione, androsterone and dehydroepiandrosterone) reached their highest levels on day 4, by day 10 only a small quantity of dehydroepiandrosterone was detected. From the daily milk intake Sas *et al.* (1969) calculate that the infant ingests in the milk nearly 300 µg of total oestrogen on day 5, nearly 200 µg of pregnanediol on day 4 and almost 12 mg of the 17-ketosteroids on day 7. The presence of 5β-pregnane-3α, 20β-diol in the milk of healthy women on day 2 is of interest since this steroid has been implicated in the cause of 'breast-milk jaundice' in infants (for references see Sas *et al.*, 1969).

5

MILK REMOVAL

WHEN milk has been secreted by the cells of the alveolar epithelium it is not readily available to the demands of the suckling or milker. The removal of milk from the mammary gland can be divided into two phases in the first of which, termed passive withdrawal (for terminology see Cowie, Folley, Cross, Harris, Jacobsohn & Richardson, 1951), the milk which is present in the udder cistern, sinuses or the larger ducts can be drawn off through the teat. However, the milk present within the alveoli and smaller ducts is retained in the glandular tissue until the second phase of milk removal occurs. This involves the expulsion of milk from the alveoli and ducts towards the teat, through the mediation of a complex neuro-endocrine mechanism. This process, known as the milk-ejection reflex, involves the active expulsion of milk from the alveolar tissue, and its name is more appropriate, therefore, than the terms 'let-down' or 'draught', occasionally used in dairy husbandry or clinical medicine.

THE MILK-EJECTION REFLEX

The story of the milk-ejection reflex spans much of the present century, and with the benefit of hindsight it may be difficult to appreciate just why it took so long to unfold. The field has been the subject of numerous reviews, the most recent and comprehensive of which are Denamur (1965*b*), Benson & Fitzpatrick (1966) and Bisset (1968). Only the historical highlights will be mentioned here and attention will be focused mainly on recent developments.

The occurrence of milk ejection after injection of extracts of the posterior lobe of the pituitary was reported in the goat by Ott & Scott (1910). In 1915, Gaines suggested that the milk-ejection

G

response caused by such extracts involved a mechanism of muscular contraction within the mammary gland, but he still considered the normal mechanism to be a purely neural reflex. Although the physiological importance of the posterior lobe of the pituitary in milk ejection was appreciated by Turner & Slaughter (1930) the first formulation of the modern concept of the milk-ejection reflex came from the work of Ely & Petersen (1941) in the cow. Apparent confirmation was obtained by Petersen & Ludwick (1942) and by Peeters, Massart & Coussens (1947), who showed that a substance causing milk ejection was present in blood taken from a cow during milking and subsequently perfused through an isolated cow's udder. Removal of the posterior lobe of the pituitary gland was found to abolish the milk-ejection reflex in the rat (Gomez, 1939; Harris & Jacobsohn, 1952; Benson & Cowie, 1956) although the time factor must be borne in mind since, in a subsequent lactation, sufficient reorganization of the cut end of the pituitary stalk occurred to allow release of neurohypophysial hormones (Benson & Cowie, 1956). The role of the magnocellular hypothalamic nuclei in milk ejection was established by studies involving stimulation or ablation of the hypothalamo-neurohypophysial system (Cross & Harris, 1950, 1951, 1952; Andersson, 1951*a*, *b*) and the determination of the structure and the subsequent synthesis of oxytocin (see du Vigneaud, 1956) confirmed that this was the milk-ejection hormone.

It is now generally agreed that, in most species, the stimulus of suckling or hand- or machine-milking triggers nerve impulses from receptors in the teat, which ascend to the hypothalmus and evoke the release of oxytocin. The hormone is then carried in the blood stream to the mammary gland where it acts on a contractile effector tissue and forcibly expels the milk from the alveoli and small ducts. The structures responsible for this final segment of the milk-ejection reflex are the myoepithelial cells surrounding and embracing the alveoli and small ducts. These were demonstrated convincingly for the first time by the elegant studies of Richardson (1949, 1951) in the mammary gland of the goat and of woman, and later in the cat, dog, rat and rabbit by Linzell (1952). These specialized cells were found to be present in sufficient quantity to make it reasonable to suppose that they were the effector contractile mechanism of the mammary gland, and this was substantiated by direct observation of the contraction of mammary alveoli in the mouse after topical application of oxytocin (Linzell, 1955) or posterior pituitary extract (Levitskaya, 1955; Zotikova, 1955) (for fuller discussion see Chapter 1).

Grachev (1964) quotes several papers by A. D. Vladimirova in support of an indirect role of the vascular system in the milk-ejection process. It is claimed that the act of milking is accompanied by an increased blood flow through the mammary gland, by an increase in temperature of the blood vessels, and that the increased supply of blood aids the access of oxytocin to the myo-epithelium. Findlay & Grosvenor (1969) pointed out that this was not in agreement with the report of Cross & Silver (1962) who observed a fall in intramammary oxygen tension in the anaesthetized lactating rabbit after administration of exogenous oxytocin, and this effect was attributed to a fall in blood flow. In contrast to this, the act of suckling in the human is accompanied by a rise in temperature of the breast (Abolins, 1954). Also, Vuorenkoski, Wasz-Höckert, Koivisto & Lind (1969) recorded a rise in temperature of the breast of human primiparae during the first few days post partum when a tape recording of the baby's hunger cry was played. The fact that this would appear to be an emotional control over mammary blood flow underlines the point that the injection of oxytocin into an anaesthetized animal may not necessarily mirror the total sum of humoral and neural influences which is elicited in response to the conscious act of nursing.

The tap reflex

It would be appropriate at this point to mention another mechanism which may perform a subsidiary role in the active process of milk ejection. In addition to being sensitive to the action of circulating neurohypophysial principles, the specialized myoepithelial cells of the mammary gland will also contract in response to direct mechanical stimuli. This was first noted by Cross (1954), who described a local mammary reflex in the rabbit, in which an increase in intramammary pressure occurred shortly after an abrupt tap was applied to the skin overlying the lactating gland. It appeared that the mammary myoepithelium was responding directly to mechanical stimulation since general anaesthesia or local anaesthesia of the nerve supply to the gland were without effect on the response. Cross termed the phenomenon the 'tap reflex' and it was later confirmed for the rabbit (Yokoyama, 1956) and reported to occur in the mouse, where gentle stroking of the exposed tissue with cotton wool caused contraction of myoepithelial cells (Linzell, 1955), the rat (Grosvenor, 1965a) and the goat (Zaks, 1962), where it was observed in both the normal and the denervated udder. Linzell (1955) also reported that contraction occurred after electrical stimulation of the myoepithelium. It appears, therefore, that the cellular mechanisms responsible for the release of the energy required for the contraction of these cells can be triggered by means other than oxytocin, since, in addition to oxytocin, vasopressin has inherent milk-ejection activity (approximately 1/5th that of oxytocin) and acetylcholine and related compounds are also extremely active in this respect (Peeters, Sierens & Silver, 1952; Linzell, 1955; Levitskaya, 1955; Zotikova, 1955; Bisset & Lewis, 1962; Folley & Knaggs, 1965b; Bisset, Clark, Halder, Harris, Lewis & Rocha e Silva, 1967). However, since the mammary gland does not appear to have parasympathetic innervation (see Linzell, 1959b), the physiological significance of the effects of cholinergic drugs on myoepithelial cells remains to be determined.

Inhibition of the milk-ejection reflex

It has been known since the work of Gaines (1915) on the dog that anaesthesia prevents the occurrence of milk ejection. Anaesthetics, including ethanol, exert this effect by blocking the release of oxytocin in response to suckling (Cross, 1955b); Fuchs & Wagner, 1963b, c; Wagner & Fuchs, 1968; Fuchs, 1969; Cobo & Quintero, 1969). In the conscious lactating subject the reflex has also been shown to be inhibited by emotional disturbances or stressful situations, and since the reflex can also be inhibited by injection of adrenaline, there were reasonable grounds for supposing that this might be the causative agent in the inhibition of the reflex (see Cross, 1961b). Indeed, electrical stimulation of the sympathetic discharge region of the hypothalamus in the rabbit inhibited the milk-ejection reflex. The inhibitory effect was abolished by bilateral adrenalectomy, and was restored by more prolonged electrical stimulation, implicating both the adrenal medulla and the sympathetic nervous system (Cross, 1955a). Hebb & Linzell (1951) concluded that, since adrenaline and noradrenaline each possess the same ratio of vasoconstricting and milk-ejection inhibiting properties, that the mode of action on the mammary gland was one of vasoconstriction, thus denying oxytocin access to the myoepithelium.

Topical application of adrenaline to exposed mouse mammary gland did not prevent the occurrence of the milk-ejection response when oxytocin was also applied topically to the gland (Linzell, 1955), and whereas the injection of adrenaline inhibited the milk-ejection response to injected oxytocin in the rabbit, it was without effect on the 'tap reflex' in this species (Cross, 1955a), thus supporting the concept of a vasoconstrictor role for adrenaline and sympathetic nerve endings in the mammary gland. However, this view had to be modified when it was shown that adrenaline could act directly on rabbit myoepithelium to compete for receptor sites with oxytocin, and that the vasoconstrictor activity of adrenaline *in vivo* could be dissociated from its milk-ejection inhibiting property (Chan, 1965). This finding was confirmed and extended by Bisset, Clark & Lewis (1967) who showed by means of selective pharmacological blockade that the receptor sites of mammary blood vessels and myoepithelium were both important for the inhibition of milk ejection by adrenaline. Although sympathetico-adrenal inhibition of the milk-ejection reflex may occur under extreme conditions, Cross (1955b) considered that the doses of adrenaline which must be administered to abolish the reflex may be in excess of endogenous output, and that a central, emotional inhibition of the release of oxytocin itself was a more important factor in emotional blockade of the reflex.

The relative importance of the milk-ejection reflex to lactation in various species

When considering the necessity for the milk-ejection reflex in milk removal, the ability of the mammary myoepithelium to respond to exogenous oxytocin is not, in itself, decisive proof for the essential nature of the reflex in a particular species. Bearing this reservation in mind, milk ejection has been shown to occur in response to systemic injection or to topical application to exposed mammary tissue of oxytocin or neurohypophysial extracts in a wide range of mammals including cow, goat, sheep, pig, woman, dog, cat, rabbit, guinea-pig, rat and mouse (for references see Cowie & Folley, 1961; Denamur, 1965b; Cross, 1966; Benson & Fitzpatrick, 1966; Bisset, 1968).

However, definite proof for the importance or otherwise of the reflex in milk removal has come only after careful study, and evidence is being accumulated gradually, species by species. The experimental approach to the problem has been either to prevent the release of oxytocin during suckling or milking by anaesthesia, surgical deafferentation of the mammary glands, surgical section or lesions of the spinal cord, or removal of the neurohypophysis or to determine whether or not oxytocin is released in response to suckling or milking. By such methods it has been shown that the reflex is essential for normal milk removal in the rat (Eayrs & Baddeley, 1956; Benson & Cowie, 1956; Grosvenor & Turner, 1957a; Eayrs & Edwardson, 1965; Yokoyama & Ôta, 1965; Edwardson & Eayrs, 1967), the rabbit (Cross & Harris, 1952; Cross, 1955b; Tindal, Beyer & Sawyer, 1963; Findlay, 1968), the cat (Beyer, Mena, Pacheco & Alcaraz, 1962a) and dog (Gaines, 1915; Pickford, 1960). In the pig, although experiments of the type mentioned above have not yet been carried out, there is nevertheless, a convincing weight of evidence which must be considered. Thus, in contrast to the domestic ruminants it is virtually impossible to obtain milk from the lactating sow by hand milking. This only becomes feasible after intravenous injection of oxytocin, and there is in fact a dose–response relationship between the dose of oxytocin and the yield of milk obtained at that particular milking (Braude & Mitchell, 1950; Braude, 1954). Taken with the positive finding of circulating oxytocin associated with removal of milk by suckling piglets, and the converse, negative, finding of no detectable circulating oxytocin associated with failure of the piglets to obtain milk (Folley & Knaggs, 1966; Knaggs, 1966), there can surely be little doubt as to the importance of the milk-ejection reflex in this species.

The goat and the sheep, however, present a completely different picture, since although the reflex may occur under normal conditions, it is by no means essential for milk removal. This has been shown beyond any reasonable doubt by denervation of the udder, or spinal cord section, or transplantation of the udder (Denamur & Martinet, 1954; 1959a, b, 1960; Tverskoï, 1958; Linzell, 1963), and also by the lack of effect of cyclopropane anaesthesia during milking on the lactational performance of the goat (Yokoyama & Ôta, 1965). Efficient hand milking and massage of the udder are sufficient for normal milk removal under these various conditions. No doubt the capacious cisterns and sinuses of the gland in these two species, which can store approximately half the milk present in the gland, are a contributing factor to the ease of milk removal in the absence of the reflex. This is, of course, in marked contrast to the sow, where the cistern is small and there is, therefore, very little storage capacity between the mammary ducts and the teat. The non-essential nature of the milk-ejection reflex in the goat has been given further emphasis by recent studies (to be discussed later, see p. 205) on the circulating levels of oxytocin associated with the hand-milking routine, where oxytocin was only detected in a minority of the experiments, although milk yields were normal (Folley & Knaggs, 1966; Knaggs, 1966; Cleverley, 1968b; see Cleverley & Folley, 1970). Furthermore, it has been accepted cowshed routine that efficient milk ejection in the cow is an essential part of dairy husbandry. However, a series of experiments carried out in this Department over a number of years (summarized by Cleverley & Folley, 1970) indicates that this, in fact, may not be entirely true, since in 32% of experiments cows did not appear to release oxytocin during the entire process of machine milking, despite normal milk yields at the experimental milkings.

Of necessity, the status of the milk-ejection reflex in the human has been evaluated by a combination of comparatively gentle experimental procedures and careful observation. Knowledge of the forceful expression of milk from one breast in response to suckling the other, which we now know to be a consequence of the milk-ejection reflex, extends back into mythology (see Folley, 1969b). The reflex is extremely important in man if the baby is to obtain more than a small fraction of the milk present in the gland (see Newton, 1961; Newton & Newton, 1967). Both natural and synthetic oxytocin have been used clinically in an attempt to relieve engorgement of the breast caused by failure of milk-ejection, and in this connexion mention should be made of the introduction of the intra-nasal application of oxytocin by Newton & Egli (1958), a therapy which has yielded mixed results (see Benson & Fitzpatrick, 1966).

In the marsupials it has long been held that the lactating mother pumps milk into the throat of the young attached to the teat by contraction of the ventral musculature in the region of the mother's pouch. This assumption, however, has been queried over the years (for references see Merchant & Sharman, 1966; Enders, 1966). It was put in doubt when it was found that removal of one

The physiology of lactation

of two or more young suckling brush possums from the pouch did not result in expulsion of milk from the vacated teat by the supposed muscular compressor action (Sharman, 1962). More recently, it has finally been disproved, at least for the opossum, since electrical stimulation of the motor nerves supplying the muscles of the pouch and surrounding region, both singly and in combination, failed to cause expulsion of milk from the lactating gland (Enders, 1966). The mechanism of milk expulsion must, therefore, reside within the mammary gland and further work will be necessary to demonstrate the occurrence of the milk-ejection reflex. A start in this direction has already been made at the very bottom of the mammalian scale, in the Prototheria or Monotremata. Griffiths (1968), working with echidnas, observed a change in shape of the mammary lobules, accompanied by the exudation of milk from the areolae, after injection of oxytocin (Figs. 5.1 and 5.2). More recently, the presence of myoepithelial cells (Fig. 5.3) was reported in these animals (Griffiths, McIntosh & Coles, 1969). While this in no way proves the normal occurrence

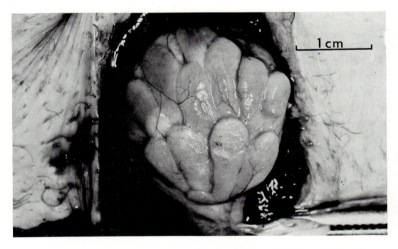

FIG. 5.1. Portion of mammary gland of the echidna, *Tachyglossus*, exposed. Photograph taken 3 min after i.m. injection of synthetic oxytocin (9 i.u./kg). Note the flaccid appearance of lobules (from Griffiths, M., 1968, *Echidnas*. International series of monographs in pure and applied biology, zoology division, edited by Kerkut, G. A., vol. 38. Oxford: Pergamon Press).

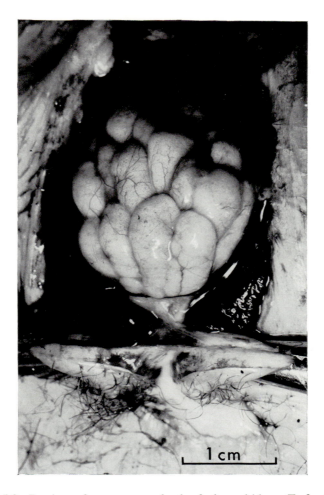

FIG. 5.2. Portion of mammary gland of the echidna, *Tachyglossus*, exposed. Photograph taken 7·75 min after i.m. injection of synthetic oxytocin (9 i.u./kg). The lobules have now assumed a swollen, mottled appearance and milk can be seen flowing at the areola (from Griffiths, M., 1968, *Echidnas*. International series of monographs in pure and applied biology, zoology division, edited by Kerkut, G. A., vol. 38. Oxford: Pergamon Press).

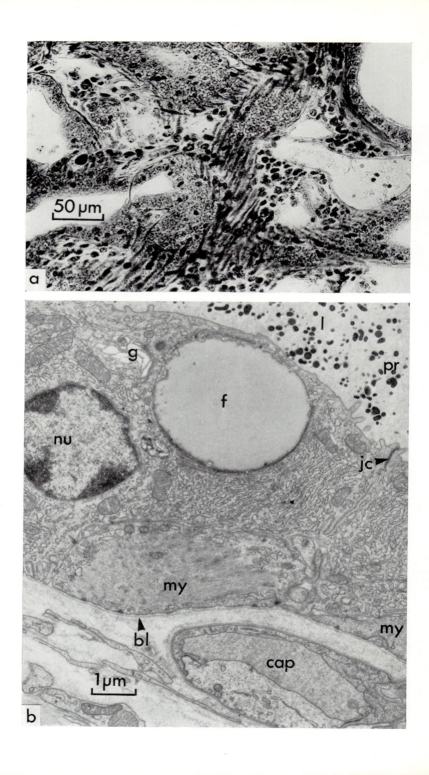

of the milk-ejection reflex in these animals, it at least shows that the necessary mechanisms are present for oxytocin to exert a milk-ejecting effect.

When considering the marine mammals, the Cetacea and Sirenia present a specialized case in having to provide suckling facilities in the water, a problem which the Pinnipedia, who come ashore for a brief breeding season, do not have to face. It has been assumed, without any justification, that the marine mammals pump the milk out of the mammary gland into the mouth of the suckling young by contraction of subcutaneous musculature over-lying the mammary glands (see Turner, 1939). However, until direct evidence is available it might be wise to treat this interpreta-tion with a certain degree of caution, since, as we have just seen, an analagous mechanism was proposed at one time for the mar-supial and has since been disproved. In view of the widespread occurrence of the milk-ejection reflex among the terrestrial mammals there seems no valid reason why the reflex should not be just as important for the seals and walruses, which also suckle on land, and even more important for the Cetacea which, suckling their young under water, require a rapid and efficient mechanism of milk removal. Indeed the presence of myoepithelial cells has been demonstrated in the mammary gland of the whale by W. A. Smit (personal communication quoted by Slijper, 1966). In the Cetacea, however, there could well be mechanisms ancillary to and operating during the latent period of the milk-ejection reflex, the combination of which might make the milk more readily and continuously available to the submerged suckling during each brief suckling period. Thus, the occurrence of the tap reflex, accom-

---

FIG. 5.3. (*a*) Section through portion of a lobule of mammary gland of echidna, *Tachyglossus* (soon after young had hatched in the pouch) showing myoepithelial cells investing surface of the alveoli (from Griffiths, M., McIntosh, D. L. & Coles, R. E. A., 1969, *J. Zool., Lond.* **158**, 371–386).

(*b*) Electron micrograph of alveolar cells of mammary gland of lactating echidna showing myoepithelial cells.

nu = nucleus   l = lumen
pr = protein granules   f = fat droplet
g = Golgi apparatus   jc = junctional complex
my = myoepithelial cell   bl = basal lamina
cap = capillary.

(Unpublished photograph, by courtesy of Dr. Gutta I. Schoefl.)

panied by contractions of teat musculature and a change in tonus of any smooth musculature which might be present in the wall of the large central lactiferous duct (see p. 9) in response to the mechanical stimulation of suckling, might assist in the removal of milk already present in the large central duct immediately prior to the onset of the neurohormonal milk-ejection reflex. There are reports of milk spurting from the teats of whales on the decks of whaling ships (see Lennep & Utrecht, 1953) and of milk continuing to spurt from the nipple after cessation of suckling (Slijper, 1966) while Harrison (1969) states that 'there is some evidence that the "let-down" [*sic*] is sudden and that much milk is ejected in a short time'. These facts would indicate that a powerful ejection mechanism does indeed exist, the exact nature of which is unknown at present. It is to be hoped that the increasing number of large aquaria throughout the world which specialize in the marine mammals, particularly the porpoises and dolphins, will make it possible to study these mechanisms in what are some of the most fascinating and specialized mammalian species.

The mechanism of suckling

The physical processes involved in the removal of milk from the teat or nipple by the suckling were, for a long time, little understood, partly because of a lack of appreciation of the significance of the milk-ejection reflex in milk removal, and hence an undue emphasis was placed on the role attributed to suction (see Ardran, Kemp & Lind, 1958*a*, *b*; Cowie & Folley, 1961). The use of the cineradiographic technique made it possible to visualize the events occurring during suckling. Ardran, Kemp & Lind (1958*b*) showed that in the human the baby sucks the nipple to the back of the mouth, thus forming a 'teat' from the mother's nipple and areolar region. When the jaw is raised this 'teat' is compressed between the upper gum and the tip of the tongue resting on the lower gum. The tongue is applied to the lower surface of the 'teat' from before backwards, pressing it against the hard palate. Suction might assist the flow of milk expressed in this manner, but is believed to be only of secondary importance. In these studies the nipple and areola were coated with a paste of barium sulphate in lanoline. In related studies in the goat, however (Ardran, Cowie & Kemp, 1957, 1958), the observations were extended since, by prior injection of barium sulphate into the udder cistern it was possible to follow the passage of milk from the udder into the mouth of the suckling. As in the case of the infant, the goat kid obliterated the neck of the teat between tongue and palate and the milk present in the teat sinus was expelled into the buccal cavity by movement of the tongue, after which the jaw and tongue were lowered to allow refilling of the teat sinus.

As far as bottle feeding is concerned, human babies, goat kids and lambs have been shown to be able to obtain milk through rubber teats by suction alone if the orifice is large enough (Ardran, Kemp & Lind, 1958*a*). However, this method is only used when the rubber teat is too rigid, in which case the suckling is unable to obliterate the neck of the teat and cannot strip the contents of the teat by positive pressure, which rises to 120 mm Hg in the goat (Ardran, Cowie & Kemp, 1958).

When considering the aquatic mammals, Slijper (1966) points out that the young Cetacean lacks proper lips, and cannot grip the nipple as firmly as the young of terrestrial mammals. According to Slijper (1966) the young Cetacean grips the nipple between the tongue and the tip of its palate, except possibly the sperm whale calf which is believed to seize it with the corner of the mouth. The tongue of the young is more muscular than that of the adult and the free tip presses the nipple from beneath and from the sides, against the palate, to form a tube leading to the throat.

Suckling and nursing behaviour

Patterns of suckling behaviour vary widely throughout the mammals, ranging over the whole gamut from very frequent to extremely infrequent episodes of suckling. In the most primitive mammals, the monotremes, it was believed until recently that the milk exuded passively from the mammary glands and dripped down the large mammary hairs of the areolar region, from where it was merely licked off by the young. However, at least in the echidna, the young sucks vigorously and audibly at the areola, and a 500 g baby can imbibe between 40 and 50 g of milk in a matter of minutes (Griffiths, 1968). The young echidna remains in the pouch until its spines reach a length and sharpness which the mother will, apparently, no longer tolerate, after which it is barred from the pouch. The pouch then regresses and disappears until the next breeding season, the mammary glands continue to grow, and the mother continues to nurse the young and to look after it for about 3 months, visiting it in a burrow to do so. She appears to feed her young about once a day, both during pouch life and also when the young is living free (Griffiths, 1968).

The new-born young of the marsupial makes its way to the mother's pouch and attaches itself to one of the teats. In the red kangaroo the infant weighs 750 mg, being outweighed by its mother by a factor of 30,000 : 1, and makes the journey from urogenital opening to pouch in about three minutes without receiving any direct assistance from the mother (Sharman & Pilton, 1964). It is aided in this Herculean task by its precociously developed forelimbs, each digit of which ends in a claw. The young have been observed to make characteristic alternate movements with the forearms and to grasp the mother's fur with the clawed digits, crawling in the direction in which the hairs point, and moving over the fur rather than through it (Lyne, Pilton & Sharman, 1959; Hughes, 1962; Sharman & Pilton, 1964). Since the mother cleans the interior of the pouch by licking and also licks the urogenital opening just before parturition, a sense of smell may have a role to play in guiding the neonate to the pouch, since this faculty happens to be particularly well developed in new-born marsupials (see Sharman & Pilton, 1964).

Once the baby has attached itself to a particular teat, it remains there for a variable length of time, depending on the species. The tip of the teat becomes bulbous, which presumably assists the neonate to maintain the teat in the mouth. A teat which is suckled undergoes gradual enlargement during lactation, while unsuckled teats remain small and vestigial. When the young have outgrown the pouch they are fed at intervals by the mother, who may come to visit them in a 'nest' in the case of the smaller species such as the opossum and bandicoot (Enders, 1966; Stodart, 1966), while in the case of the kangaroos, when the young, usually single, leaves the pouch, it is fed in the open and continues to suckle the same teat which it suckled when in the pouch. By this time the teat may have enlarged to 7·5 cm in length and may be left dangling over the lip of the pouch in the interval between feeds (Sharman & Pilton, 1964).

The Cetacea have, of necessity, to suckle their young under water, although they may do so very close to the surface. According to Slijper (1966), the mother moves very slowly during suckling and the calf approaches the nipple from behind. The young dolphin (*Tursiops*) has been reported to suckle approximately once every 26 minutes day and night by McBride & Kritzler (1951), and about 2 or 3 times each hour by R. J. Harrison (unpublished observations quoted by Harrison, 1969). Each suckling episode is brief, since the young calf cannot stay under water for more than half a minute at a time (Slijper, 1966). The amount of milk imbibed each day by the Cetacean calf is unknown, but it has been estimated that for the large whales this may be of the order of 600 kg (Slijper, 1962).

The Pinnipedia feed their new-born young on land and remain with them for a short time, after which the mothers go to sea and return to feed the young at intervals of up to a week (see Harrison, 1969). The Sirenia, like the Cetacea, suckle their young under water, and as Harrison (1969) points out, there appears to be no truth in the legend that the manatee cow suckles its young in a vertical position with the calf's head above water and embraced in the mother's flipper, since suckling takes place under water in a horizontal position.

The frequency of natural suckling is, of course, irrelevant in those domestic ruminants which are hand- or machine-milked. In the sheep, where milking is the exception rather than the rule, ewes appear to allow their lambs to suckle on demand for the first few weeks, but eventually the mother determines the times of the start and finish of suckling (Munro, 1956). The interval between successive sucklings increases as the lambs grow older. The frequency of suckling at six weeks of age has been variously reported to be 22 times in 16 daylight hours (Munro, 1956) and six times (Ewbank, 1964) and ten times (Ewbank, 1967) in a day. In both the latter papers, Ewbank corrected his figures to allow for increasing daylength during the observation period and presented data in terms of a theoretical 12-hour day.

An interesting case is presented by the pig, where the young piglets suckle the sow at intervals of approximately one hour (see Braude, 1954) and usually suckle the same teats at each feed (McBride, 1963). Suckling is accompanied by a particular pattern of behaviour which has been described in detail by Gill & Thompson (1956). At the start of a suckling period, the sow lies on her side to allow the young access to the teats and there is then a phase of 'initial massage' in which each piglet vigorously massages the area of mammary gland immediately surrounding its selected teat by bunting with its snout. This phase, which lasts 1–2 min is followed immediately by the 'milk-ejection phase', during which the young obtain milk and appear to swallow extremely rapidly rather than to suck. This phase is comparatively brief, lasting for an average of only 14 sec according to Gill & Thompson (1956) although Folley & Knaggs (1966) observed a range of 13–58 sec for this stage. The cessation of milk flow is followed by the third phase, 'final massage', which has a slower rhythm than the initial massage, lasts for 5–15 min and is usually terminated by the mother turning over on to her udder or moving away.

While the small laboratory rodents such as the rat, mouse and guinea-pig are suckled at frequent intervals, the rabbit presents an entirely different situation, since, with the possible exception of the first day or two of life, the young are allowed to suckle only once per day and obtain their daily ration of milk in a few minutes (Cross & Harris, 1952; Zarrow, Denenberg & Anderson, 1965). A more extreme case is exhibited by the nursing behaviour of the tree shrew, *Tupaia*, where the young remain in a special 'nursery' nest constructed by the male, and the parents sleep together in a separate nest. The mother visits the young and allows them to suckle for 4–10 min once every 2 days (Martin, 1966). Neither the tree shrew nor the rabbit mothers exhibit retrieving behaviour, and the brief suckling period does not permit any parental grooming. Zarrow *et al.* (1965) suggested that the long interval between suckling in the rabbit may have survival value, since the fewer visits the mother makes to the nest, the less chance there will be of predation.

When the decision as to when the young will be allowed to suckle is taken by the mother, as it must be in these two species, what makes the mother decide to nurse? In the rabbit, Cross (1952) concluded that mammary distension was the chief factor in the motivation of nursing, while in a later study Findlay (1969) observed that mammary distension was a sufficient but not a necessary condition for the induction of nursing behaviour. When a rabbit litter is only allowed to suckle once a day for several days while the mother is under deep barbiturate anaesthesia, milk secretion continues quite normally provided exogenous oxytocin is given to ensure milk removal. At the end of such a regime when normal nursing is resumed, the mother displays normal, or sometimes exaggerated, maternal behaviour (Tindal, Beyer & Sawyer,

1963). However, if such a regime is begun at the time of parturition and normal nursing is permitted from the eighth day post partum, when the doe is presented with her young she does not display nursing behaviour. Furthermore, if the suckling during anaesthesia is not begun until the fifth day post partum and the mammary glands are emptied by foster young, when the mother regains consciousness each day she will display normal nursing behaviour towards her young, despite the fact that her mammary glands are empty (Findlay & Roth, 1970). In contrast to the previous study (Findlay, 1969) it was concluded from this more recent work that distension of the mammary glands with milk is not, in fact, a sufficient condition either for the induction or for the long-term maintenance of nursing behaviour in the rabbit, and that there is a critical post partum period during which contact with the young is vital for the initiation of nursing behaviour.

Milk-ejection activity in circulating blood

Perhaps the most cogent evidence for the occurrence of the milk-ejection reflex has been obtained by the detection of milk-ejection activity in the blood of animals during suckling or milking. Such evidence has been slow to come because progress in this field had to await the development of improved blood-extraction techniques and more sensitive and specific bioassay methods. Early work on milk ejection in perfused cows' udders has already been mentioned (see p. 186), in which a substance with milk-ejection activity was detected in the blood of the cow during the milking process. However, in themselves, these experiments did not differentiate between neurohypophysial peptides and other substances such as plasma kinins which we know more about today (see p. 213). There have been several reports of measurements of oxytocin levels in the blood during milking in the cow and goat (Hawker & Roberts, 1957; Hawker, 1961; Bílek, Janovský, Makoč & Kozlík, 1963; Gorokhov & Trofimov, 1965; Ivanov, Kichev, Gendzhev & Khristov, 1966; Lawson & Graf, 1968) which, in the light of present knowledge are unrealistic either in the amount of oxytocin claimed to be present in the blood or in the pattern of release of the hormone in relation to the milking process. These results need not detain us since they are open to the serious criticism that the bioassay techniques used were of poor specificity and precision (see Cleverley, 1968b).

One is then left with results obtained with what might be considered adequate and modern techniques. By the use of the intra-arterial milk-ejection assay in the lactating rabbit, Fitzpatrick (1961) detected a transient release of oxytocin during suckling in the ewe. The maximum level of activity observed was 114 μu. oxytocin/ml. plasma, and this fell to a very low level within two minutes after the start of suckling. The intra-arterial milk-ejection assay was adapted for the guinea-pig, with an accompanying increase in sensitivity (Tindal & Yokoyama, 1960, 1962) and was later modified and its use combined with dextran gel-filtration extraction of blood plasma, a mild procedure in which little or no artefacts are produced and which gives an excellent recovery (Folley & Knaggs, 1965*a*, *b*). Using these techniques, Folley & Knaggs (1966), Knaggs (1963, 1966), Cleverley (1968*b*) and Cleverley & Folley (1970) have investigated the release of oxytocin into external jugular vein blood in response to suckling or milking in sows, cows and goats.

Releases of oxytocin in the sow (Fig. 5.4) were, with one exception, associated with the initial massage of the mammary gland by the piglets and with the milk-ejection phase. The amounts released ranged from 5 to 132 μu. oxytocin/ml. plasma. In most of the cases where no hormone was detected the piglets did not obtain any milk, as judged by their behaviour (Folley & Knaggs, 1966).

In the cow (Fig. 5.5), the stimulus most consistently followed by a transient appearance of oxytocin in the blood was the application of the teat cups of the milking machine, although in some cases there was a second release of oxytocin, later in the milking process, unrelated to any apparent stimulus. The range of releases of oxytocin in the cow was 15–2000 μu./ml. plasma. The blood extract containing the highest milk-ejection activity (2000 μu./ml.) was further subjected to paper chromatography, and good evidence was obtained to warrant attributing the milk-ejection activity of the extract to oxytocin (Knaggs, 1963; Folley & Knaggs, 1966). However, in subsequent work in which the cows were more carefully trained to the experimental routine, the release of oxytocin was no longer preferentially associated with application of the teat cups, and releases of oxytocin (9–889 μu./ml. plasma) occurred in response to all stimuli associated with the milking routine (Cleverley & Folley, 1970). It is of interest that in the latter study,

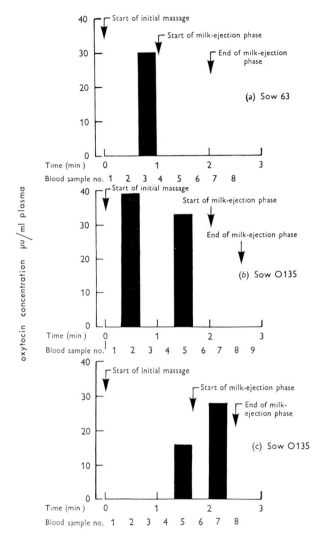

Fig. 5.4. Oxytocin concentration in jugular vein blood of sows during suckling (from Folley, S. J. & Knaggs, G. S., 1966, *J. Endocr.* **34**, 197–214).

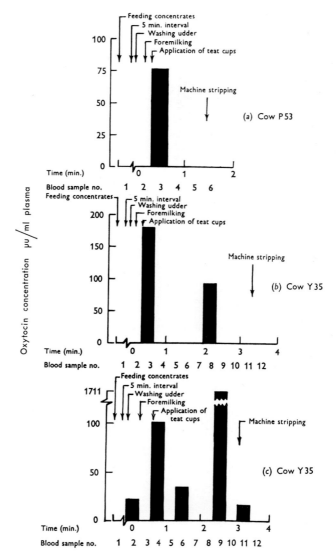

FIG. 5.5. Oxytocin concentrations in jugular vein blood of cows during machine milking (from Folley, S. J. & Knaggs, G. S., 1966, *J. Endocr.* **34**, 197–214).

and in the previous work (Folley & Knaggs, 1966), no release of oxytocin was detected in 32% of experimental machine milkings, although in most cases milk yields were normal (see p. 191).

In the goat (Fig. 5.6), Folley & Knaggs (1966) and Knaggs (1966) detected oxytocin in the blood in only a minority of experimental hand milkings, the individual releases of oxytocin ranging from 7 to 142 μu./ml. plasma. Whether or not oxytocin

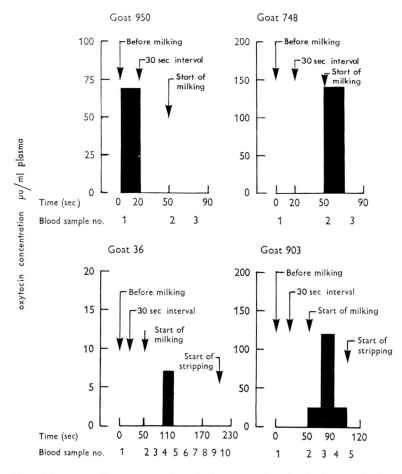

FIG. 5.6. Oxytocin concentrations in jugular vein blood of goats during hand milking (from Folley, S. J. & Knaggs, G. S., 1966, *J. Endocr.* **34**, 197–214).

was found in the blood, the milk yield at the experimental milking did not differ appreciably from the value to be expected from comparable milkings for the preceding week. In later work (Cleverley, 1968*b*), essentially similar results were obtained, and the combined results of Folley & Knaggs (1966) and Cleverley (1968*b*) (see Cleverley & Folley, 1970) showed that oxytocin release occurred in only 8 out of 25 experimental hand milkings in the goat (32%). In contrast, recent studies by A. S. McNeilly (unpublished work) in this laboratory indicate that release of oxytocin in the goat occurs more readily when the animal is suckled by her kids. Thus, in a series of 18 experiments on 6 goats which were suckled by their twin kids, 16 of these experiments (89%) were positive for oxytocin release (6–55 μu./ml. plasma) and 2 were negative. Subsequently, in the same six animals McNeilly detected oxytocin release (8–63 μu./ml. plasma) in 12 out of 22 experimental hand milkings (59%), a figure which is considerably higher than that found in the previous work described above (see Addendum 5).

The relatively low levels of oxytocin detected in jugular blood of the ruminant during suckling or milking do not reflect an inability of the neurohypophysial system to release larger quantities. It has been shown in the goat that whereas electrical stimulation of many sites in the hypothalamus will cause release of oxytocin in amounts similar to those observed during suckling or milking, stimulation of two particular sites evoked much greater releases, equivalent to 1·26 and 20·90 mu. oxytocin/ml. plasma. This would indicate that the neurohypophysis of the goat is potentially capable of releasing more oxytocin than is normally released in response to natural stimuli (Cleverley, Knaggs, Tindal & Turvey, 1968).

In the lactating rabbit, Kaveshnikova, Chudnovskiĭ & Shenger (1969) studied the release of oxytocin in response to suckling. In a series of experiments on three animals, the level before suckling ranged from 0·5 to 500 and during suckling from 4 to 4500 μu. oxytocin/ml. plasma, a finding which no doubt reflects the use of the *in vitro* rat mammary cube assay (see p. 215). More recently, Bisset, Clark & Haldar (1970) reported levels of 31–375 μu. oxytocin/ml. blood during suckling in the rabbit. However, although a reliable bioassay method was used, from the description given in their paper of the cannulation procedure it is not possible to conclude whether the blood samples were pituitary venous effluent blood, peripheral blood, or a mixture of the two.

Conditioning of the milk-ejection reflex

Although the event which normally triggers the milk-ejection reflex is the tactile stimulation of the teat, nevertheless, under appropriate conditions the reflex can be conditioned so that oxytocin is released in response to certain auditory or visual stimuli. This has been shown in the rat, where the reflex has been conditioned to occur when the lactating mother is placed within sound of another rat suckling her young (Deis, 1968). In the human, the reflex can be conditioned to occur in response to the sound of the baby crying at the scheduled time of feeding, or even such extraneous stimuli as the habit of drinking a glass of water or smoking a cigarette before nursing (see Newton, 1961). Also, milk-ejection pressure responses have been recorded from the cannulated mammary gland of the lactating woman in response to the mother seeing the baby or hearing it cry in a nearby room (Sica-Blanco, Sala & Caldeyro-Barcia, unpublished results, quoted by Caldeyro-Barcia, 1969).

However, it is in the cow that conditioning of the milk-ejection reflex is most commonly said to occur in response to the appearance of the accustomed milkers or to the sounds of dairy equipment, although this has not been the case with Soviet workers who regard the provision of food as being the most potent stimulus associated with the milking process (see Zaks, 1962). Surprisingly, there has until recently been a lack of incontrovertible evidence to prove the point one way or the other. A contribution to the problem was made by Peeters, Stormorken & Vanschoubroek (1960), who classified the efficacy of various stimuli in eliciting the milk-ejection reflex. In ascending order of potency (i.e. the weakest first, the most effective last) these stimuli were found to be: showing the calf to the mother, washing the udder with water at 40°C, washing the udder plus showing the calf, and finally, suckling itself.

In our laboratory, the experiments of Folley & Knaggs (1966) were not designed specifically to show conditioning of the reflex, but rather to see whether oxytocin release could be easily demonstrated, so further work was carried out with a refined milking routine. A series of 24 carefully controlled experiments were carried out on 8 cows, which were accustomed to a strict daily afternoon milking routine, including the presence of the experimenter, for 10 days before blood sampling began. Control blood samples were taken before the approach of the milker, and serial 25 ml. blood samples were taken during the entry and approach of the milker and throughout the entire milking routine, from an indwelling polyethylene cannula placed in an external jugular vein the day before blood sampling. All blood samples were extracted and bioassayed individually. In 9 experiments, transient releases of oxytocin were detected in blood plasma at the time of the entry and approach of the milker into the stall (Fig. 5.7). The

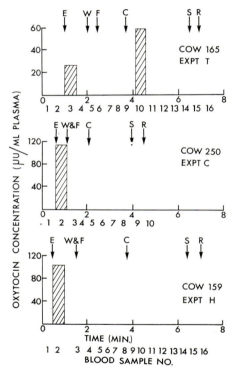

FIG. 5.7. Oxytocin concentrations in jugular vein blood of cows, after conditional stimulation, during machine milking. E = entry of milker; W = washing udder; F = foremilking; C = teat cup application; S = stripping; R = removal of teat cups (from Cleverley, J. D. & Folley, S. J., 1970, *J. Endocr.* **46**, 347–361).

amount of individual releases varied from 20 to 210 μu. oxytocin/ ml. plasma, and there was no release of oxytocin during the remainder of the milking routine in 5 of these 9 experiments. In addition to blood sampling, in some of the experiments intra-mammary pressure was recorded from a cannulated teat by means of a pressure transducer and portable recorder; increases in intra-mammary pressure were found to occur, associated with the detection of oxytocin in the plasma following the entry of the milker (Cleverley, 1968a, b; Cleverley & Folley, 1970). These findings, therefore, provided direct experimental evidence that the reflex release of oxytocin can be conditioned to auditory and visual stimuli associated with a strict milking routine.

However, not only in the cow, but also in the goat, the release of oxytocin can be conditioned to occur in response to the visual and auditory stimuli associated with milking or suckling, and condi-tioned release of the hormone occurred after 7–10 days habituation to the experimental routine (Cleverley, 1968b). Out of a total of 12 experiments carried out on 9 goats, oxytocin release occurred during hand milking in 4 cases in 4 different animals. In three of these four positive cases there was also a conditioned reflex release of oxytocin in response to the approach and entry of the milker into the pen in the range 19–177 μu./ml. plasma. More recently in this laboratory, in the comparison of hand milking versus natural suckling mentioned earlier (A. S. McNeilly, un-published results), it was found that the release of the hormone can be conditioned to occur in response to sight or sound of the kids since, in 6 of the 16 positive experiments, release of oxytocin occurred before the start of suckling in addition to further release during suckling. The amount of oxytocin released in response to conditioned stimuli (8–50 μu./ml. plasma) was similar to that released during suckling.

Milk-ejection reflex in man

It has been known for some time that the suckling of the human infant at one breast evokes rhythmic changes in intramammary pressure which can be recorded *via* cannulae inserted in the milk ducts of the unsuckled breast (Sica-Blanco, Méndez-Bauer, Sala, Cabot & Caldeyro-Barcia, 1959). These changes in pressure, which terminate abruptly at the cessation of suckling are presumably caused by waves of contraction of the mammary myoepithelium in response to circulating oxytocin, and Sica-Blanco *et al.* (1959) were able to evoke a similar type of contraction pattern by i.v. infusion of oxytocin, at a rate of 4 mu./min. It was shown later that the intramammary pressure changes evoked by natural suckling could be mimicked more closely by periodic, discrete injections of oxytocin (Sica-Blanco & Sala, personal communication quoted by Cobo, Bernal, Gaitan & Quintero, 1967) and this finding was confirmed by Cobo *et al.* (1967). The latter group of workers illustrated one particular case (Fig. 5.8) where intramammary pressure was recorded during an 8·5 min suckling period and in which there were three distinct rises and falls of pressure. These were paralleled to a quite remarkable extent by the subsequent i.v. injection of three separate doses of oxytocin, of 30, 20, and 20 mu. respectively. A single i.v. injection of the sum of these three doses (70 mu.) resulted in a different type of response, consisting of a succession of contractions of decreasing magnitude, reminiscent of the type of multiple response to oxytocin occasionally seen at the start of the assay by the lactating guinea-pig method (Tindal & Yokoyama, 1962). This type of response has also been reported in the sow, sheep and rat (Whittlestone, 1954; Debackere, Peeters & Tuyttens, 1961; Bisset, Clark, Haldar, Harris, Lewis & Rocha e Silva, 1967) and usually occurs after fairly large doses of oxytocin. Cobo *et al.* (1967) found that a continuous i.v. infusion of oxytocin at the rate of 4 mu./min yielded a series of small, regular waves of myoepithelial contraction, unlike the more irregular, repetitive response to natural suckling. Both Cobo *et al.* (1967) and Caldeyro-Barcia (1969) have concluded that oxytocin is released in the woman in response to suckling, in spurts, and in variable amounts, thus confirming and extending to the woman the concept of the quantal release of oxytocin in response to suckling put forward by Folley & Knaggs (1966) on the basis of experiments carried out on farm animals.

Direct evidence for the presence of circulating oxytocin in the woman in response to suckling has been obtained recently by Coch, Fielitz, Brovetto, Cabot, Coda & Fraga (1968). Samples of what were claimed to be internal jugular blood were treated with trichloroacetic acid and Amberlite IRC 50, and were subjected either to paper electrophoresis or paper chromatography. The electrophoretic or chromatographic strips containing oxytocin were eluted and the eluates were bioassayed either on the lactating

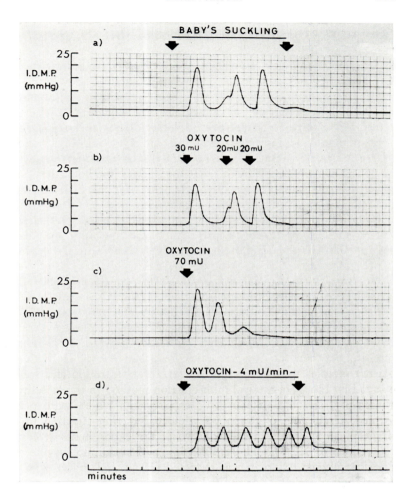

Fig. 5.8. Intramammary pressure records from a lactating woman. I.D.M.P. = intraductal mammary pressure. The changes in pressure evoked by an 8·5 min suckling episode by the baby at the other nipple (*a*) are closely mimicked by the subsequent i.v. injection of separate doses of 30, 20 and 20 i.u. synthetic oxytocin (*b*). Different types of responses were obtained in (*c*) by injecting the total amount used in (*b*) as a single i.v. injection of 70 i.u. synthetic oxytocin and in (*d*) by giving a continuous i.v. infusion of synthetic oxytocin at the rate of 4mu./min (from Cobo, E., Bernal, M. H. de, Gaitain, E. & Quintero, C. A., 1967, *Am. J. Obstet. Gynec.* **97**, 519–529.

rabbit mammary gland *in vivo* or rat mammary strips *in vitro*. Levels of 12–25 μμ. oxytocin/ml. plasma were detected. Coch *et al.* (1968) reasoned that since milk ejection can be elicited in the lactating woman by i.v. infusion of synthetic oxytocin at the rate of 4 mu./min (Sica-Blanco *et al.*, 1959), and that since they found a level of 30μu. oxytocin/ml. in peripheral plasma during i.v. infusion of synthetic oxytocin at the rate of 128 mu./min, then the concentration of oxytocin in peripheral plasma during suckling in the woman should be approximately 1 μu./ml. Allowing for a factor of 10 for the difference in concentration of oxytocin between peripheral and jugular blood, then, they argue, the concentration of oxytocin in jugular blood during suckling could, on theoretical grounds, be expected to lie somewhere in the region of 10 μu./ml. plasma—in good agreement with the levels found by them during suckling of 12–25 μu./ml. plasma. Coch *et al.* (1968) also suggest that, in the light of their findings, their previous report (Coch, Brovetto, Cabot, Fielitz & Caldeyro-Barcia, 1965) of circulating levels of oxytocin in man during suckling of 200–300 μu./ml. plasma now appears unrealistic. However, their earlier findings may not have been misleading since Fox & Knaggs (1969) have recently detected circulating oxytocin in peripheral venous blood of a lactating woman during natural suckling at levels intermediate between the two extremes described above. Individual plasma samples were subjected to dextran gel-filtration and were assayed by the intra-arterial milk-ejection method in the lactating guinea-pig, and out of the three experiments which were performed, circulating oxytocin was detected during suckling in a single plasma sample in each of two of the experiments at concentrations of 122 and 11 μu./ml. plasma. In addition, in one of the experiments oxytocin was detected (19 μu./ml. plasma) in a control sample taken one minute before the start of suckling.

The pattern of oxytocin release in response to suckling or milking

These recent studies in man serve to emphasize that it is the advent of more sophisticated extraction and assay methods which has revealed not only the transient appearance but also the extremely low levels of circulating endogenous oxytocin which are capable of eliciting normal milk ejection. Equally, however, it should be pointed out that the careful studies which have made these facts available have been carried out up till now in the large domestic animals and man, where the withdrawal of a considerable number of blood samples of sufficient size presents no problem. It would be prudent to defer assuming a more general occurrence of the pattern of release observed during suckling or milking in these larger species until similar experiments have been performed on the smaller laboratory animals. In particular, the rabbit could possibly present an extreme case, where, after the first three or four days of life the young suckle only once per day and obtain all the milk in as little as three or four minutes (Cross & Harris, 1952; Zarrow, Denenberg & Anderson, 1965). The studies of Cross (1955*b*) and Fuchs & Wagner (1963*a*) both suggest an 'all-or-nothing' type of release in response to suckling in this species, rather than a series of discrete spurts, and it is to be hoped that the relatively large body size, and hence reasonably large blood volume, of certain breeds of rabbit will enable this question to be resolved in the near future. The studies of Kaveshnikova *et al.* (1969) and Bisset, Clark & Haldar (1970) are not really relevant to this particular problem, since only one blood sample was taken at each experimental suckling period. The estimation of oxytocin in serial blood samples will be essential if the pattern of release of oxytocin in response to suckling in the rabbit is to be determined.

Plasma kinins and milk ejection

Recent studies by the Belgian group of G. Peeters have indicated that, at least in the ruminant, substances other than oxytocin may have to be considered as having a role to play in the removal of milk from the udder. Plasma kinins are known to be produced in the blood by the breakdown of plasma protein, brought about by the action of enzymes known as kallikreins. It has been shown that the mammary gland of the goat and sheep is extremely sensitive to the action of at least one of these kinins since bradykinin, given by the intravenous route, evoked a rise in intramammary pressure or an ejection of milk, according to the parameter being studied. Milk ejection occurred after as little as 1 µg. bradykinin i.v., and the response was matched by 1 mu. oxytocin i.v. The minimum effective dose for eliciting a rise in intramammary pressure was slightly higher, being 5 µg. and 5 mu. i.v. respectively (Houvenaghel & Peeters, 1968). The interesting point is made that the myoepithelium of the lactating small ruminant is more sensitive to bradykinin than that of the guinea-pig or rabbit, since as little as 0·1 µg./kg was effective. The goat and sheep were also found to be sensitive to the action of kallikrein, while the cow was relatively insensitive to bradykinin but sensitive to kallikrein (Houvenaghel, Peeters, Vandaele & Djordjevic, 1968), suggesting, perhaps, that a kinin or kinins other than bradykinin might be active in the cow. In the sheep it was also found that when oxytocin or bradykinin were injected intravenously the relative potencies for milk-ejection activity were of the order of 450 : 1, on a weight basis. However, when injected into the mammary artery, this ratio dropped to 40 : 1, and responses could be obtained with as little as 0·5 ng of bradykinin (Reynaert, Peeters, Verbeke & Houvenaghel, 1968).

Since high kallikrein activity is known to occur in salivary glands and pancreas, it is natural to ask what role plasma kinins, released by kallikreins, have to play in the normal processes of milk ejection in the ruminant. While it is too soon to draw any conclusions, the fact that kallikrein activity has also been extracted from the udder tissue of cows and sheep (Reynaert *et al.*, 1968) would indicate that this aspect of mammary gland physiology merits further study.

Bioassay of milk-ejection activity (oxytocin)

A review of bioassay methods for oxytocin would be out of place here since the subject has already been covered extensively (Sawyer, 1966; Bisset, 1968; Fitzpatrick & Bentley, 1968; Stürmer, 1968; Cleverley, 1968*b*). Suffice it to say that, at the time of writing, the assay preparations combining the properties of maximum sensitivity with maximum specificity, stem from the intra-arterial intra-mammary pressure method in the lactating animal. This was originated by Fitzpatrick (1961) in the rabbit, and was developed to a higher level of sensitivity in both the guinea-pig (Tindal & Yokoyama, 1960, 1962; Folley & Knaggs, 1965*a*, *b*) and the rat (Bisset, Clark, Haldar, Harris, Lewis & Rocha e Silva, 1967). The guinea-pig and rat preparations have similar sensitivities to oxytocin and to vasopressin, but differ slightly in their responses to other agents, the rat being more sensitive to bradykinin and 5-hydroxytryptamine, and the guinea-pig being more sensitive to angiotensin (Folley & Knaggs, 1965*b*; Bisset, 1968; Cleverley, 1968*b*). Both methods are far more specific than assays depending on the contraction of isolated strips of mammary gland or the isolated uterus (see Bisset, 1968; Cleverley, 1968*b*).

However, the recent development of a simple *in vitro* assay procedure for oxytocin (Van Dongen & Hays, 1966) warrants consideration. The principle of the method is to drop cubes of mammary gland obtained from a freshly-killed lactating rat, into standard solutions containing known amounts of oxytocin, or into the 'unknown' solutions being tested. The time elapsing between addition of the mammary cube to the solution and the appearance of milk in the solution is inversely related to the concentration of oxytocin present. The technique has the advantage of simplicity and does not require specialized recording equipment. However, in an extensive series of experiments designed to compare the performance of this *in vitro* technique with the *in vivo* lactating guinea-pig preparation, Cleverley (1968*b*) found, as did Van Dongen & Hays (1966), an unsatisfactory value for the index of precision of the *in vitro* assay, and found that the mean error of the estimate of potency, 29·4%, was also high. In agreement with Van Dongen & Marshall (1967) the *in vitro* preparation was found to be highly sensitive to acetylcholine and vasopressin. However, whereas Van Dongen & Marshall (1967) reported the *in vitro* preparation to be insensitive to histamine, 5-hydroxytryptamine and bradykinin, Cleverley (1968*b*) found that it responded to the first two substances at concentrations slightly higher than those used by Van Dongen & Marshall. In contrast to this, however, the *in vitro* preparation was found to be highly sensitive to bradykinin responding to 0·01 µg./ml. which means that the *in vitro* method is 100 times as sensitive as the *in vivo* guinea-pig method to this substance. It should also be pointed out that the assay of blood samples from the ruminant by the rat mammary cube preparation may be particularly misleading in studies of milk-ejection activity during the milking process; since the threshold concentration for the effective dose of bradykinin in this assay was found to be 0·01 µg/ml. (Cleverley, 1968*b*) then it is within the bounds of possibility that what has, on occasion, been reported in the literature as 'oxytocin' activity may in fact have been at least partly due to circulating kinins.

Although the rat mammary cube assay has the advantages of being simple to set up, and of having great sensitivity to oxytocin, these are outweighed by the lack of specificity and poor inherent precision. The *in vivo* assays are the methods of choice where a combination of sensitivity, specificity and accuracy are required. In agreement with this view, Fabian, Forsling, Jones & Lee (1969) compared the performances of the *in vivo* rat mammary gland and the *in vitro* rat mammary strip bioassays for oxytocin and concluded that when the concentration of hormone is low the method of choice is the *in vivo* mammary gland.

However, the *in vivo* methods are fairly tedious to set up and are dependent on a regular supply of first-class lactating animals. There seems little doubt that the next few years will see the rise of radioimmunoassays for oxytocin with the advantages of rapidity, specificity and application to the investigation of a wide range of species. This possibility was foreshadowed by reports of radio-iodination of oxytocin, of production of antibodies to this octa-peptide hormone, and the first preliminary accounts of radio-immunoassay procedures (Gilliland & Prout, 1965a, b; Gusdon, 1967; Glick, Kumaresan, Kagan & Wheeler, 1969; Chard, Forsling & Kitau, 1969). It became a reality with the definitive publication of a radioimmunoassay for oxytocin (Chard, Kitau & Landon, 1970; Chard, Forsling, James, Kitau & Landon, 1970).

SEGMENTAL REFLEXES

In addition to the neurohormonal milk-ejection reflex, there are other mechanisms which may assist in the removal of milk from the lactating mammary gland. Mention has already been made of the 'tap reflex', in which the motor effector mechanism of the milk-ejection reflex, the myoepithelial cells, may themselves contract in response to mechanical stimuli. In addition, however, Soviet workers have postulated the existence in ruminants of purely neural, segmental reflexes, involving pathways from mammary gland to spinal cord and back to mammary gland, the evidence for which has been reviewed by Baryshnikov (1959, 1965) and Zaks (1962). It has been postulated that the process of milk ejection comprises a complex, two-stage act, in the first stage of which, commencing within a few seconds of the application of the milking stimulus, there is a relaxation of cisternal musculature and a change in tone of the larger ducts, thus facilitating the movement of milk from ducts to cistern in preparation for the expulsion of milk from the alveoli under the influence of oxytocin during the second, neurohormonal stage of milk ejection. The initial, purely neural phase precedes the second phase by 30–60 seconds owing to the time required for oxytocin to be carried in the blood stream from the neurohypophysis to the mammary gland. Moreover, there appear to be species differences in the manifestation of the initial, neural phase of milk ejection, since it is said to be accompanied by a temporary drop in intramammary pressure in the cow, while in the goat the opposite situation prevails, since there is said to be a rise in intramammary pressure at this stage of milking (Gofman, 1955). Gofman (1955) suggests that this may be due to the difference in the relative capacity of the cisternal region of the udder in these two species. A mechanism similar to this first phase of milk ejection is also said to operate more gradually between milkings in response to stimulation of baroreceptors in the duct system by the rising intramammary pressure, thus aiding the redistribution of milk within the udder. Soviet work has also emphasized the role of reflex control of smooth muscle in the walls of the udder cistern to explain the ability of the cistern to contain, within limits, increasing quantities of milk without appreciable increase in intramammary pressure.

However, these theories are open to serious criticism. In particular, the presence of adequate numbers of interoceptors within the mammary parenchyma is an essential part of the proposed reflexes. Although electrophysiological evidence for the existence of a few isolated pressure receptors within the mammary gland of the rabbit was presented by Findlay (1966), histological, and, more recently, electron microscopical studies (see Cross, 1961*b*; Cross & Findlay, 1969) have demonstrated, unequivocally, that while the teat and the neighbouring region are profusely endowed with sensory nerve endings, these are so sparse as to be virtually absent within the parenchyma of the gland. The latter authors consider it more reasonable to regard the few parenchymal receptors, found by them in the rabbit, as part of the normal dermal innervation of the area which has become enmeshed in the mammary parenchyma during its development. As regards the claim for an initial fall in intramammary pressure which is said to occur at the start of the milking process in the cow, this is not substantiated by the experiments of Cleverley & Folley (1970) in this species, in which no such drop in intramammary pressure was found to occur.

H

Another essential requirement for the operation of segmental reflexes is the existence of efferent motor nerves to the mammary gland and suitable musculature within the gland, yet such is not the case. It is now known, beyond any reasonable doubt, that the efferent innervation of the mammary gland is represented by the sympathetic division of the autonomic nervous system (see Cross, 1961*b*), and, as Findlay & Grosvenor (1969) have pointed out, the properties of the sympathetic nervous system, which tends to discharge *en masse* rather than discretely, and where postganglionic sympathetic fibres greatly outnumber preganglionic sympathetic fibres, are not what is required for the operation of the reflex arcs proposed by various Soviet workers (see Zaks, 1962), in which precise localization would be essential for the fine control of muscle within the mammary gland. Furthermore, smooth muscle is concentrated almost entirely in the teat, and becomes extremely sparse away from this region, where the main physical support is provided by elastic tissue (see Cross, 1961*b*).

Zaks (1962) admits the hypothetical nature of the assumed efferent innervation of the parenchyma, but maintains that it should exist on the basis of physiological observations. Even on physiological grounds, however, the arguments in favour of the segmental nature of these reflex mechanisms are not entirely convincing. Thus, cooling of the spinal cord (Pavlov, 1955) blocked the ascent of impulses to the neurohypophysis and eliminated the second (neurohormonal) phase of milk ejection in the goat without affecting the first (neural) phase. This has been taken as evidence by Zaks (1962) for the segmental nature of the reflex, yet, by the nature of the experiment itself, it was not possible to conclude whether the mechanism under investigation was segmental, or purely intramammary, in nature. In the same year, Astrakhanskaya (1955) reported on the absence of the first stage of the reflex after mammary denervation in the goat, although, as Zaks (1962) commented, the existence of the first stage had not been established before section of the nerves. In a later study, Aminov (1961) also reported on the absence of the first stage of the reflex after denervation, but since, of the six animals which were investigated over a period of two years, the first stage was absent in three animals, in one animal this phase was said to merge with the second phase in the first year of observation and was absent in the second year, and the pattern of milk ejection in another animal was not described, Aminov (1961) appears to base his conclusions on the effects of denervation in only one goat.

Evidence which militates against the segmental nature of reflex mechanisms which are involved in the first phase of milk ejection in the ruminant has come from recent studies of milk flow in the Prèalpes du Sud breed of sheep during machine milking. When lactating ewes of this breed are machine-milked without pre-liminary massage of the mammary gland, they can be divided into two categories, based on the pattern of milk flow into the milking machine. In one type, the ewe gives most of her milk in one rapid emission at the start of the milking process, while in the other type, the ewe gives it in two quite distinct emissions, separated in time by 30–40 sec. Those ewes exhibiting the double peak in milk flow were found to have a total milk production 25–30% higher than those having only the single peak, and furthermore, pre-liminary massage of the udder in animals having the double peak resulted in the second peak shifting into and merging with, the first peak (Labussière & Martinet, 1964; Labussière, 1966). It was concluded from later studies (Labussière, Martinet & Dena-mur, 1969) that the second peak in milk flow, which occurred in only a proportion of the animals, was attributable to the neuro-hormonal milk-ejection reflex, and it was also shown that the first peak in milk flow persisted after bilateral denervation of the udder, thus denying the participation of segmental reflexes. From this it may be concluded that at least in this breed of sheep, any movement of milk which precedes the neurohormonal milk-ejection reflex, can be effected by mechanisms entirely within the mammary gland alone.

It would be appropriate at this point to mention that Soviet workers have also proposed the occurrence of liposecretory reflexes in which, it was claimed, direct innervation of the alveoli was concerned with discharge of pre-formed fat from the milk-secreting cells into the alveolar lumen (see Zaks, 1962). Much of the evidence for this hypothesis came from studies on the goat (see Zaks, 1962) and the mouse (Zotikova, 1955). However, Zotikova (1962) later withdrew some of her earlier claims for discharge of fat droplets after stimulation of the mammary nerve in the mouse, and others have reported on the lack of effect of mammary denervation both on the secretion of milk fat in the goat (Denamur & Martinet, 1959a; Tverskoĭ, 1962; Linzell, 1963) and sheep (Labussière *et al.*, 1969) and on the fatty acid composition of milk fat from the goat, assessed by gas–liquid chromatography (Ward & Huskisson, 1966). The more recent work, therefore, suggests that if liposecretory reflexes exist at all, they seem to be of doubtful physiological significance.

However, the above observations do not mean that efferent innervation, represented by the sympathetic division of the autonomic nervous system, has no part to play in the control of mammary function. Indeed, these sympathetic fibres exert considerable influence over the smooth musculature of the teat, cistern and large ducts, sparse though it is. It has been shown that electrical stimulation of the inguinal nerve of the isolated perfused bovine udder elicited strong contractions of the smooth musculature of the teats, which were abolished by the anti-adrenergic drug dibenamine (Peeters, Coussens & Sierens, 1949). In the sheep and goat, stimulation of the external spermatic nerve was followed by contraction of teat musculature, and this was also inhibited by dibenamine (Linzell, 1959*a*). Denervation of the mammary gland of the goat, guinea-pig and rabbit caused dilatation of the mammary ducts (Astrakhanskaya, 1955; Hebb & Linzell, 1966), while in the rat, denervation of the mammary gland or the intraductal injection of local anaesthetic decreased the resistance to filling the gland with fluid (Grosvenor & Findlay, 1968), which also indicated a relaxation of ductal tonus. In this connexion, there have also been claims for the presence of sphincters in a layer of circular muscle fibres at the mouths of the ducts of the cow's udder (Bogdashev & Eliseev, 1951) and of annular constrictions at the mouths of the small ducts of the mouse's mammary gland (Levitskaya, 1955; Zotikova, 1955), whose relaxation or contraction may assist or retard the movement of milk from alveoli to teat. In the mouse, these sphincters were observed to contract after electrical stimulation of the mammary nerve or after topical application of adrenaline (Levitskaya, 1955; Zotikova, 1955). It was already known that in the goat and guinea-pig (Barȳshnikov, Zaks, Zotikova, Levitskaya, Pavlov, Pavlov, Tverskoĭ, Tolbukhin & Tsakhaev, 1951) electrical stimulation of the external spermatic nerve inhibited the removal of milk through a catheter for varying lengths of time. In later chronic experiments, when electrical stimulation was applied to the nerve of one half-udder through permanently-implanted electrodes prior to milk ejection in the goat, milk ejection was prevented on the side being stimulated (Barȳshnikov, Borsuk, Zaks, Zotikova, Pavlov & Tolbukhin, 1953), and it has been proposed that constriction of sphincters at the mouths of mammary ducts under the influence either of sympathetic innervation or circulating adrenaline, may have a role to play in the peripheral inhibition of milk ejection (see Barȳshnikov, 1965).

The unilateral denervation of the udder in the small ruminant has yielded divergent results in terms of the subsequent location of milk within the gland. Thus, in the goat, the operation was reported to cause an increase in the proportion of alveolar, or residual, milk to cisternal milk in the denervated udder half, the ratio changing from 20 : 80 before operation to 48 : 52 after operation on the denervated side, and this was attributed to a reduction in the tone of the smooth muscle of the ducts (Tsakhaev, 1953*b*). In contrast to this, in their previously mentioned study in the sheep, Labussière *et al.* (1969) made the observation that after unilateral denervation, although there was no change in the level of secretion, there was a slight increase in the proportion of cisternal milk, accompanied by a corresponding decrease in the volume of alveolar milk, indicating that transfer of milk from alveolar tissue to the cistern between milkings in the sheep had been facilitated by denervation. It seems clear that the sympathetic system exerts control over the tonus of mammary ducts, and that denervation of the mammary gland results in a decreased duct tonus. The reason for the difference in response between goat and sheep to denervation may well be a reflection of subtle and as yet unrecognized morphological differences in the mammary gland of these two species.

When considering the relaxation of tonus of the walls of the udder cistern in response to an increasing volume of milk contained within the udder, the control exerted by the sympathetic nervous supply may well be important. However, it has been shown that when the udder cistern of the cow was filled in steps of 200 ml, there was a slow rise, accompanied by periodic small falls in pressure as the cistern walls relaxed in response to increasing volume of milk, and this was demonstrated both in the intact and in the isolated udder (Peeters, Coussens & Oyaert, 1949). This would indicate that simple physical adjustment of the elastic tissue in the walls of the cistern may be responsible for at least a part of the response of the cistern to the accumulation of milk in the udder between milkings.

In conclusion, it is clear that the mechanisms governing removal of milk from the mammary gland are complex and are not fully understood at the present time. Although the details of the classical neurohormonal reflex of milk ejection are now clearly outlined, the role of purely neural mechanisms in milk removal, especially in the ruminant, is more difficult to interpret. This applies particularly to the segmental reflexes, discussed above, whose existence has not been proved beyond reasonable doubt and whose role in milk removal remains questionable. In the present state of knowledge it would appear that non-hormonally-induced transfer of milk within the gland may be effected by an interplay of the alteration of ductal and cisternal tone mediated by the sympathetic system, aided, perhaps, by the contraction of at least some myoepithelial cells in response to mechanical stimuli.

6

THE NEUROENDOCRINE REGULATION
OF MAMMARY GLAND FUNCTION

CENTRAL PATHWAYS OF THE MILK-EJECTION REFLEX

IN addition to the removal of milk from the mammary gland, the act of suckling or milking also triggers complex neuroendocrine mechanisms which are concerned with the normal functioning of the gland. This control over mammary function is exerted by an ascending nervous pathway which originates in sensory receptors in the teat and passes up the spinal cord to the brain and pituitary body, and by a descending vascular pathway which conveys both adenohypophysial and neurohypophysial secretions to the mammary gland. The trophic hormones released from the adeno-hypophysis act both directly, and indirectly through target organs, on the mammary gland to ensure the continuation of milk secretion, while the neurohypophysial polypeptide hormone, oxytocin, is necessary in most species for the active removal of preformed milk from the gland. This latter mechanism, the milk-ejection reflex, was described in the preceding chapter with particular reference to events occurring at the level of the mammary gland. In the present chapter the neural mechanisms mediating the release of hormones in response to suckling or milking will be considered.

Sensory receptors in the mammary gland

If the stimuli associated with the act of suckling or milking are to be transformed into nerve impulses which ascend in the central nervous system to cause release of pituitary hormones, there must be a suitable system of receptors at the mammary level. These receptors are distributed profusely in the teat, and in the human at least, Cathcart, Gairns & Garven (1948) considered the nipple to be one of the most highly innervated tissues of the body. The sensory innervation of the mammary gland is confined almost entirely to the teat, as demonstrated in the lactating rabbit by the blockade of the milk-ejection reflex in response to suckling after local anaesthesia of the teats (Findlay, 1968). Cross (1961*b*) pointed out that earlier claims for a more widespread sensory innervation of the mammary gland were based on unreliable histological techniques. Recent histochemical investigations in the cow (Lukášová & Lukáš, 1965) and rabbit (Ballantyne & Bunch, 1966; Hebb & Linzell, 1966) have not demonstrated any innervation of the mammary parenchyma and have also shown that while extensive innervation occurs in the teat, it is more attenuated in the surrounding mammary skin. Recent electron-microscope observations in the rabbit (Cross & Findlay, 1969) (Fig. 6.1) are in agreement with these histochemical findings and have also indicated that the sensory receptors consist of bundles of unmyelinated nerve fibres. Changes in electrical activity were recorded from fibres of the afferent nerve supply of the mammary gland in the lactating rabbit in response to mechanical stimulation of the teat. In addition, distension of mammary lobules by intraductal injection of saline evoked an afferent discharge in some cases. However, the majority of the receptors which were sensitive to mammary distension were found to be in the teat or skin and were responding to transmitted pressure from within the gland. A few receptors were, apparently, present within the mammary parenchyma, since the response to mammary distension was not inhibited by anaesthesia of the teat or removal of skin, but only by intraductal injection of local anaesthetic (Findlay, 1966; Cross & Findlay, 1969). Earlier support for the presence of at least some interoceptors in the mammary gland of the goat was presented by Grachev (1949, quoted extensively by Grachev, 1964). In his experiments, the udder was separated from the body, except for the nervous supply which remained intact, and the gland was perfused with oxygenated Tyrode's solution. Artificial distension of the udder cistern with air or the injection of 0·1% KOH solution into the cistern both elicited a rise in systemic blood pressure, which was taken to indicate the presence of baroreceptors and of chemoreceptors within the gland.

    In addition to the degree of innervation, there are also differences in the pattern of innervation and in the type of skin to be found over the mammary gland. Thus, in the human, although

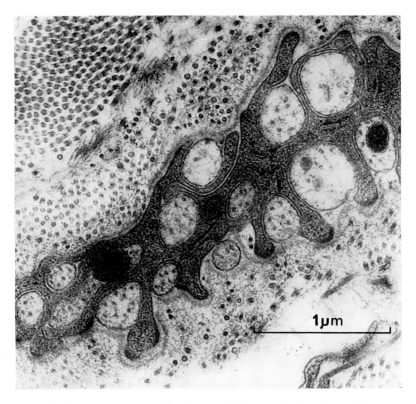

FIG. 6.1. Electron micrograph showing Schwann cell invaginated by non-myelinated nerve fibres, lying in connective tissue at tip of rabbit teat (from Cross. B. A. & Findlay, A. L. R., 1969, in *Lactogenesis: The Initiation of Milk Secretion at Parturition*, edited by Reynolds, M. & Folley, S. J., pp. 245–252. Philadelphia: University of Pennsylvania Press).

the hair follicles are small, the breast skin peripheral to the areola is essentially hair-covered skin and is largely innervated by the free fibres and circular and palisade fibres which are normally associated with hair follicles. Within the areolar region, hair follicles are sparse, while they are absent in the nipple, and in both these regions the most frequently occurring nerve terminals are free-fibre endings concentrated in the deeper portions of the dermis. In addition, there is very little innervation associated with the superficial dermis or epidermis, in marked contrast to the mammary skin peripheral to the areola where such innervation does occur (Miller & Kasahara, 1959).

Ascending path of the milk-ejection reflex in the spinal cord

The ascending pathways in the spinal cord which are activated by suckling or milking to evoke the release of pituitary hormones are not clear at the present time, and what little is known may be complicated by species differences. In the goat, which was the first species to be studied in this context, Tsakhaev (1953a) found that hemi-section of the spinal cord abolished the milk-ejection reflex if milking was confined to the ipsilateral mammary gland, but that it occurred quite normally when the gland contralateral to the spinal cut was milked. When hemi-section was combined with section of the dorsal funiculus of the opposite side, the milk-ejection reflex was abolished in response to milking both halves of the udder (Tsakhaev, 1953a). Similar experiments in the goat (Popovici, 1963) confirmed these findings, since unilateral removal of $1-1\frac{1}{2}$ cm of the dorsal spinal funiculus blocked the reflex in response to ipsilateral, but not to contralateral, milking. However, Popovici (1963) made two additional observations. The first was that if the mammary gland was fully distended with milk, milking the ipsilateral gland did cause a very feeble milk-ejection reflex, and that complete blockage of the reflex occurred only after removing portions of both the dorsal and lateral spinal funiculi. His other observation was that if one hypothalamic paraventricular nucleus was destroyed with a radio-frequency lesion, the milk-ejection reflex only occurred in response to milking the contra-lateral gland. The conclusions drawn from these studies were that, in the goat, the milking-induced impulses pass along that side of the cord ipsilateral to the mammary gland of their origin, that they travel almost entirely within the dorsal funiculus, and that the impulses from each mammary gland travel to the hypothalamus exclusively on their side of origin, without decussation. In the rat, Eayrs & Baddeley (1956) carried out an elegant study in which they first of all sectioned the dorsal spinal roots, determined the area of abdominal wall which was insensitive, and removed all teats outside this region. When the pups were allowed to suckle the remaining teats within the insensitive area, there was a failure both of milk ejection and milk secretion, yet, in a subsequent lactation, when partial sensitivity had returned, normal lactation was restored. They then showed that complete hemi-section of the cord combined with removal of teats on one side or the other resulted in almost complete failure of lactation when only the teats ipsilateral to the cut were suckled, while lactation continued when contralateral teats were suckled. In addition, cuts which extended deep into the lateral funiculus, but which spared the dorsal and ventral funiculi, virtually blocked lactation when only the teats ipsilateral to the lesion were suckled. Unlike the goat therefore (Tsakhaev, 1953*a*), damage to spinal pathways in the rat led not only to disruption of milk ejection, but also to loss of milk secretion, indicating impairment of both neurohypophysial and adenohypophysial function. From their experiments, Eayrs & Baddeley (1956) concluded that the ascending path in the cord of the rat was mainly ipsilateral, with a minor contralateral component, and that it lay in the lateral funiculus. They also suggested the possibility that the pathway may be related to the spino-thalamic system of fibres.

This apparent difference in the routes traversed by impulses from the teat in the ruminant and rodent has recently been extended to the rabbit, where the ascending path associated with the milk-ejection reflex was found to lie not in the dorsal, but in the ventrolateral column of the spinal cord (Mena & Beyer, 1968*a*). A common factor in all three species studied so far was that the pathway appeared to be either completely or principally ipsilateral to the side being suckled or milked. However, these views may require modification, at least in the ruminant, in the light of recent investigations carried out in the sheep by the group at Jouy-en-Josas. Two types of experiments were carried out, in the first of which, Richard (1970) recorded potentials in the pituitary stalk of sheep in response to electrical stimulation of the inguinal nerves, which innervate the mammary glands. It was found that the tracts conveying impulses from the mammary gland to the pituitary stalk were chiefly contralateral, with a minor ipsilateral component. The dorsal funiculi were not found to be necessary for transmission of impulses to the pituitary stalk, and the fibres involved were distributed diffusely in the lateral and ventral parts of the spinal cord.

This, of course, was in marked contrast to previous findings in the goat, yet, in the second type of experiment, Richard, Urban & Denamur (1970) found in the sheep, as had Tsakhaev (1953*a*) and Popovici (1963) in the goat, that section of the dorsal funiculi blocked the milk-ejection reflex, and unilateral section only blocked the reflex when the ipsilateral mammary gland was milked. At the cervical level, however, interruption of the dorsal funiculus was ineffective. This suggested the possible involvement of the spino-cervico-thalamic tract, which has already been demonstrated in the sheep (Richard & Urban, 1969) and which is situated ventrally at the cervical level before relaying with the lateral cervical nucleus. Richard *et al.* (1970) proposed that, in the sheep, whereas the spinothalamic system carries the impulses of the milking stimulus to the diencephalon, there is an over-riding control mechanism which resides in the spino-cervico-thalamic system, and that the site of interaction of the two path-ways may lie in the diencephalon. With respect to the diffuse nature of the pathway reported by Richard (1970) in the spinal cord of the sheep, it may be relevant to mention recent studies in the pig. While the spinothalamic tract does exist in the latter species, it is secondary in prominence to a large spinoreticular fibre system, and the spinal fibre systems of the pig which sub-serve pain are more diffuse than those found in carnivores or primates (Breazile & Kitchell, 1968*a*, *b*). More recently, the dis-tribution and termination of spinoreticular afferent fibres has been studied in the brainstem of the sheep (Rao, Breazile & Kitchell, 1969).

The present state of knowledge of the pathways in the spinal cord, therefore, is a little confusing, and the problem will require considerable experimental ingenuity if it is to be solved satis-factorily. While not contributing data on the ipsi- or contralateral nature of the path, studies on the release of oxytocin by localized, discrete, electrical stimulation of various regions of the spinal cord should prove rewarding in pin-pointing the trajectory of the pathway.

Ascending path of the milk-ejection reflex in the brain

Although as far as the spinal cord is concerned, the ascending path of the milk-ejection reflex cannot yet be defined with any degree of certainty, this is not the case further rostrally in the brainstem, for which a reasonably complete account can now be given. In the goat, there was a single report of milk ejection following electrical stimulation of the medial lemniscus (Andersson, 1951*b*). Ten years later, studies in the rabbit indicated that milk ejection occurred after stimulation of a wide variety of sites, including central grey, reticular formation, medial lemniscus, subthalamus, supramammillary area, mammillary peduncle, septum and fimbria of the fornix (B. A. Cross & I. A. Silver, unpublished work quoted by Cross 1961*a*). Also in the rabbit, two brief reports in which no details of quantitative or qualitative aspects of hormone release were given, indicated the occurrence of milk ejection after stimulation of the gracilis and cuneate nuclei, internal arcuate fibres, medial lemniscus, ventral posterolateral and reticular thalamic nuclei, reticular formation, central grey, subthalamus and lateral hypothalamus, while more rostrally, effective sites were also found in pyriform cortex, amygdala, hippocampus, fornix and septum (Holland, Woods & Aulsebrook, 1963; Holland, Aulsebrook & Woods, 1963). Using a different experimental approach, Beyer, Mena, Pacheco & Alcaraz (1962*b*) blocked lactation in the cat by making extensive lesions in the region of the extreme rostral central grey and the posterior hypothalamus but because lactation was not restored by replacement therapy with oxytocin, Beyer *et al.* (1962*b*) concluded that the prime cause of lactation failure was inhibition of milk secretion. However, this claim was later withdrawn and the disturbance of lactation was attributed to blockade of oxytocin release (Beyer & Mena, 1965*b*), a conclusion which had been reached by Stutinsky & Terminn (1964*a*) after similar lesions in the lactating rat. In a related study in which removal of teats from one side of the body was combined with either an ipsilateral or contralateral posterior hypothalamic lesion, Stutinsky & Terminn (1964*b*) suggested that the ascending path from teat to hypothalamus for oxytocin release might be both ipsilateral and contralateral, or that there might even be a double decussation.

While the studies involving lesions indicated that the pathway for oxytocin release probably entered the hypothalamus through the posterior hypothalamus, no clearly defined pathway, if indeed one existed, had emerged from the electrical stimulation studies. Some of the problems attending the latter technique, such as inhibition of the mammary response to oxytocin by sympathetico-adrenal activation, the correct choice of stimulus parameters and the fact that vasopressin also possesses inherent milk-ejection activity, were pointed out by Cross (1966). The first evidence of a

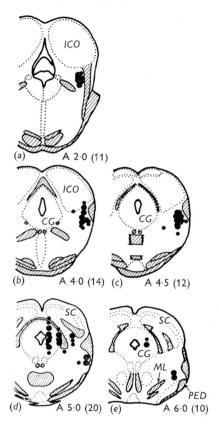

Fig. 6.2. The ascending path of the milk-ejection reflex in the guinea-pig. Drawings of transverse sections through the brain showing sites where electrical stimulation evoked milk-ejection responses. Planes are labelled as mm anterior to the interaural (APO) plane, passing rostrally a–e. Sites where stimulation caused milk-ejection responses equal to or greater than those caused by i.v. injection of 200 μu. synthetic oxytocin are shown as large closed circles, sites where stimulation caused responses equivalent to less than 200 μu, as small closed circles. Numbers in parentheses refer to the number of electrode tracks studied in each plane. Note the compact ascending path of the milk-ejection reflex in the caudal midbrain (from Tindal, J. S., Knaggs, G. S. & Turvey, A., 1967*c*, *J. Endocr.* **38,** 337–349).

definitive ascending path in the brain concerned with oxytocin release came from studies in the guinea-pig (Tindal, Knaggs & Turvey, 1967*a*, *c*). However, although the techniques of spinal cord section or adrenalectomy were used in the rabbit to prevent sympathetico-adrenal activation caused by electrical stimulation of the brain (see Cross, 1961*a*), they were found to be unsuitable for the guinea-pig, in which the same end-result was achieved by transection of the brain at the mid-cerebellar level (Tindal *et al.*, 1967*c*). In the guinea-pig, the afferent path of the milk-ejection reflex in the caudal mid-brain was found to be compact and lay in the lateral wall of the tegmentum (Fig. 6.2). Most of the milk ejection responses obtained by stimulation of this region were relatively large, equivalent to i.v. injection of 200–800 μu, synthetic oxytocin, and the effective sites were in the form of a vertical band. More rostrally, while the main responsive area still lay in the lateral tegmentum, other sites were also found in the tectum and mesencephalic central grey. However, the main pathway continues forward until it comes to lie just medioventral to the medial geniculate body, in a region with ill-defined boundaries, the posterior thalamic complex, with a group of less responsive sites extending vertically up the tegmentum to reach the tectum. As the pathway is traced forward in the diencephalon, this single major pathway on each side of the brain divides into two (Fig. 6.3). One part, the dorsal path, passes forward close to the rostral central grey, parafascicular nucleus and periventricular region, while the other part, the ventral path, extends medioventrally into the subthalamus between the medial lemniscus and cerebral peduncle to involve the substantia nigra and zona incerta. The dorsal and ventral paths enter the hypothalamus close to the 3rd ventricle, and in the lateral hypothalamus, respectively. Within the hypothalamus, milk-ejection responses were elicited after stimulation of many sites, and the two ascending pathways appeared to pass to the pituitary stalk. The recording of intra-mammary pressure alone does not, of course, differentiate between milk-ejection responses caused by oxytocin alone and those caused by vasopressin or a mixture of the two hormones. In a later study, discrete portions of the ascending pathway found by Tindal *et al.* (1967*c*) were investigated further, using both intra-mammary pressure and arterial blood pressure recording to differentiate between release of the two hormones. It was found

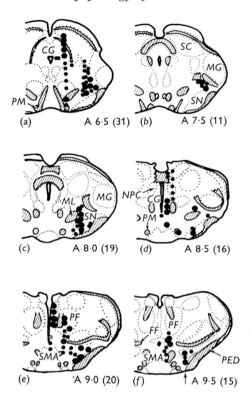

FIG. 6.3. The ascending path of the milk-ejection reflex in the guinea-pig. See legend to Fig. 6.2. for details. At the level of the rostral mid-brain the path lies medioventral to the medial geniculate body (a, b). Further rostrally, the path bifurcates into dorsal and ventral paths (c–f) in the periventricular region and subthalamus, respectively (from Tindal, J. S., Knaggs, G. S. & Turvey, A., 1967c, *J. Endocr.* **38**, 337–349).

FIG. 6.4. The ascending path of the milk-ejection reflex in the rabbit. Drawings of transverse sections through the brain showing sites where electrical stimulation evoked release of oxytocin (solid circles), of vaso-pressin or vasopressin + oxytocin (solid triangles) or no release of oxy-tocin or vasopressin (open circles). In this, and the following two figures, planes are labelled as mm posterior (P) or anterior (A) to the anterior–posterior zero (APO) plane, and pass rostrally, a, b, ... in each figure. Note the compact ascending path of the milk-ejection reflex in the mid-brain (from Tindal, J. S., Knaggs, G. S. & Turvey, A., 1969, *J. Endocr.* **43**, 663–671).

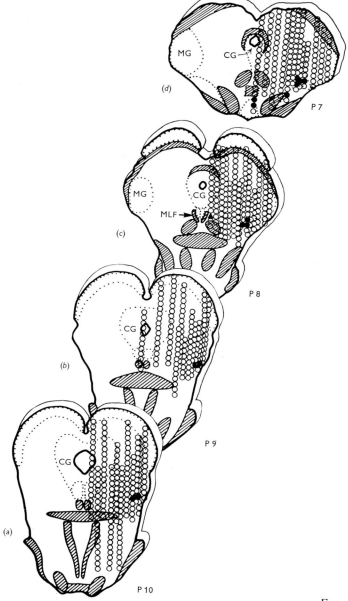

FIG. 6.4

that in the guinea-pig, the common ascending path in the mid-brain and the dorsal and ventral paths were concerned with the preferential release of oxytocin. Milk-ejection responses which occurred as a result of electrical stimulation of these pathways were found to be caused entirely by oxytocin since there was no associated elevation of arterial blood pressure. Intravenous doses of exogenous vasopressin which were large enough to elicit a milk-ejection response always betrayed themselves by a concomitant pressor response (Tindal, Knaggs & Turvey, 1968). Although it cannot be stated that no endogenous vasopressin was released in response to these stimulations, the amount must have been far less than that of oxytocin. It should be emphasized that this was not due to failure of the technique to detect vasopressin release in guinea-pig since stimulation of the rostral tuberal region adjacent to the pituitary stalk evoked release of a mixture of oxytocin and vasopressin in the ratio of approximately 3 : 1 (Tindal *et al.*, 1968).

In the lactating rabbit the mesencephalon and diencephalon were explored with stimulating electrodes, both intramammary pressure and arterial blood pressure were monitored, and it was found that the same paths for the milk-ejection reflex occurred in the rabbit as in the guinea-pig (Tindal, Knaggs & Turvey, 1969). Thus, in the mesencephalon the ascending pathway for oxytocin release again lay in the lateral tegmentum (Fig. 6.4). Further forward it was found medio-ventral to the medial geniculate body, and as it was traced rostrally it divided into dorsal and ventral paths which merged again in the posterior hypothalamus (Fig. 6.5). Within the hypothalamus (Fig. 6.6), as in the guinea-pig, the pathway lost much of its identity, since oxytocin release was observed after stimulation of a wide range of sites which could be traced both to the paraventricular nucleus and to the pituitary stalk (Tindal *et al.*, 1969).

Although the possibility that small quantities of vasopressin were released together with oxytocin is not excluded, it is of interest that significant release of vasopressin did occur after stimulation of sites in the brain other than the afferent path of the milk-ejection reflex. Effective sites for evoking vasopressin release in the rabbit were found close to the medial longitudinal fasciculus and in the reticular formation and subthalamus, in agreement with findings in the dog and monkey (Mills & Wang, 1964; Hayward & Smith, 1964), while in the hypothalamus a mixture of oxytocin

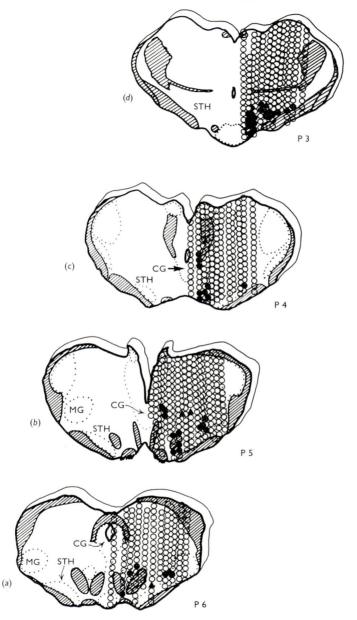

FIG. 6.5. The ascending path of the milk-ejection reflex in the rabbit. See legend to Fig. 6.4 for details. As the path enters the diencephalon it bifurcates into dorsal and ventral paths (from Tindal, J. S., Knaggs, G. S. & Turvey, A., 1969, *J. Endocr.* **43**, 663–671).

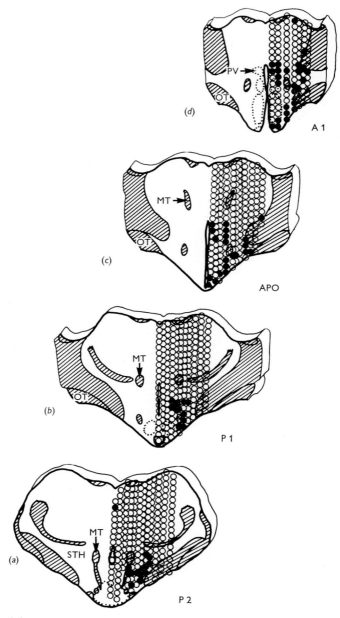

Fig. 6.6.

and vasopressin, ranging in ratio from 1 : 1 to 3 : 10, was released after stimulation of the region of the supraoptic nucleus and a mixture of unknown ratio (>2 mu. oxytocin plus >5 mu. vasopressin) after stimulation of a site in the tuberal region (Tindal *et al.*, 1969).

While the technique of exploring the brain stem with a stimulating electrode has proved invaluable for the study of ascending pathways involved in the release of oxytocin, within the hypothalamus the method has definite limitations. This region of the brain contains a veritable feltwork of fibres, and release of oxytocin after stimulation of a particular point does not necessarily indicate that the rostral continuation of any one particular pathway is being investigated. There could be many paths converging on this region, not to mention the efferent tracts which pass from the magnocellular hypothalamic nuclei and sweep down to the neurohypophysis. Two problems in particular remained unresolved, the first of which was whether the ascending path of the milk-ejection reflex passed out of the diencephalon at any stage of its trajectory. This possibility existed because it had been claimed that the reflex path passed through the amygdala, since the reflex was reported to be absent in the lactating rat after destructive lesions were placed in this complex (Stutinsky & Terminn, 1965; Stutinsky & Guerne, 1967). However, in the anaesthetized lactating guinea-pig electrical stimulation of the amygdala did not lead to release of oxytocin (Tindal *et al.*, 1967c). Furthermore, oxytocin is released in this species in response to electrical stimulation of the reflex path in the mesencephalon after the entire cerebral cortex, hippocampus, amygdala and structures rostral to the hypothalamus have been removed by suction (Tindal & Knaggs, 1971). Also, in the anaesthetized sheep, potentials recorded from the pituitary stalk in response to electrical stimulation of the inguinal nerve were not diminished by removal of cerebral cortex or amygdala (Richard, 1970). Unless the rat proves to be a special case, it is difficult to reconcile these findings with the interpretations of Stutinsky & Terminn (1965) and Stutinsky & Guerne

FIG. 6.6. The ascending path of the milk-ejection reflex in the rabbit. See legend to Fig. 6.4 for details. The dorsal and ventral paths reunite in the posterior hypothalamus, while further rostrally the pathway intermingles with efferent fibres from the paraventricular nucleus (from Tindal, J. S., Knaggs, G. S. & Turvey, A., 1969, *J. Endocr.* **43**, 663–671).

(1967), especially since no illustrations of the effective lesion sites in the amygdala were given. Two obvious possibilities exist, either that the lesion in the amygdala extended sufficiently far medial to damage the hypothalamic pathway, or that the lesion blocked oxytocin release not by cutting the afferent path but by activating an emotional inhibition of oxytocin release, a process which appears to occur only too readily in the rat (Grosvenor & Mena, 1967).

It must be remembered that the milk-ejection reflex involves ascending tactile pathways, and it is not denied that other fore-brain structures outside the diencephalon may be involved in release of oxytocin by means other than the suckling stimulus or electrical stimulation of ascending tactile pathways. In this con-nexion, milk ejection has been reported in response to stimulation of a variety of structures within the forebrain including septum and fornix (B. A. Cross & I. A. Silver, unpublished work quoted by Cross, 1961*a*), periventricular region rostral to the paraventricu-lar nucleus (Tindal *et al.*, 1968; Aulsebrook & Holland, 1969*a*) and prelimbic cortex, nucleus accumbens and diagonal band (Aulsebrook & Holland, 1969*a*). Not all these reports necessarily reflect the sole release of oxytocin, since some may have resulted from the simultaneous release of both the neurohypophysial hormones. Nevertheless, they do underline the fact that the afferent path of the milk-ejection reflex is but one path, a tactile path, to the neurohypophysis.

The second problem which remained to be answered concerns the site of action of the suckling stimulus. Since electrical stimula-tion both of the paraventricular nucleus and of the pituitary stalk and its environs can evoke the release of oxytocin (Tindal *et al.*, 1967*c*, 1968, 1969; Aulsebrook & Holland, 1969*a*), these studies did not indicate whether suckling-induced impulses travel directly to the pituitary stalk, or whether they must first pass to the paraventricular nucleus, and then down the efferent fibres to the pituitary stalk. Neither was an answer provided by Brooks, Ishikawa, Koizumi & Lu (1966) or Ishikawa, Koizumi & Brooks (1966) who correlated milk-ejection responses in the cat, evoked by applying suction to a nipple, with electrical activity both in the paraventricular nucleus and the pituitary stalk. Even the demon-stration of evoked potentials of 7 msec latency or less in hypo-thalamic nuclei in response to electrical stimulation of more caudal points in the brain stem (Beyer, Tindal & Sawyer, 1962;

Woods, Holland & Powell, 1969) and of fibre degeneration in the paraventricular nucleus after placement of lesions in the posterior hypothalamus (Woods *et al.*, 1969) did not decide the matter one way or the other. The only satisfactory manner in which to attack the problem is to use the functional approach, in terms of release or non-release of oxytocin. Such a study has recently been carried out in the anaesthetized lactating guinea-pig in which the afferent path of the milk-ejection reflex in the mesencephalon was stimulated both before and after surgical interruption of hypothalamic pathways (Tindal & Knaggs, 1971). It was found that transection of the hypothalamus just rostral to the paraventricular nuclei was without effect on oxytocin release, while a similar cut made immediately caudal to these nuclei, yet rostral to the pituitary stalk, abolished the release of oxytocin in response to stimulation of the path in the mid-brain. Furthermore, by the use of a special brain knife to undercut and isolate the paraventricular nuclei from the ventral hypothalamus, it was shown that these nuclei do lie on the ascending path of the reflex. Also, at least from the mid-brain forwards, the pathway does not decussate, since under-cutting the paraventricular nucleus of one side blocks the release of oxytocin only when the ipsilateral path in the mid-brain is stimulated (Tindal & Knaggs, 1971). It is believed that this consti-tutes sufficient proof for this final afferent link in the pathway, especially when the studies of Brooks *et al.* (1966) and Ishikawa *et al.* (1966) are taken into account. In this connexion it should be noted that not all the cells in the paraventricular nucleus innervate the neurohypophysis. Cross, Novin & Sundsten (1969) reported that only about 50% of paraventricular nucleus cells in the rabbit, whose electrical activity was recorded, were activated by anti-dromic stimulation from an electrode in the neurohypophysis, and that 75% of these responsive cells did not discharge spontaneously. This recent finding may make it easier to appreciate the conflicting reports concerning which neurohypophysial hormone is released after stimulation of the paraventricular nucleus. Thus, stimulation of this nucleus in the cat has been reported to cause the release of small amounts of vasopressin alone (Bisset, Hilton & Poisner, 1967), variable mixtures of vasopressin and oxytocin (Bisset, Clark & Errington, 1970) and oxytocin alone (Brooks *et al.*, 1966; Ishikawa *et al.*, 1966). In the guinea-pig and rabbit (Tindal *et al.*, 1968, 1969; Aulsebrook & Holland, 1969*a*) stimulation of the

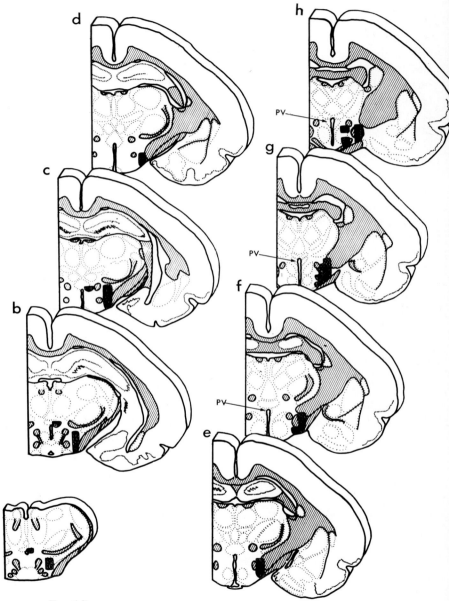

Fig 6.7.

paraventricular nucleus led to release of oxytocin alone. It can be appreciated that if only a proportion of paraventricular cells project directly to the neurohypophysis (Cross *et al.*, 1969), and if other cells project, first of all, to the supraoptic nucleus and then to the neurohypophysis, the proportion doing so varying from species to species, then there is at least a basis for understanding why stimulation administered by the tip of an electrode placed in the paraventricular nucleus should not necessarily be associated with the release of oxytocin.

The one remaining segment of the afferent reflex path in the forebrain which requires clarification is that lying between the point of entry of the dorsal and ventral pathways into the posterior hypothalamus (Tindal *et al.*, 1967c) and the paraventricular nuclei. This has now been investigated, again in the guinea-pig, by combining electrical stimulation of the ascending path in the mid-brain with surgical cuts in the forebrain, made by lowering a

---

FIG. 6.7. The ascending pathway of the milk-ejection reflex in the hypo-thalamus of the guinea-pig. The diagram is a summary of experiments in which narrow, transverse cuts were made in the hypothalamus to determine which cuts blocked and which cuts spared the afferent path of the reflex, assessed by the release or non-release of oxytocin in response to stimulation of the discrete ascending pathway further caudally (see Fig. 6.2) in the mid-brain. a–h are transverse stereotaxic planes passing rostrally at 0·5 mm intervals from A 9·5 to A 13·0. At planes A 9·5, 10·0 and 10·5 (a–c) the dorsal and ventral paths (see Fig. 6.3) are clearly seen. In separate experiments, cutting the dorsal path reduced the response by approximately one third, while cutting the ventral path reduced it by approximately two thirds. Further rostrally at A 11·0 (d) the dorsal path has swung out to reunite with the ventral path in the lateral hypo-thalamus and the combined path continues forward in the extreme lateral hypothalamus until the level of the paraventricular (PV) nucleus is reached (A 12·5, g). Here, irregularities appear on the medial edge of the path which, at the most rostral plane (A 13·0, h), move medial to the fornix and appear to form two isolated portions of the path. At this level, however, neurosecretory fibres pass laterally from the PV nucleus on their way to the pituitary stalk (see Fig. 6.8) and intermingle with the final segment of the ascending pathway which moves medially from the lateral hypothalamus to the lateral tip of the PV nucleus (see Tindal & Knaggs, 1971). This final contact between ascending pathway and PV nucleus is not shown since it occurs between plane A 13·0 (shown in this figure) and plane A 13·5 where complete hypothalamic transection does not block oxytocin release (from Tindal, J. S. & Knaggs, G. S., 1971, *J. Endocr.* **50**, 135–152).

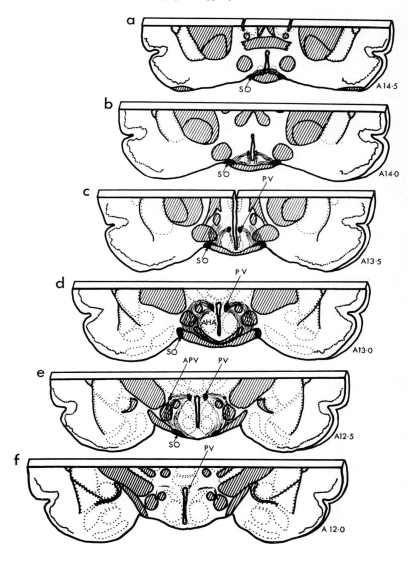

Fig. 6.8.

narrow blade in 0·5 mm steps at selected sites and determining where the cut blocks the release of oxytocin (Tindal & Knaggs, 1971). These studies (Fig. 6.7) have indicated that in the guinea-pig the ascending reflex pathway in the hypothalamus lies in the far-lateral hypothalamus, and even appears to enter the internal capsule as it approaches the level of the paraventricular nucleus. Since the efferent fibres passing from this nucleus to the neuro-hypophysis also sweep far out into the lateral hypothalamus (Arizono & Okamoto, 1957; Ford & Kantounis, 1957), it is extremely difficult to dissociate the two systems. While Arizono & Okamoto (1957) published illustrations of the course of these neurosecretory fibres in the rat, they only gave a brief, verbal description of those in the guinea-pig. However, since this exact trajectory must be known before the final segment of the ascending pathway can be determined, of necessity our work on surgical interruption of the pathway was carried out in conjunction with a histological study (Fig. 6.8) of the neurosecretory system in the guinea-pig (Knaggs, Tindal & Turvey, 1971). It was concluded that, at the level of the paraventricular nuclei, the ascending pathway swings medially from the lateral hypothalamus, at right angles to the longitudinal axis of the brain stem, to relay with the lateral tip of the ipsilateral paraventricular nucleus (Tindal & Knaggs, 1971), thus affording an explanation for the finding that surgical isolation of the basal hypothalamus from the remainder of the brain does not block milk ejection in the rat if the cut is left incomplete at one side (Yokoyama, Halász & Sawyer, 1967).

FIG. 6.8. Diagram showing neurosecretory pathways from the para-ventricular (PV) nucleus in the brain of the guinea-pig. a–f are drawings of transverse stereotaxic planes through the brain passing caudally from A 14·5 to A 12·0. The main part of the PV nucleus, with the magnocellular neurosecretory neurones concentrated in its lateral tip, lies between A 13·0 and A 12·5. Neurosecretory fibres from the main part of the PV nucleus pass ventral to the fornix at A 13·5, both dorsal and ventral to the fornix at A 13·0 and mainly dorsal to this structure at A 12·5. After passing round the fornix these fibres merge to form a broad band of fibres at A 13·0 which constitutes the main paraventricular-hypophysial tract. This tract curves around the lateral edge of the anterior hypo-thalamic area (AHA) and turns caudo-medially over the dorsal surface of the optic chiasma towards the median eminence. An accessory PV nucleus (APV) is present at A 12·5 (from Knaggs, G. S., Tindal, J. S. & Turvey, A., 1971, *J. Endocr.* **50**, 153–162).

The neural basis for the afferent path of the milk-ejection reflex

For almost twenty years there has been speculation as to the fibre systems which are responsible for conveying the impulses initiated by the suckling or milking stimulus to the hypothalamus. Andersson (1951*b*) reported milk ejection in a goat after stimulation of the medial lemniscus in the medulla, yet on later evidence this assumption must at least be queried since, in a comparative anatomical study of the medial lemniscus in the hindbrain, Verhaart (1960) showed it to be in an entirely different position in the goat from that claimed by Andersson (1951*b*). The medial lemniscus was also suggested as a pathway which mediated oxytocin release in the cat by Rothballer (1966), although this appears to have been based mainly on negative evidence. Reviewing the evidence available at the time, Cross (1961*b*) proposed that the milk-ejection reflex involved diffuse, afferent pathways, indeed this was the only reasonable conclusion to draw since no one particular ascending pathway appeared to hold the key to oxytocin release. The first clear indication came from studies in the guinea-pig, where a compact pathway was located in the lateral wall of the mid-brain, stimulation of which evoked a large milk-ejection response (Tindal *et al.*, 1967*a*, *c*) later shown to be attributable to release of oxytocin (Tindal *et al.*, 1968). After their spinal investigations in the rat, Eayrs & Baddeley (1956) had hinted at the possibility of spinothalamic fibres being involved in the release of oxytocin caused by suckling, but the studies in the guinea-pig (Tindal *et al.*, 1967*a*, *c*) provided the first direct evidence to allow the conclusion that the spinothalamic system carries the burden of sensory information from the mammary gland which is destined to activate hormone-releasing mechanisms in the hypothalamus, a view which has since been endorsed by others (Mena & Beyer, 1968*a*; Richard *et al.*, 1970). The justification for this belief has already been given in detail (Tindal, 1967; Tindal *et al.*, 1967*c*), the major points of which are the position of the pathway in the mid-brain and the fact that further rostrally at the level of the meso-diencephalic boundary it can be traced to a characteristic position medioventral to the medial geniculate body (see Mehler, Feferman & Nauta, 1960) as it passes close to the posterior thalamic complex, whose principal afferent input is provided by the spinothalamic tract (Poggio & Mountcastle, 1960; Whitlock & Perl, 1961; Scheibel & Scheibel, 1966). Further forward, the oxytocin-release path, on each side of the brain, divides into two portions (Tindal *et al.*, 1967c). One of these, the dorsal path, passes through the parafascicular nucleus and extreme rostral central grey, both of which receive contributions from the spino-thalamic system (Gerebtzoff, 1940; Nauta, 1960), while the other portion passes ventromedially to enter the subthalamus, which also receives spinothalamic innervation (Scheibel & Scheibel, 1967; Denavit, 1968). The further onward course of the pathways to the hypothalamus must obviously involve relay with other fibre tracts which take origin at or about this level, and it seems probable that the two systems involved are the dorsal longitudinal fasciculus and the medial forebrain bundle, respectively. As mentioned previously, the final link in the oxytocin-release path is represented by the paraventricular nucleus and its neurosecretory fibres in the hypothalamus.

It is unknown at present whether the ascending reflex path relays with cells of the posterior thalamic complex, or whether spinothalamic collaterals in the tegmentum (Nauta, 1960; Scheibel & Scheibel, 1967) bypass this structure *en route* to the hypothalamus. However, this point is of minor importance. What is significant is that the pathway which is activated by suckling is associated with the afferent path to the posterior thalamic complex which is known to receive tactile information mainly from spinothalamic fibres (Fig. 6.9). The fact that such information is essentially non-specific, giving little or no topographic localization from stimuli which impinge on the body surface (Poggio & Mountcastle, 1960; Perl & Whitlock, 1961; Calma, 1965a) is not surprising in view of the fact that, in general, the spinothalamic system is activated by stimuli of an abrupt or alerting nature. This is in marked contrast to the response to fine touch and the ability to give accurate localization of sensation which resides in the medial lemniscal-thalamocortical sensory mechanism (see Perl & Whitlock, 1961; Albe-Fessard, 1967; Horridge, 1968). Moreover, at the thalamic level, there is also an association between one of two patterns of presynaptic dendritic arborization with either somatotopic function, in the case of lemniscal afferents, or integrative function, in the case of spinothalamic afferents (Scheibel & Scheibel, 1966).

The difference in the type of sensory information which is

The physiology of lactation

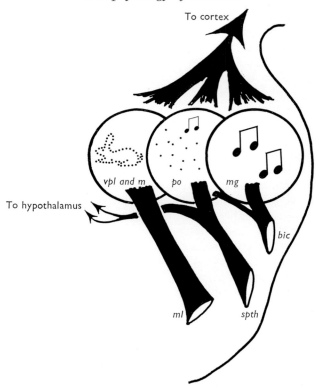

FIG. 6.9. Simplified diagram of a transverse section through the brain, at the level of the caudal diencephalon, to illustrate the relationship between the ascending path for impulses triggered by the suckling stimulus and the sensory thalamic nuclei. Note the topographic representation conveyed to the ventroposterior lateral and ventroposterior medial (vpl and m) thalamic nuclei by the medial lemniscus (ml) (for simplicity, facial representation is shown as being conveyed by ml), the purely auditory input to the medial geniculate body (mg) and, between them, an ill-defined and fairly primitive region, the posterior thalamic complex (po), in which there is little or no topographic representation of the body surface and which receives a small auditory input from the brachium of the inferior colliculus (bic) and its major tactile input from the spino-thalamic system (spth). In general, the latter system is activated by more powerful and abrupt stimuli than the medial lemniscal system, which can respond to such delicate stimuli as movement of hairs. It is now known that the spinothalamic system also provides the ascending path in the brain for impulses triggered by the suckling stimulus which are destined to activate neuroendocrine mechanisms, and that within the diencephalon the spinothalamic path relays with other ascending fibre systems to reach the hypothalamus (from Tindal, J. S., & Knaggs, G. S., 1970a, *Mem. Soc. Endocr.* **18**, 239–258).

carried by the two tactile sensory systems is also mirrored at the periphery by the arrangement of sensory receptors. Thus, in the teat, which has only limited powers of sensory discrimination (Wood-Jones & Turner, 1931), the profuse innervation is confined essentially to the dermis (Cathcart *et al.*, 1948; Miller & Kasahara, 1959). However, in areas of the body, such as the hands, where sensory discrimination is highly developed, the nerve endings are concentrated in the epidermis and superficial dermis (Miller, Ralston & Kasahara, 1958). It is the functional characteristics of the receptors in the teat, and of the spinothalamic system as a whole, therefore, which appear to hold the key to the problem of why casual tactile stimuli are ineffective and why the normally vigorous onset of the act of suckling is effective in triggering the milk-ejection reflex. This system would enable the body to select from the constant barrage of tactile stimuli the stimulus which satisfies the requirements for activation of an ascending pathway which is now known to project to hormone-releasing mechanisms in the forebrain, a view which becomes even more logical when phylogenetic considerations are also borne in mind (see Tindal & Knaggs, 1970*a*).

Central aspects of conditioning of the milk-ejection reflex

Peripheral aspects of the release of oxytocin in response to conditioned stimuli have already been described in the preceding chapter. However, consideration of the central mechanisms which govern such a release is hampered by a general lack of knowledge of brain function. While the pathways to the neurohypophysis which are activated by the stimulus of suckling or milking are now known in some detail, there is, as yet, no clear-cut indication of the neural basis for the conditioned release of oxytocin. The only reasonable approach at present is to consider those structures in the forebrain which do not lie on the ascending path activated by the suckling stimulus, stimulation of which will evoke release of the hormone. These include the hippocampus, fimbria of the fornix, pyriform cortex and septum (B. A. Cross & I. A. Silver, unpublished work quoted by Cross, 1961*a*; Holland, Aulsebrook & Woods, 1963) and cingulate cortex (Beyer, Anguiano & Mena, 1961; Cleverley, Knaggs, Tindal & Turvey, 1968). Indeed, Cross (1961*b*) proposed that limbic structures such as these may well be concerned with the conditioned release of oxytocin. More recently, oxytocin release has been reported in the rabbit after stimulation of a small area in the rostral pole of the forebrain, encompassing the prelimbic cortex and parts of the nucleus accumbens, hippocampal rudiment, diagonal band and periventricular system, and the responsive region extended caudally, close to the mid line, to reach the paraventricular nucleus (Aulsebrook & Holland, 1969a). Degeneration studies in the rabbit after placement of lesions in the hippocampal rudiment indicated a caudally-directed pathway, which passed via the septum and fornix to the paraventricular nucleus, and it was suggested that the hippocampal rudiment may lie on the oxytocin-release pathway from cingulate cortex to paraventricular nucleus (Woods *et al.*, 1969). However, against this interpretation must be set the findings of Domesick (1969), who, in an extensive degeneration study of projection fields of the cingulate cortex in the rat, found no evidence of direct cingulate projections to either the septal region or the hypothalamus.

The mechanisms, therefore, by which a particular auditory or visual stimulus can trigger the release of oxytocin are still unknown. Both auditory (Poggio & Mountcastle, 1960; Perl & Whitlock, 1961) and visual (Calma, 1965a; Suzuki & Kato, 1969) information can reach the posterior thalamic complex, which itself is in close proximity to the ascending path of the milk-ejection reflex, and this would suggest the possibility that this route might be involved in a conditional reflex release of oxytocin. However, it would seem equally probable that the pathways of special sense would lead to the temporal lobe, and thence to the limbic system, indeed it has been proposed that visual information can pass from the lateral geniculate body direct to the hippocampal gyrus, and possibly from there to the hippocampus (MacLean, 1966). Structures in the limbic system could then activate the release of oxytocin, as suggested by Cross (1961b). In the final analysis, the solution of the mechanisms underlying the conditioned release of oxytocin is dependent on a more sophisticated understanding of the intangible processes of memory, and of maternal, as distinct from purely sexual, behaviour, than is available at the present time.

Central inhibition of the milk-ejection reflex

Although peripheral mechanisms may prevent oxytocin manifesting its galactokinetic effect on the mammary myoepithelium, it is believed that the most usual cause of milk-ejection failure is a central inhibition of the release of oxytocin itself (Cross, 1955*b*). Relatively little is known of the neural basis which underlies this inhibition, and there is no reason to suppose that only a single mechanism is responsible. The inhibitory process may well attack the ascending pathway for oxytocin release at several levels, dependent on the circumstances. It is known that general anaesthesia (see Cross, 1966), and also ethanol narcosis (Fuchs & Wagner, 1963*b*, *c*; Wagner & Fuchs, 1968; Cobo & Quintero, 1969; Fuchs, 1969), can block the release of oxytocin in response to suckling, yet it is equally true that electrical stimulation of ascending pathways in the brain of the anaesthetized animal can evoke the release of oxytocin (see Tindal & Knaggs, 1970*a*). The conclusion which must be drawn from this, therefore, is that the site of action of general anaesthesia, in terms of blockade of oxytocin release, must lie caudal to the brain. Since the processes of the manifestation of pain and the release of oxytocin evoked by suckling both appear to involve the spinothalamic tracts, recent studies on pain mechanisms may assist in the interpretation of the inhibition of the milk-ejection reflex by general anaesthesia.

It has been proposed that pain may be controlled by a presynaptic gating mechanism situated near the point of entry of each dorsal root in the spinal cord. Administration of pentobarbitone produces a progressive closure of this gate, thus inhibiting the ascent of impulses of cutaneous origin (Melzack & Wall, 1965; Wall, 1967). Wall (1967) suggested that cutaneous anaesthesia may be dependent on a selective depression of transmission across the first spinal synapse of the cutaneous sensory pathways located in lamina 4 of the dorsal horn. This view has been confirmed and extended to the volatile anaesthetic halothane by De Jong & Wagman (1968), who consider that the mechanism concerns cells in lamina 4 whose axons enter the non-lemniscal afferent pathways. Since this would apply to the spinothalamic system of fibres, which is now believed to be the major carrier of cutaneous impulses from the mammary gland to the hypothalamus (Tindal *et al.*, 1967*c*), there is good reason for believing that the inhibitory action of anaesthetics on oxytocin release may well be exerted at the level of the dorsal horn of the spinal cord.

Although not strictly an inhibitory phenomenon, it would be pertinent to mention that the length of discharge of cells in lamina 4 produced by stimulation of unmyelinated peripheral fibres

I

increases with each subsequent stimulation, if the repetition rate is greater than 1 every 2 to 3 sec. In addition, the discharge is more susceptible to inhibition by barbiturate than that produced by stimulation of myelinated fibres (Mendell, 1966). This type of discharge, appropriately termed 'windup' (Mendell, 1966), appears to be reflected in the observation of Richard (1970) that whereas a single pulse applied to the inguinal nerve of the sheep did not evoke potentials in the pituitary stalk, a train of impulses was effective. This would suggest that the total size of the sensory barrage which ascends from the mammary gland is important in overcoming a synaptic resistance in order to achieve reflex activation of the neurohypophysis, and recalls the observations of Fuchs & Wagner (1963a) in the rabbit where the suckling by a single pup evoked only a trivial release of oxytocin compared with the amount released when the whole litter was suckling. It is of interest that this type of spatial summation has also been reported to apply to the suckling-induced release of oxytocin and of prolactin in the rat (Edwardson & Eayrs, 1967; Mena & Grosvenor, 1968).

When central blockade of oxytocin release is evoked by means other than anaesthesia, that is to say by factors such as pain or emotional stresses, which, in the case of the rat can be as mild as human conversation (Grosvenor & Mena, 1967), the point of attack probably lies further rostrally within the brain. Inhibition of oxytocin release in the lactating rat which was caused by pain was overcome by cortical spreading depression (Taleisnik & Deis, 1964) in which the application of KCL to the cortical surface is followed by a temporary 'pharmacological decortication'. A logical site for such a mechanism to act would be where the ascending pathway for oxytocin release bifurcates in the diencephalon into dorsal and ventral paths, which presumably involves a spinothalamic relay with other fibres (Tindal *et al.*, 1967c). Indeed it is in this region that corticofugal fibres are believed to exert an inhibitory action on non-specific ascending sensory pathways (Calma, 1965b).

In the rabbit, the release of oxytocin following stimulation of rostral forebrain structures was inhibited by simultaneous stimulation of other subcortical regions of the brain (Aulsebrook & Holland, 1965, 1969b). The inhibitory sites were found in the central grey, superior colliculus, raphe and posterior commissural nuclei, pretectum, parafascicular and dorsomedial thalamic nuclei and pyriform cortex. In addition to inhibiting the release of oxytocin, stimulation of some of these sites also evoked release of vasopressin, and Aulsebrook & Holland (1969*b*) discussed their results in terms of two opposing limbic systems, one concerned with preservation of self which responded to noxious stimuli, and the other concerned with preservation of the species which operated when the environment was tranquil. However, it should be noted in passing that their conclusions were based on the inhibition of oxytocin release, which itself was elicited by stimulation of a region in the medial forebrain rostral to the paraventricular nuclei. Since, at least in the guinea-pig, the afferent path of the milk-ejection reflex does not ascend to structures rostral to these nuclei (Tindal & Knaggs, 1971) it remains to be shown whether this inhibitory scheme bears any functional relation to blockade of suckling-induced release of oxytocin or whether it is, perhaps, more concerned with control of conditioned release of the hormone.

Within the striatum, the caudate nucleus has been shown to inhibit the firing of cells of the posterior hypothalamus in response to peripheral stimulation (Dafny & Feldman, 1968), while at the thalamic level the thalamic reticular nucleus has been implicated in the blockade of ascending peripheral stimuli at the level of the posterior diencephalon (Scheibel & Scheibel, 1967). The structural and functional complexity of the diencephalon makes it difficult to determine whether such mechanisms can modulate neurohypophysial function and whether they can be linked directly with the blockade of tactile pathways which are concerned specifically with the release of oxytocin. A mechanism of this latter type could well have been involved in the finding that administration of 5-hydroxytryptamine (5-HT) abolished the milk-ejection reflex in rats by means of a central blockade of oxytocin release (Mizuno, Talwalker & Meites, 1967). Interpretation of this action of 5-HT is aided by a consideration of studies on the neuropharmacology of sleep mechanisms, since an agent which interferes with 5-HT synthesis, p-chlorophenylalanine, not only inhibits sleep in the cat, as does the destruction of the raphe nuclei in the mid-brain, whose cells are known to contain 5-HT (see Jouvet, 1969), but has also been shown to cause hyperalgesia in the rat (Tenen, 1968). It has been suggested (Vogt, 1969) that the raphe nuclei send fibres to the dorsal spinal columns where they exert an effect by reducing the transmission of sensory impulses. If this assumption is valid, then the action of 5-HT on the release of oxytocin could well be one of inhibition of ascending sensory pathways at the spinal cord level. However, this is mere supposition, since the work of Mizuno *et al.* (1967) did not localize the site of action of 5-HT in the blockade of the milk-ejection reflex.

It would not be surprising if an inhibitory mechanism was associated with the synapses at the input to the paraventricular nucleus, the pharmacology of which has been reviewed by Bisset (1968), at the start of the final common path to the neurohypophysis. This site would presumably present the final opportunity for the brain to modify the effect of incoming sensory information on the release of oxytocin. Little is known of mechanisms which can influence oxytocin release at this level, save for the ultrastructural study of Klein, Porte & Stutinsky (1968) which showed axo-axonal synaptic contacts in the supraoptic and paraventricular hypothalamic nuclei which were believed to be of an inhibitory nature.

From this brief survey of the field, it will be evident that a detailed knowledge of inhibitory mechanisms and their sites of action within the brain is not yet available. Thus, there is no immediate explanation for the findings of A. S. McNeilly, described earlier (see p. 206), that the natural suckling of a goat by her kids is a more potent stimulus for oxytocin release than is hand milking. Whether one considers the natural suckling to represent a facilitation or the hand milking to represent a failure to lift an inhibition is immaterial, since both presumably represent different aspects of the same process. Now that the basic mechanisms concerning the release of oxytocin are beginning to be understood, it is surely the inhibitory processes, whose actions presumably exert a tonic braking effect, which will provide the most rewarding field of study in the near future (see Addendum 5).

CENTRAL NERVOUS CONTROL OF PROLACTIN SECRETION

The secretion of milk by the mammary gland is governed by a galactopoietic complex of pituitary trophic hormones. Although the composition of this complex varies from species to species the most frequently occurring constituent is prolactin, indeed in the rabbit it appears to be the single galactopoietic hormone (see p. 149). For this reason, studies of the neuroendocrine control of milk secretion are mainly, although not entirely, concerned with the central nervous control of prolactin secretion. Extensive coverage of earlier aspects of the subject may be found in the reviews of Desclin (1962), Meites, Nicoll & Talwalker (1963), Everett (1966, 1969), Meites & Nicoll (1966), Meites (1966, 1967), McCann, Dhariwal & Porter (1967), Pasteels (1967) and Tindal (1967).

Inhibitory influence of the brain on prolactin secretion

In contrast to the mechanisms governing the secretion of most of the pituitary trophic hormones, the brain appears to exert an over-all inhibitory influence on the secretion of prolactin. Thus, when the normal connexion between pituitary and hypothalamus is severed by transplanting the gland under the renal capsule, secretion of the majority of the trophic hormones virtually ceases, while the secretion of prolactin continues and may even be enhanced (Everett, 1954, 1956). Indeed, in a site such as this where the graft can become well vascularized, sufficient prolactin can be secreted to maintain milk secretion in the hypophysecto-mized rat, provided ACTH and oxytocin are administered (Cowie, Tindal & Benson, 1960) and also to initiate milk secretion in the oestrogen-primed rat (Meites & Hopkins, 1960). If the disconnexion between pituitary and central nervous system is made by surgical stalk section in the lactating goat, with the insertion of an impervious plate to maintain the patency of the separation, milk yield falls to approximately 30% of the preoperative level. Considerable restoration of milk yield occurs when hormone combinations which contain ox STH, corticoid and tri-iodothyronine, but which do not contain prolactin, are administered (Cowie, Daniel, Knaggs, Prichard & Tindal, 1964). In this study, the composition of the milk was found to be normal, whether or not exogenous hormones were administered, in contrast to the report of Donovan & Van der Werff ten Bosch (1957) that stalk section in the lactating rabbit resulted in the secretion of milk of a reduced nutritive value.

Although the technique of stalk section with the insertion of an impervious barrier across the cut ends of the stalk ensures that there will be no regeneration of pituitary portal blood vessels, it is accompanied by severe necrosis of the anterior lobe of the pituitary and hence a reduction in the amount of viable secretory tissue (Daniel & Prichard, 1958). A method of overcoming this difficulty is to destroy, either partially or completely, the tuberal region and median eminence at the top of the pituitary stalk. When this region was damaged surgically in the goat (Tverskoy, 1960) or by electrolytic lesions in the rat (McCann, Mack & Gale, 1959) lactation was inhibited, and was restored to 70–80% of normal in the rat by treatment with cortisol plus oxytocin, and exogenous prolactin was not required (Gale, Taleisnik, Friedman & McCann, 1961). Lesions in this region in the oestrogen-primed ovariectomized rabbit caused activation of mammary glands and this was accompanied in some cases by the onset of copious milk secretion (Haun & Sawyer, 1960, 1961). Also, surgical damage to the anterior tuberal region in the post-partum cat, whose mammary glands had been allowed to regress [*sic*] over a period of up to 2 months before operation, was reported to result in mammary growth and milk secretion (Grosz & Rothballer, 1961). However, it should be noted that since the onset of milk secretion occurred within a few days after the operation, it seems doubtful whether the mammary glands could have regressed to any great extent. Lesions in the median eminence of the goat caused a drop in milk yield which could be restored by hormonal mixtures which omitted prolactin (Gale & Larsson, 1963; Gale, 1963), while mammary activation was reported in male rats after the placement of tuberal lesions (De Voe, Ramirez & McCann, 1966). These studies offer a basis for understanding the occurrence of milk secretion in nonparturient women after section of the pituitary stalk, performed to alleviate mammary carcinomas (Ehni & Eckles, 1959) although it should be pointed out that these patients were also receiving regular cortisone therapy.

More interesting, perhaps, is the rare condition of women with spontaneous and persistent milk secretion. In some cases there is no obvious reason for the condition, while in others the state of galactorrhoea can be associated with a pituitary tumour (see Folley, 1960). Three distinct syndromes have, in fact, been reported in the literature. The Chiari–Frommel syndrome occurs post partum after a normal pregnancy and lactation, and here the definition is one of persistent lactation associated with amenorrhoea and a normal sella turcica. In addition, Argonz & del

Castillo (1953) described an entirely distinct syndrome in which the onset of milk secretion is not associated with pregnancy and which can occur in nulliparous women. Here, as in the Chiari–Frommel syndrome, the sella turcica appears normal, but there is a decreased level of urinary gonadotrophin (FSH) and evidence of oestrogenic insufficiency. Forbes, Henneman, Griswold & Albright (1954) described a related syndrome where lactation was, again, spontaneous, but was associated with an enlarged sella turcica, and a pituitary tumour was found to be present in 7 out of the 15 cases investigated by them. This latter syndrome is characterized not only by amenorrhoea, but, as in the Argonz–del Castillo syndrome, also by a decreased urinary FSH level. In a control study on 15 normal post-partum women 9 of whom were nursing, while 8 of the 9 mothers had amenorrhoea, their FSH excretion was normal, and Forbes *et al.* (1954) concluded that the galactorrhoea could be ascribed to overproduction of prolactin at the expense of FSH.

Only in those cases of galactorrhoea, therefore, where a pituitary tumour is present is it possible to arrive at any conclusion as to the cause of the syndrome. In the others, where there appears to be no physical abnormality of the hypothalamus or pituitary, it can only be assumed that the delicate hypothalamic mechanisms which control the pituitary have, in some way as yet unknown, been deranged. Finally, a note of caution should be introduced against too rigid a classification of cases of galactorrhoea into the various syndromes, since Young, Bradley, Goldzieher, Myers & Lecocq (1967) reported on two patients who evolved from the supposedly benign Chiari–Frommel syndrome, through the Argonz–del Castillo syndrome, to the Forbes–Albright syndrome associated with a pituitary tumour.

Activation of prolactin-release mechanisms has been shown to occur after administration of certain steroids and tranquillizing drugs, whose principal site of action appears to be within the hypothalamo-hypophysial system (see Tindal, 1967). Local implants of oestrogen placed in the anterior pituitary of the rabbit (Kanematsu & Sawyer, 1963*a*, *b*) or placed in either the median eminence or anterior pituitary of the rat (Ramirez & McCann, 1964) evoked release of prolactin. However, the tranquillizing drugs reserpine and perphenazine appear to act exclusively at the level of the median eminence (Kanematsu & Sawyer, 1963*c*;

Mishkinsky, Lajtos & Sulman, 1966). More recently, studies in the rabbit have shown that oestrogen can also act at various sites within the amygdaloid complex to evoke prolactin release (Tindal, Knaggs & Turvey, 1967*b*) (see p. 279).

Hypothalamic neurohumours

The earlier studies on transplantation of the pituitary or section of the pituitary stalk suggested that the brain exerted an inhibitory control over prolactin secretion and that the mechanism might involve a substance which was produced in the brain and was conveyed to the anterior pituitary via the hypophysial portal system. As often happens, advance in this particular field had to await the technical development of a suitable system in which this problem could be studied. The answer lay in the *in vitro* culture of the anterior pituitary gland of the rat, and under these conditions it was found that the pituitary could be maintained in a viable state for a considerable period, and that over several days it could produce far more prolactin than was present at the time of autopsy (Meites, Kahn & Nicoll, 1961; Pasteels, 1961*a*). In addition, the secretion of prolactin was enhanced by the presence of oestrogen in the culture medium, which suggested that the steroid could act directly on the pituitary of the rat (Nicoll & Meites, 1962*a*). Indeed, an augmentation of prolactin secretion was also observed if the cultured pituitary was taken from an oestrogen-primed rat (Ratner, Talwalker & Meites, 1963). However, although the facilitatory effect of oestrogen on the pituitary *in vitro* was confirmed by Ben-David, Dikstein & Sulman (1964), Pasteels (1963) found that oestrogen was without effect, while Gala & Reece (1964) reported inhibition of prolactin release *in vitro* by oestrogen. It has also been claimed that the stage of the oestrous cycle at which the donor rat is killed has an influence on the subsequent performance of the pituitary *in vitro*. Thus, pituitaries removed from rats during pro-oestrus or oestrus were reported to release more prolactin *in vitro* than pituitaries removed from rats during dioestrus (Sar & Meites, 1967). In reviewing this field of the *in vitro* secretion of prolactin by the pituitary, Rivera & Kahn (1970) concluded that although oestrogen can modify the secretion of prolactin at both levels of the hypothalamo-hypophysial system, the details of the interactions are far from clear. Recent studies *in vivo* in the rat have shown that the serum level of prolactin during the oestrous cycle is highest during oestrus and lowest during dioestrus, and that low doses of exogenous oestrogen in the ovariectomized rat are more effective than high doses in elevating the level of serum prolactin (Amenomori, Chen & Meites, 1970; Chen & Meites, 1970).

The discovery that the addition of hypothalamic extract or tissue to the incubation medium could inhibit the secretion of prolactin by the cultured pituitary represented the first positive evidence for the nature of the central nervous inhibition of prolactin secretion (Pasteels, 1961*b*, 1963; Danon, Dikstein & Sulman, 1963; Talwalker, Ratner & Meites, 1963). It was also found that the inhibitory action of the hypothalamus on prolactin secretion *in vitro* was itself inhibited by perphenazine, either by adding the drug directly to the incubation medium or by using hypothalami from perphenazine-primed rats (Danon *et al.*, 1963), an effect later extended to reserpine (Ratner, Talwaker & Meites, 1965). The, as yet, unknown substance in hypothalamic tissue has been termed prolactin-inhibiting factor (PIF), and is not identical with oxytocin, vasopressin, adrenaline, noradrenaline, acetylcholine, 5-hydroxytryptamine, histamine, substance P or bradykinin (Talwalker, Ratner & Meites, 1963). There is some doubt as to whether PIF is identical with luteinizing hormone-releasing factor (LRF). Although Schally, Meites, Bowers & Ratner (1964) and Arimura, Saito, Müller, Bowers, Sawano & Schally (1967) could find no PIF activity in purified LRF preparations, Dhariwal, Grosvenor, Antunes-Rodrigues & McCann (1968) were not able to demonstrate a clear-cut separation between LRF and PIF activity in highly purified hypothalamic extract. If these two factors are small molecules with similar molecular weights and possibly even similar structures, this obviously poses great problems in their separation from each other.

As regards the effect of the suckling stimulus on the hypothalamus, Ratner & Meites (1964) could not detect PIF activity in the hypothalamus of suckled rats, and concluded that suckling depleted the hypothalamic concentration of PIF. In contrast to this, crude hypothalamic extracts prepared from as little as one third of a rat hypothalamus, taken from rats either before or after they were suckled, inhibited suckling-induced release of prolactin in the rat, and it was suggested that the suckling stimulus elicited prolactin release in the rat, not by destroying, but by

hypothalamus exerted a facilitatory, rather than an inhibitory, effect on prolactin secretion in the sheep and goat. This claim was based on the fact that lesions of the ventromedial hypothalamus caused a fall in milk yield, which could not be restored by prolactin alone but which could be restored by administration of the hormonal combination of prolactin, somatotrophin and ACTH. However, it had previously been shown that both prolactin and somatotrophin are essential members of the galactopoietic complex in the hypophysectomized lactating goat (Cowie & Tindal, 1961*b*; Cowie, Knaggs & Tindal, 1964). In addition, after lesions of the median eminence or after surgical stalk section in the goat, the pituitary gland is capable of producing considerable quantities of prolactin, and under these conditions hormonal combinations which contain somatotrophin but which exclude prolactin can restore milk secretion (Gale, 1963; Cowie, Daniel, Knaggs, Prichard & Tindal, 1964). Since Domański *et al.* (1967) did not administer hormonal combinations which excluded prolactin, their claim in support of a hypothalamic facilitation of prolactin release in the ruminant is based on faulty reasoning and can be dismissed.

Evidence of an indirect nature has been marshalled to support the idea of prolactin releasing activity in the hypothalamus of the rat to explain the extremely rapid drop in pituitary prolactin content which has been reported to occur within less than one minute following stress, or within two minutes of the start of suckling (Grosvenor, McCann & Nallar, 1965; Grosvenor, Mena & Schaefgen, 1967). Grosvenor, Mena, Dhariwal & McCann (1967) concluded from this that inhibition of PIF action alone did not offer a satisfactory explanation and that certain stimuli may activate a prolactin releasing factor (PRF) of hypothalamic origin which may overide the inhibitory action of PIF. However, it would seem that a more detailed analysis of the role of PIF in the processes of prolactin synthesis and prolactin release will be necessary before this view could be accepted without reservation.

Another claim for the presence of prolactin-releasing activity in rat hypothalamus was based on the observation that extracts of hypothalami or pituitaries taken from lactating rats exert a greater mammogenic action in oestrogen-primed virgin rats than similar extracts prepared from virgin rats (Mishkinsky, Khazen & Sulman, 1968). However, crude extracts of rat hypothalamus had previously been shown to initiate lactation in the rat (Meites, Talwalker & Nicoll, 1960), yet in restrospect this effect was considered to be non-specific, or at best indirect, possibly caused by the FSH-RF content of the extract evoking release of oestrogen, which itself could cause release of prolactin (see Meites, 1966). As regards the greater mammogenic activity of the pituitary glands taken from lactating, as against virgin, rats (Mishkinsky *et al.*, 1968), it is known that suckling, as well as oestradiol or reserpine will deplete the rat's hypothalamus of PIF (Ratner & Meites, 1964; Ratner, Talwalker & Meites, 1965) which suggests that the pituitary glands taken from lactating rats would have been in a more active state of prolactin elaboration than those from virgin animals and might, therefore, have been expected to elicit greater mammogenic activity than those taken from virgin rats.

Recently, it has been reported (Desclin & Flament-Durand, 1969) that when a pituitary gland was transplanted into the hypothalamus of the rat, the systemic administration of reserpine only stimulated the acidophil cells when the graft was placed in a discrete midline region. This included, but extended slightly more dorsal and rostral than the hypophysiotrophic area of Halász, Pupp & Uhlarik (1962). Desclin & Flament-Durand (1969) considered that their results could not be explained solely on the basis of a depression of PIF activity and that they seemed to imply the presence of a stimulating factor. This may well be so, but the possibility should be borne in mind that the reserpine might gain access to the graft more readily in medial sites by diffusion from the CSF in the third ventricle. At this stage of knowledge it would be wise, perhaps, to keep an open mind on the subject, at least until a purified extract of mammalian hypothalamic tissue has been demonstrated to possess specific prolactin-releasing activity. Indeed the whole problem of the neurohumoral control of adenohypophysial function can be fully understood only when the structures of the neurohumours are known and when pure, synthetic material is available for investigation.

It should be noted that in contrast to the now well-established concept of hypothalamic inhibition of prolactin secretion in the mammal, this is not so in the bird. Thus, prolactin secretion is not stimulated by *in vitro* culture of the pituitary (Nicoll & Meites, 1962*b*), by transplantation of the pituitary (Ma & Nalbandov, 1963) or by pituitary stalk section (Assenmacher & Tixier-Vidal,

1964). Also, the hypothalamus of the bird does not possess prolactin-inhibiting activity, but does contain prolactin-releasing activity. This has been demonstrated in the pigeon (Kragt & Meites, 1965), the tricoloured blackbird (Nicoll, 1965*b*), the duck (Gourdji & Tixier-Vidal, 1966), the chicken and the quail (Kragt, 1966) and turkey (Chen, Bixler, Weber & Meites, 1968). The implications of this paradox are not yet fully understood. Of particular interest, of course, are the central nervous mechanisms by which environmental stimuli trigger the release of prolactin, since this hormone plays such an important role in incubation and rearing of the young in certain avian species (see Lehrman, 1965, 1967; Friedman & Lehrman, 1968; Bern & Nicoll, 1968).

As regards the mode of action of hypothalamic neurohumours, McCann & Porter (1969) pointed out that a principal action of releasing factors might be the specific depolarization of the pituitary cell membrane by a particular releasing factor, a process associated with the uptake of Ca^{++} which could activate the release of storage granules. Conversely, they suggest that in the case of prolactin-secreting cells, the action of PIF might be a hyperpolarization and hence an inhibition of release. Whatever differences may exist between the release mechanisms of prolactin on the one hand and the remaining anterior pituitary hormones on the other, the final step would appear to be similar, since the presence of Ca^{++} has been shown to be vital for the release not only of the gonadotrophins but also of prolactin (Wakabayashi, Kamberi & McCann, 1969; Parsons, 1969). McCann & Porter (1969) acknowledge that their view of the mode of action of releasing and inhibiting factors may be grossly oversimplified. Nevertheless, it has the merit of underlining the fact that the hypothalamus is, after all, a part of the central nervous system and serves as a reminder that basal hypothalamic mechanisms may well be activated by action potentials just as much as by circulating target-organ hormones.

More recently, this concept of the mode of action of releasing factors has been strengthened by the report of Milligan & Kraicer (1970), who incubated rat adenohypophyses in a medium containing potassium ion in sufficient concentration to provoke release of several of the trophic hormones. This release was accompanied, in more than half the cells investigated, by a reversed, positive transmembrane potential. They concluded that this finding was consistent with a process of 'stimulus-secretion coupling' in which hypothalamic releasing factors act by selective depolarization of their 'target' cells and that the positive potentials may be due to a prolonged preferential permeability to calcium ions, triggered by an initial depolarization of the cell membrane to a threshold value by increased external potassium ion.

Feedback control of prolactin secretion

Whereas target organ hormones are released into the circulation in response to several of the pituitary trophic hormones, in the case of prolactin there is no known hormone produced by its principal target, the mammary gland, and hence no target-organ feedback effect for the control of the output of prolactin. However, in recent years it has become clear that another type of feedback mechanism exists, termed a 'short' feedback, in which a particular trophic hormone can act on the hypothalamus to limit its own rate of secretion and/or release (see Martini, Fraschini & Motta, 1968; Motta, Fraschini & Martini, 1969). The first evidence to suggest that there may be a 'short' feedback for prolactin came from studies on rats bearing transplanted prolactin-secreting tumours. In such animals the prolactin concentration in the pituitary, assessed by gel electrophoresis, was greatly reduced, while in rats bearing transplanted somatotrophin-secreting tumours, the level of pituitary somatotrophin was reduced (MacLeod, Smith & DeWitt, 1966). A similar reduction in host pituitary prolactin content in rats bearing transplanted prolactin-secreting tumours was reported by Chen, Minaguchi & Meites (1967) who also found an elevated level of PIF in the hypothalamus of the tumour-bearing animals. The concept that a high circulating level of prolactin, produced by the tumours, may have been responsible for depressing the synthesis of prolactin by the pituitary and raising the concentration of PIF in the hypothalamus was supported by a similar effect following prolonged systemic adminis-tration of prolactin (Sinha & Tucker, 1968), or the presence of transplanted pituitary glands (Mena, Maiweg & Grosvenor, 1968; Welsch, Negro-Vilar & Meites, 1968). The 'short' feedback mechanism for prolactin received conclusive proof when it was found that a local implant of prolactin in the median eminence of the rat depressed pituitary prolactin concentration and raised the level of PIF in the hypothalamus (Clemens & Meites, 1968).

Furthermore, while an implant of prolactin in the median eminence depressed lactation, the depression was even more severe when the implant contained both prolactin and ACTH (Clemens, Sar & Meites, 1969). This indicated that the secretion of both of the two trophic hormones known to be essential for milk secretion in the hypophysectomized rat (Bintarningsih, Lyons, Johnson & Li, 1957, 1958; Cowie, 1957) can exert a negative-feedback effect on their own release, at least under these experimental conditions. It has also been found that when exogenous oestrogen is administered to a rat bearing an implant of prolactin in the median eminence, that a low level of oestrogen (1 μg oestradiol benzoate/day) was unable to counteract the effect of the prolactin implant on the content of pituitary prolactin. A dose of 5 μg/day was only partially effective, while 10 μg/day was as effective in increasing anterior pituitary prolactin levels whether a prolactin implant was present in the median eminence or not. The prolactin implant had apparently raised the threshold for the action of oestrogen on prolactin secretion and it was suggested that circulating levels of prolactin might also alter the action of oestrogen on the anterior pituitary and hypothalamus (Welsch, Sar, Clemens & Meites, 1968). In addition to causing an increase in hypothalamic PIF level, the local implantation of prolactin in the median eminence of the rat has also been reported to lead to reduced mammary development in the oestrogen-primed virgin rat (Mishkinsky, Nir & Sulman, 1969) and to elicit release of FSH and to cause the onset of precocious puberty in the young female rat (Clemens, Minaguchi, Storey, Voogt & Meites, 1969; Voogt, Clemens & Meites, 1969).

Sgouris & Meites (1953) suggested that removal of prolactin from the circulation by the lactating mammary gland might be a factor in the stimulation of prolactin synthesis by the pituitary, in the sense of the removal of a negative feedback. Prolactin undoubtedly can exert control over its own secretion under the experimental conditions outlined above, but it remains to be proved whether such a mechanism has a role to play in the control of prolactin secretion in the normal animal. It has not yet been shown that the level of circulating prolactin in the normal animal reaches a sufficiently high level to elicit a negative-feedback effect, which may possibly only be manifested under extreme conditions, and may be a type of emergency mechanism.

While the mechanisms involved in the release of prolactin have been the subject of intense investigation, the re-charging of the pituitary gland with prolactin following suckling has received scant attention. Recent work, however, suggests that this may not be an entirely passive process. In the intact rat, two hours of suckling reduced the pituitary prolactin content by 88·5%, and the prolactin content of the pituitary increased gradually during the post-suckling interval, to achieve the pre-suckling level after 8 hours. However, if the pituitary gland is removed from a rat immediately after suckling and cultured *in vitro* for two hours, prolactin repletion does not occur (Convey & Reece, 1969), which suggested that some influence is exerted *in vivo* to favour the post-suckling synthesis of prolactin. In this respect it has been noted that if hypothalamic extract is injected into a rat immediately after suckling, then there is an increased rate of post-suckling reaccumulation of prolactin (Grosvenor, Maiweg & Mena, 1969a). While the effect of the hypothalamic extract could be mimicked by a single subcutaneous injection of 2 mg ovine prolactin given after suckling, the injection of 4 mg ovine prolactin increased pituitary prolactin concentration to a level considerably higher than that observed before suckling. Also, whereas purified PIF had the ability to block suckling-induced release of prolactin if given before suckling, when it was injected after suckling it had no effect on the rate of reaccumulation of prolactin by the pituitary. Since the effect of prolactin implants in the median eminence is to decrease prolactin secretion, it should be pointed out that this facilitatory effect of circulating prolactin on the rate of re-accumulation of the hormone appears to be a short-term phenomenon, operating over a period of hours. Grosvenor *et al.* (1969a) concluded that prolactin regulates its own rate of synthesis in the post-suckling period through the mediation of a factor or factors in the hypothalamus. This may be the correct interpretation, but nevertheless there is an alternative explanation. In the light of present knowledge concerning the negative feedback action of high circulating levels of prolactin on the release of this hormone, the results of Grosvenor *et al.* (1969a) could be explained on the basis of an inhibition of a succession of trivial releases, or a continuous low-level release, of prolactin in response to non-specific environmental stimuli in the inter-suckling period, and hence an apparent increase in the rate of reaccumulation.

The suckling and milking stimulus

In 1934, Selye proposed that the act of suckling stimulated the production of prolactin. Subsequently, this was confirmed by reports of a fall in prolactin content of the pituitary when a lactating rat was suckled by her litter after being isolated from them for 10 hours (Grosvenor & Turner, 1957b, 1958b). The suckling stimulus has also been found to cause discharge of ACTH in the rat (Grégoire, 1946; Voogt, Sar & Meites, 1969), goat and sheep (Denamur, Stoliaroff & Desclin, 1965), STH in the rat (Grosvenor, Krulich & McCann, 1968; Tucker & Thatcher, 1968; Sar & Meites, 1969), melanophore-stimulating hormone in the rat (Taleisnik & Orías, 1966), but not of TSH in the rat (Sar & Meites, 1969). In addition, cytological evidence has indicated that the anterior pituitary is activated by the suckling stimulus (Pasteels, 1963). After lactating rats had been separated from their litters for 10 hours, the erythrosinophil prolactin cells were observed to become engorged with granules. A brief period of suckling after the 10-hour separation led to severe degranulation without affecting the size or number of these cells. Electron microscopy revealed that prolactin granules were excreted from the pole of the cell into the perisinusoidal spaces (Pasteels, 1963) and prolactin granules continued to be excreted for about one hour after the end of nursing (R. E. Smith, quoted by Grosvenor, McCann & Nallar, 1965). The release of prolactin in the lactating rat is related to the intensity of the suckling stimulus since two pups are insufficient to trigger measurable release of prolactin from the pituitary, although it is not denied that some may be released (Mena & Grosvenor, 1968). Similarly, the suckling of only two teats by two pups is insufficient to maintain lactation in the rat (Edwardson & Eayrs, 1967). At the hypothalamic level, suckling has been shown to depress the release both of luteinizing hormone-releasing factor and prolactin-inhibiting factor, leading to inhibition of LH release and facilitation of prolactin release from the pituitary, respectively (Minaguchi & Meites, 1967; Sar & Meites, 1969). The most direct and unequivocal evidence for release of prolactin during suckling or milking would, of course, be the measurement of levels of the circulating hormone. For many years this goal remained unattainable owing to the relatively poor sensitivity of existing assay methods for prolactin, but the recent development of highly sensitive and specific radioimmunoassay techniques (see p. 74) has at last made it possible to measure, in several species, the level of circulating prolactin in the blood.

In the sheep, Arai & Lee (1967) found a control level of 100 ng prolactin/ml. plasma in samples taken from 8 non-pregnant animals. A further 6 sheep were each sampled a total of 6 times at intervals varying from 1 to 3 months from the beginning of pregnancy to the end of lactation. Prolactin titres fell to low levels by the end of pregnancy, rose at parturition and continued to rise, reaching a peak of approximately 300 ng prolactin/ml. plasma in the third month of lactation, and declined thereafter to the control level by the fifth month of lactation. There was considerable variation in the prolactin content of samples taken at the same reproductive stage in the different animals, as evidenced by the high values given for the standard deviations. In the cow, Schams & Karg (1969) took blood samples 4 times a day for several weeks in the period preceding parturition, and reported a rapid rise at parturition to a level of 300–350 ng prolactin/ml. plasma. During the first two weeks of lactation prolactin levels were lower than at parturition, and there appeared to be a random variation in plasma prolactin titres, ranging from extremely small amounts up to 130 ng/ml. plasma, which suggests the necessity for known and accurate timing of blood samples in relation to environmental stimuli.

Bryant, Greenwood & Linzell (1968) measured plasma prolactin levels in the goat by radioimmunoassay. In 28 random blood samples taken from intact and castrated goats of both sexes, the levels ranged from less than 4 to 300 ng/ml. plasma. This emphasizes the need for information on the causes of fluctuation in the plasma level of prolactin, and on what is the baseline level, if any, of this hormone. In a later study (Bryant, Linzell & Greenwood, 1970), the effect of hand milking was studied in 4 lactating goats. This stimulus caused a rise in plasma prolactin concentration in all 4 animals between one and ten minutes after milking. In one of them, 7 venous samples taken at approximately hourly intervals throughout the day had prolactin concentrations between 55 and 275 ng/ml. plasma, except for an additional sample taken 10 minutes after the afternoon milking, when the level rose to 735 ng/ml. plasma. In two of the animals the apparent rise in plasma prolactin level following milking was less than had occurred spontaneously one hour before milking, and Bryant *et al.* (1970) point out that continuous blood sampling before, during and after teat stimulation will be necessary for a quantitative assessment of prolactin release.

The relationship between the milking process and the level of circulating prolactin in the ruminant has been investigated in the greatest detail, up to now, by Johke (1969*a*) in a series of experiments involving 9 cows and 2 goats. Seven cows were machine milked, while the other two, and the two goats, were hand milked. Venepuncture and the insertion of an indwelling polyethylene cannula in an external jugular vein was carried out approximately one hour prior to milking. Blood samples were taken from this time until $1\frac{1}{2}$–2 hours after milking, the frequency of sampling being greatest during the milking procedure. In seven of the cows (Fig. 6.10) (including the two hand-milked animals), and both

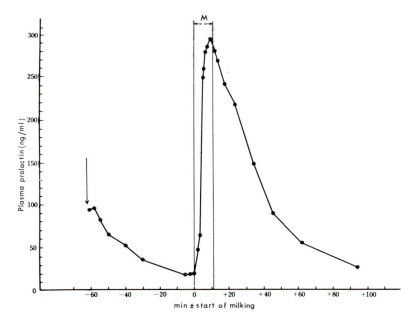

Fig. 6.10. Effect of machine milking (M) on plasma prolactin concentration in the cow. Venepuncture and cannulation of an external jugular vein, denoted by vertical arrow, was performed 60 min before milking. Note the abrupt rise in plasma prolactin during milking; also the smaller, apparent, rise associated with venepuncture and cannulation (from Johke, T., 1969*a*, *Endocr. jap.* **16**, 179–185).

goats, plasma prolactin levels increased abruptly within 1–2 min of the start of milking, while in the other 2 cows the prolactin level rose shortly before the onset of milking (Fig. 6.11). The

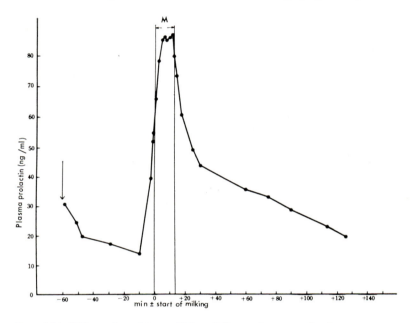

FIG. 6.11. Effect of machine milking (M) on plasma prolactin concentration in the cow. Venepuncture and cannulation of an external jugular vein, denoted by vertical arrow, was performed 60 min before milking. In this animal, stimuli other than milking itself, but presumably associated with preparation for the milking routine, appeared to trigger the release of prolactin (from Johke, T., 1969a, *Endocr. jap.* **16**, 179–185).

goats, which were in mid-lactation, showed maximum prolactin levels of 545 and 290 ng/ml. plasma (Fig. 6.12). In the group of cows, the stages of early, middle and late lactation were all represented. Their maximum prolactin levels ranged between 26 and 293 ng/ml. plasma with a marked tendency for there to be a much smaller release of prolactin towards the end of lactation. This latter feature bears a similarity to earlier findings in the lactating rat in which, after 10 hours isolation from the mother, suckling by the litter will induce a drop in pituitary prolactin content, at least up to the 14th day of lactation, but will not do so on the 21st day

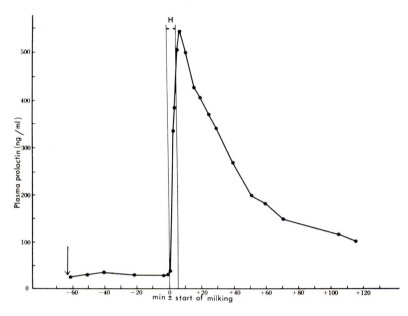

Fig. 6.12. Effect of hand milking (H) on plasma prolactin concentration in the goat. Venepuncture and cannulation of an external jugular vein, denoted by vertical arrow, was performed 60 min before milking. Note the abrupt rise in plasma prolactin level during and immediately after milking (from Johke, T., 1969*a*, *Endocr. jap.* **16**, 179–185).

(Grosvenor & Turner, 1958*b*). Also, suckling will cause this drop in pituitary prolactin content after 8 hours isolation, but not if the 7-day-old pups have been isolated from the mother for 16 hours, and it has been suggested that there may be a link between an increasing length of period between natural sucklings and the decline of lactation (Grosvenor, Mena & Schaefgen, 1967). However, not only the timing, but also the quality of the stimulus, may be important. Thus, in the rabbit, where lactose synthesis has been correlated with the amount of circulating prolactin, natural suckling is more potent than hand milking in stimulating the synthesis of lactose, and hence, by inference, the release of prolactin (Gachev, 1968*a*).

Until recently, investigation of the release of prolactin in response to suckling in the rat has been confined to measurements of pituitary prolactin content. The development of a radio-immunoassay for rat prolactin (see p. 77) has now made it possible to measure the level of serum prolactin directly. Removal of litters from rats on the 4th day post partum for 3 hours resulted in a rapid decline in serum prolactin to a level of 8·3 ng/ml. When litters of 10 pups each were returned to their mothers for a 30-minute suckling period after being isolated from their mothers for 12 hours, the serum prolactin level rose to 130 ng/ml. and pituitary prolactin content fell. Regular suckling by litters which remained with their mothers was found to maintain both high pituitary and high serum prolactin levels (Amenomori, Chen & Meites, 1970).

Release of prolactin in response to conditioned stimuli

As is now known to be the case for oxytocin (see Chapter 5), the release of prolactin can occur in response to stimuli other than, although associated with, the suckling or milking stimulus. Thus, the two cows in which release of prolactin occurred just before the start of milking (Johke, 1969a) illustrate this point very neatly (see Fig. 6.11), although it is not clear whether the tactile stimuli of washing the udder and foremilking, or visual or auditory stimuli arising from the milking personnel was the actual trigger in these cases.

More than twenty years ago, Freud & Uyldert (1948) reported on the existence of conditioned reflexes in the lactating rat. Rats were brought into lactation by treatment with oestrogen and were given litters to nurse. It was found that animals which had recently undergone a normal lactation had a better lactational performance than those which had either not littered previously, or had not done so for some time. This difference in performance during the subsequent artificially-induced lactation was also apparent when primiparous rats were either allowed to rear their litter normally or were separated from their pups at parturition. This association of a better lactational performance with recent suckling experience in the rat foreshadowed more recent work in this species, in which the release of prolactin in response to conditioned stimuli was assessed by measuring changes in pituitary prolactin content. When a primiparous lactating rat was isolated from her 14-day-old litter for several hours and was then placed over them, but separated physically by a wire-mesh screen, the mere presence of the pups triggered the release of prolactin, just as if the mother had been suckled (Grosvenor, 1965*b*). This conditioned release of prolactin in response to, as yet, unidentified stimuli which could be visual, auditory or olfactory, does not occur if the rat pups are only 7 days old (unpublished observations, quoted by Grosvenor & Mena, 1967). The critical time for the appearance of the conditioned release appears to be when the pups are about 10 days old, and studies carried out over two successive lactations showed that the conditioned release mechanism was retained and carried over into the 2nd lactation (Grosvenor, Maiweg & Mena, 1969*b*, 1970). The external cue which triggers the onset of the conditioned release at about the 10th day of the first lactation has not yet been identified. It might, of course, be associated with increasing vigour and activity of the pups, although auditory stimuli do not appear to be vital since freshly-killed non-moving pups can trigger the release of prolactin (Grosvenor, 1969).

In a related study, Moltz, Levin & Leon (1969) claimed that in the post-partum rat which had been thelectomized before its first pregnancy, the physical presence of the pups or contact with the mother will cause release of prolactin. This was assessed by the deciduoma response and by the arrest of the oestrous cycle. However, the experimental design did not include a group of thelectomized animals deprived of pups, and hence did not exclude the possibility of post-surgical irritation of the proximal ends of the severed afferent nerves which had innervated the teats. It is known that physical irritation of afferent paths within the central nervous system can evoke release of prolactin (Relkin, 1967; Tindal & Knaggs, 1969) and until proved otherwise the interpretation of Moltz *et al.* (1969) warrants a degree of caution. There is little doubt that problems such as this will be resolved now that circulating levels of prolactin can be measured, and what appear to be major differences at present may well prove to be a matter of degree. The preliminary study of Bryant *et al.* (1968) in the goat gave some indication of the, apparently, random variations in blood prolactin levels in response to unknown stimuli of external or internal origin, and a more complete picture will be necessary before deciding whether the amounts of prolactin released in the experiment of Moltz *et al.* (1969) would have been sufficient to maintain lactation, or whether they represented relatively trivial amounts which may be associated with non-specific stimuli, as was found to be the case for venepuncture in the cow, where prolactin levels rose to one third of the value seen during the subsequent milking (Johke, 1969a).

Other signals concerned with prolactin release

In addition to suckling or milking and environmental stimuli associated with them, prolactin release can occur in response to other stimuli. In the rabbit, for instance, the act of mating leads to a depletion, not only of LH, but also of prolactin and ACTH from the pituitary (Desjardins, Kirton & Hafs, 1967). Of more immediate interest, perhaps, was the earlier observation that massage of the mammary gland of the sow before the first service caused significant development of the mammary glands (Kudryav-stev & Glebina, 1941). A quarter of a century later similar findings were made in the rat, where self-licking of the nipples during preg-nancy led to a greater degree of mammary development at parturition than occurred if licking was prevented by a collar (Roth & Rosenblatt, 1966, 1968), which suggested a licking-induced release of prolactin. The failure of self-licking in the rat to deplete pituitary prolactin stores by a measurable amount (Grosvenor & Mena, 1969) does not invalidate this concept, since a small but continuous release may not be detectable by bioassay, when compared with the dramatic fall in pituitary prolactin content which is caused by suckling. Parallel observations in the goat have shown that regular application of the 'milking' stimulus to the teats of the virgin animal causes mammary development to occur, followed by the onset of milk secretion (Cowie, Knaggs, Tindal & Turvey, 1968) which, again, is indicative of a significant level of circulating prolactin, and possibly other pituitary hor-mones, in response to manipulation of the teat (see p. 118).

Thus, the prolactin-release mechanism casts its sensory net not merely over the suckling stimulus, but includes quite a repertoire of stimuli. Indeed, as far as the female rat is concerned, the sug-gestion has been made that she may utilize different stimuli in succession as her physiological status changes, moving from self-licking in pregnancy to the suckling stimulus post partum, which, in turn, is replaced by exteroceptive stimuli other than suckling later on in lactation (Grosvenor & Mena, 1969).

Another mechanism for prolactin release which has been pro-posed was that of Benson & Folley (1956, 1957), who suggested oxytocin as a possible prolactin-releasing agent. The balance of evidence at the moment seems not to favour this concept, although there is a certain amount of evidence to suggest that oxytocin administration can, at least in cattle, alter pituitary function with respect to gonadotrophin secretion (for reviews see Folley, 1963; Meites, Nicoll & Talwalker, 1963; Benson & Fitzpatrick, 1966; Meites & Nicoll, 1966; Hansel, 1967).

While discussing the stimuli which can affect the release of prolactin, it would be appropriate to mention a central nervous mechanism which can inhibit release of this hormone in the mouse. Thus, when a mouse, which is in the first four days of pregnancy to a particular male, is brought into proximity with another male of either the same or another strain of mouse, pregnancy is blocked (Bruce, 1959, 1960). This block was later found to be the result of the failure of prolactin secretion and to be caused by olfactory stimuli emanating from the male (see Parkes & Bruce, 1961). This mechanism, which appears to be restricted to the mouse, is rather a special case, since, in general, environmental stimuli stimulate rather than inhibit prolactin secretion. It is noteworthy that in the lactating rat, while apparently trivial environmental stresses such as human conversation will inhibit the release of oxytocin in response to the suckling stimulus, the release of prolactin remains unimpaired (Grosvenor & Mena, 1967). In the natural state, such an arrangement would have obvious survival value, since although milk ejection and feeding the young may have to be postponed temporarily in the presence of adverse conditions, the secretion of milk, governed to a large extent by the circulating level of prolactin, must go on.

In recent years the dividing line between the effects of stress and of the suckling or milking stimulus has become increasingly blurred. At one extreme, the exposure of oestrogen-primed female rats to various noxious stimuli such as cold, heat, restraint or injection of formalin, all of which are known to release ACTH, caused initiation of milk secretion, which suggested that prolactin had been released as well as ACTH (Nicoll, Talwalker & Meites, 1960). Also, the stresses of laparotomy and bleeding under ether anaesthesia or stunning and decapitation were found to be just as effective as the suckling stimulus in causing discharge of prolactin from the rat's pituitary, and careful handling prior to killing the animals was essential if unintentional prolactin depletion of the pituitary was to be avoided (Grosvenor, McCann & Nallar, 1965).

This latter point is underlined by the fact that the olfactory-induced pregnancy block in mice can itself be inhibited by appropriate daily handling of the mice (Bruce, Land & Falconer, 1968). Even the relatively mild procedure of venepuncture in the cow appeared to be a sufficient stimulus to cause elevation of the prolactin level in the plasma (Johke, 1969a).

At the other extreme, we are faced with the fact that in the species studied so far not only does the milking or suckling stimulus cause elevation of blood prolactin levels in both the cow and the goat and depletion of the pituitary prolactin content in the rat (Johke, 1969a; Grosvenor & Turner, 1957b), but it also evokes a rapid discharge of ACTH from the pituitary of the rat (Voogt, Sar & Meites, 1969), sheep and goat, which is claimed to be proportionally as great in the latter two species as that caused by stress in the rat (Denamur, Stoliaroff & Desclin, 1965). Thus, the release of ACTH, which was originally thought to be the preserve of stressful stimuli, is now seen to apply equally to the application of the suckling or milking stimulus.

This apparent paradox appears more logical when considered in the context of a recent attempt to explain why the suckling or milking stimulus was effective in triggering the neuroendocrine milk-ejection reflex, while other tactile stimuli were generally ineffective. When the neuroanatomical and neurophysiological evidence was examined in detail it became clear that, of necessity, the tactile stimulus to the teat must be of an alerting or mildly stressful nature if it was to succeed in eliciting release of oxytocin from the neurohypophysis (see Tindal & Knaggs, 1970a). The nature of the stimulus has to be such as to overcome a considerable physiological 'resistance' in order to achieve oxytocin release, and in the light of present knowledge once this level of stimulation is employed it is hardly surprising that both prolactin and ACTH are released concomitantly. As far as the lactating animal is concerned, this might be considered as a rather appropriate stress response to the demands imposed on the body by a metabolic emergency, lactation.

The suckling stimulus and the maintenance of lactation

The importance of the neuroendocrine milk-ejection reflex for the removal of milk in different species has already been described. Having considered some of the factors governing release of prolactin from the anterior pituitary it would be appropriate at this point to consider how important the suckling or milking stimulus is for anterior pituitary activation to occur in those species so far investigated. There is now convincing evidence that the suckling stimulus is essential for the maintenance of lactation both in the rat (Eayrs & Baddeley, 1956) and cat (Beyer, Mena, Pacheco & Alcaraz, 1962*a*). Lactation was arrested in both species after spinal cord section, and was not restored in the cat even when milk ejection was induced with exogenous oxytocin (Beyer *et al.*, 1962*a*). After detailed studies of mammary gland innervation in the rat, it was found that severance of the appropriate spinal roots led to the complete failure of both milk ejection and milk secretion (Edwardson & Eayrs, 1967; J. A. Edwardson, unpublished results, quoted by Edwardson & Eayrs, 1967). There had been a report that lactation could continue at a reduced level in the cord-sectioned rat, provided that the operation is performed at mid-lactation when the pups are vigorous, and that oxytocin is administered (Grosvenor, 1964). However, in view of the later finding that release of prolactin can occur in response to stimuli arising from the litter, other than the suckling stimulus (see Grosvenor, Maiweg & Mena, 1969*b*), there seems little doubt that such a mechanism could have accounted for Grosvenor's (1964) findings. Since the view taken by the present authors is that the question of necessity or otherwise for the suckling stimulus must apply from the start of lactation, then the suckling stimulus is vital for the maintenance of milk secretion in the rat.

As previously stated (see p. 190) the milk-ejection reflex is not essential for milk removal in the sheep and goat, and may be less important than considered hitherto in the cow. As regards the maintenance of milk secretion, the release of anterior pituitary hormones also does not depend on the suckling or milking stimulus in these species. In the goat (Tverskoï, 1953) and cow (Mielke & Brabant, 1963), normal milk yields are obtained if the teats are permanently cannulated and the mammary glands are evacuated by regular administration of posterior pituitary extract or oxytocin. Furthermore, in the goat and sheep, lactation can continue in the absence of any nervous connexions between mammary gland and central nervous system (see p. 190 for references).

The rabbit appears to occupy an intermediate position between the rat and cat on the one hand and the ruminants on the other, since although the milk-ejection reflex is necessary for milk removal (see p. 190) the suckling stimulus may not be essential for anterior pituitary activation to occur. Provided exogenous oxytocin is administered to eject the milk, milk secretion continues quite normally when the lactating rabbit is anaesthetized deeply with barbiturate immediately prior to and during the once-daily suckling period (Tindal, Beyer & Sawyer, 1963), and the same holds true when such a regime is begun at parturition (Findlay & Roth, 1970). Although lactation in the rabbit is inhibited by spinal section and is only partially restored by oxytocin, the milk yield can be restored if, in addition to oxytocin, either prolactin or ACTH are injected for a few days (Mena & Beyer, 1963). Furthermore, once milk secretion is restored, it is maintained even after the trophic hormone is withdrawn (Mena & Beyer, 1963). It is clear, therefore, that in at least three species so far investigated, the goat, sheep and rabbit, a mechanism exists within the body which acts independently of the suckling or milking stimulus to ensure the secretion of the trophic hormones essential for the maintenance of milk secretion. While such a mechanism may not be the sole endocrine regulator of milk secretion in these species and may merely serve as an auxiliary mechanism in the normal animal, its nature must now be considered.

Possible internal mechanisms regulating trophic hormone release in the lactating animal

Many years ago it was suggested that the lactating mammary gland might destroy prolactin, and that by doing so, the reduced level of circulating prolactin might favour the further secretion of prolactin (Sgouris & Meites, 1953; Tverskoĭ, 1957). While it is now known that high circulating levels of prolactin can exert an effect at the hypothalamic level to depress release of prolactin from the pituitary (Clemens & Meites, 1968) it is by no means certain, at present, that the reverse is the case and the question can best be answered by detailed studies of the circulating level of prolactin in lactating and non-lactating animals. Another suggestion which has been made is that the mammary gland releases an unknown humoral agent into the blood stream which might exert a positive feedback action at the hypothalamic level (Sgouris & Meites, 1953; Grosvenor, 1964). Again, there is no evidence either to support or refute this.

A more general approach to the problem was proposed by Denamur & Martinet (1960), who suggested that systemic stimuli might be associated with the physiological mechanism involved in the demands of the mammary gland for water, metabolites and hormones, and that such stimuli might act either directly on the anterior pituitary or at the level of the hypothalamus. A more specific proposal was put forward by Cowie & Tindal (1965), in terms of the great demands made on the body's resources by the abstraction of milk precursors from the blood stream. Such a view is not unrealistic, indeed Kronfeld (1969) even considers that the mammary gland can be seen as an aggressive commensal whose demands on the host's metabolism may be excessive. Cowie & Tindal (1965) envisaged that the increased maternal food intake accompanying a high level of milk secretion might be the key, since appetite-regulating mechanisms are known to reside in the hypothalamus. If the 'hunger centre' in the lateral hypothalamus and the 'satiety centre' in the ventromedial region can be controlled metabolically, there seems no valid reason, in theory, why metabolic activation should not also apply to the trophic hormone-release mechanisms in the hypothalamus, and even possibly the limbic system. Tindal (1967) pointed out that the study of Mena & Beyer (1963) on the cord-sectioned rabbit supported this view since, once lactation was restored either by ACTH or prolactin, it became self-maintaining, suggesting that above a certain critical level of milk synthesis, metabolite utilization may be able to elicit the release of prolactin and/or ACTH.

In the goat, it is interesting that both prolactin and somatotrophin (STH) are of equal importance in the maintenance of milk secretion (Cowie & Tindal, 1961*b*; Cowie, Knaggs & Tindal, 1964). It may be relevant that STH is now known to be released in response to the metabolic needs of the body, at least in man (Roth, Glick, Yalow & Berson, 1963*a, b*; see Pecile & Müller, 1966). However, much remains to be learnt of the physiological factors which govern the secretion of somatotrophin (see Baylis, Greenwood, James, Jenkins, Landon, Marks & Samols, 1968), although the final control mechanism appears to reside in the hypophysiotrophic area of the hypothalamus (Halász, 1968) and is mediated by both a releasing (Deuben & Meites, 1964) and an inhibiting factor (Krulich, Dhariwal & McCann, 1968).

There is, then, a basis for supposing that metabolic activation may play an ancillary role to the suckling or milking stimulus in causing release of the trophic hormones necessary for the maintenance of lactation. Furthermore, it may be purely coincidental, but the species to which such a mechanism might apply are the ones in which a relatively long interval between successive milk removals either occurs naturally, as in the rabbit, or can be tolerated as in the goat and sheep, and hence the frequency of suckling- or milking-induced release of prolactin will be lower than that of many other species. The metabolic interdependence of bodily organs and the mammary gland was stressed by Grachev (1964), who, in the final chapter of his book laid great emphasis on the interrelationships between the mammary gland and the digestive, vascular and endocrine systems, and made the valid point that the mammary gland should not be considered in isolation, but in the context of total bodily function.

The neural basis for the modulation of prolactin secretion: possible mechanisms of action of the suckling stimulus

At the present time, remarkably little is known about the central nervous pathways and mechanisms involved in prolactin secretion, and it would be more appropriate to speak of the present state of ignorance, rather than knowledge, in this field. Even the site or sites of PIF synthesis are unknown so that, unlike the neurohypophysial system and the magnocellular hypothalamic nuclei, there is as yet no point of attack for the study of prolactin-releasing pathways. Within the hypothalamus there is some evidence that a region dorsolateral to the paraventricular nuclei may be concerned in prolactin release. Lesions placed in this area were reported to lead to dioestrus in the rat and to favour deciduomata formation after trauma of the uterus (Flament-Durand & Desclin, 1964). On the other hand, lesions in this region prevented lactogenesis in the rat (Averill & Purves, 1963) yet were without effect on established lactation (McCann, Mack & Gale, 1959; Averill, 1965). Electrolytic lesions of the paraventricular nuclei led to lobulo-alveolar development in male rats (deVoe *et al.*, 1966), although care must be exercised when attributing positive effects to this type of lesion in view of the possibility of chemical irritation at the periphery of the necrotic area (Everett & Radford, 1961). Also in the rat, stimulation of the premammillary complex, dorsomedial nucleus and part of the ventromedial nucleus caused the onset of pseudo-pregnancy (Everett & Quinn, 1966).

An indication that the hypothalamus may not be the sole arbiter of prolactin secretion came from the report that removal of the entire telencephalon caused lactogenesis in the oestrogen-primed ovariectomized rabbit (Beyer & Mena, 1965a). These authors were careful to point out, however, that the response may have been due to the release of ACTH and corticosteroids (see Talwalker, Nicoll & Meites, 1961; Chadwick & Folley, 1962). Evidence to implicate the limbic system in prolactin secretion came from studies on the effect of local implantation of oestradiol monobenzoate in the amygdaloid complex of the pseudopregnant rabbit. Release of prolactin, assessed by the lactogenic response, occurred when implants were placed in the medial nucleus, in the central nucleus, and in the basomedial part of the basal nucleus of the amygdala, as well as in the stria terminalis (Tindal & Knaggs, 1966; Tindal, Knaggs & Turvey, 1967b). Also, lesions of the base of the temporal lobe which destroyed the ventral amygdala caused lactogenesis in the oestrogen-primed ovariectomized rabbit (Mena & Beyer, 1968b). Tindal *et al.* (1967b) suggested that, on existing anatomical knowledge (Ban & Omukai, 1959), the lactogenic responses were caused by oestrogen-sensitive neurones in the amygdala acting via the stria terminalis on the preoptic area and/or the basal hypothalamus to cause the release of prolactin, and that since maximal lactogenic responses were not obtained, that this might be a fine-control mechanism, rather than an all-or-nothing modulation.

This concept of steroid-sensitive neurones which are remote from the immediate vicinity of the basal hypothalamus has received support from more recent studies on the regulation of ACTH secretion in the rabbit. Local implants of corticosterone placed in the central, lateral basal and medial amygdaloid nuclei depressed endogenous corticosterone synthesis while similar implants in the cortical amygdaloid nucleus were ineffective. In the hippocampus, however, corticosterone implants placed in the cornu ammonis facilitated synthesis of the steroid, while implants in the neighbouring alveus and fascia dentata were ineffective (Kawakami, Seto & Yoshida, 1968). This differential effect of implants in different sites in the limbic system, together with the fact that the microelectrophoretic application of dexamethasone to neurones in the mid-brain of the rat results in immediate responses in unit-firing rates (Steiner, Ruf & Akert, 1969) militate against the view that steroids applied to extra-hypothalamic sites may be acting, via the ventricular system, on the basal hypothalamus (Kendall, Grimm & Shimshak, 1969).

The terminal hypothalamic distribution of the stria terminalis has been the source of some controversy in the past, but the development of an improved technique for tracing axon degeneration (Fink & Heimer, 1967) has enabled a detailed study to be made of the hypothalamic targets of this fibre bundle (Heimer & Nauta, 1969). Whereas the postcommissural component of the stria terminalis terminates principally in the anterior hypothalamus and also sends a few fibres to join the medial forebrain bundle, the supracommissural component terminates to a minor extent in the ventral premammillary nucleus and predominantly in a dense synaptic zone which surrounds the ventromedial nucleus. This zone contains a massive plexus of dendrites which protrude not only from the ventromedial nucleus but also from neighbouring cell groups such as the arcuate and dorsomedial nuclei. This latter observation led to the suggestion that the stria terminalis has synaptic contacts not only with adjacent cell bodies but also with dendrites of neurones whose cell bodies may lie well outside its synaptic fields (Heimer & Nauta, 1969). The findings of De Olmos (1969), reported in abstract, are in essential agreement with those of Heimer & Nauta (1969). The amygdala, therefore, can be envisaged as exerting an effect on a considerable part of the medial hypothalamus, in terms of endocrine function.

In such circumstances, it is natural to look for a system which could act in opposition to the amygdala. The most obvious candidate for such a role would be the hippocampus via its fibre projection, the fornix, which projects to the septum and either directly to medial hypothalamic regions in some species, such as the rat and guinea-pig, or after synaptic relay in the lateral hypothalamus in others, such as the cat and monkey (Valenstein & Nauta, 1959). There is, therefore, an anatomical basis for a homeostatic regulatory mechanism in terms of hypothalamic control of the pituitary (Nauta, 1960), operating at a higher level than the basal hypothalamus. Such a control system could be envisaged as being responsive to both exteroceptive and interoceptive stimuli such as target organ hormones; indeed Kawakami *et al.* (1968) demonstrated opposing effects of corticoid implants in the hippocampus and amygdala.

When considering prolactin secretion in the lactating animal, the most obvious exteroceptive stimulus of course is the suckling or milking stimulus. The ascending prolactin-release pathway activated by the suckling stimulus has been described in the rabbit from the mesencephalon as far forward as the posterior hypothalamus (Tindal & Knaggs, 1969). In the mesencephalon there is a common path for both oxytocin and prolactin release in the lateral tegmentum, which involves the spinothalamic system. However, upon entering the diencephalon, whereas the oxytocin-release path bifurcates into dorsal and ventral paths, the prolactin-release path appears to utilize only the dorsal path, and enters the posterior hypothalamus in the neighbourhood of, but apparently not involving, the mammillo-thalamic tracts (Tindal *et al.*, 1967*c*, 1968, 1969; Tindal & Knaggs, 1969). Further rostrally, the picture remains obscure. Although the pathway might move directly to the median eminence, there is no evidence at the moment to suggest that this is the case, and it could equally well pass elsewhere in the forebrain to an integrating centre before reaching the median eminence. Although no definite conclusions can be drawn until the diencephalic course of the tactile pathway for prolactin release is known, one possibility, suggested by Tindal (1967), was that the suckling stimulus might influence prolactin release by modulating the action of opposing limbic systems which projected to a common target in the basal hypo-thalamus. The reasoning behind this proposal was that the ascending pathway of the milk-ejection reflex and, as is now known, the ascending path for prolactin release, lies in the lateral tegmentum of the mesencephalon (Tindal *et al.*, 1967*c*, 1969; Tindal & Knaggs, 1969), and that high-frequency stimulation of this region in the cat increased the amplitude of potentials evoked in the ventromedial nucleus and tuberal region of the hypothala-mus by single-pulse stimulation of the amygdala, and decreased those caused by similar stimulation of the septum (Tsubokawa & Sutin, 1963). The activities of the two major components of the limbic system, the amygdala and hippocampus, are influenced by many factors, and their interaction could be envisaged as playing a role in determining whether particular neurohumours were released or not, dependent on which system could inhibit the

K

action of the other on the hypothalamus via stria terminalis and fornix, resulting in either a hyperpolarization or depolarization of hypothalamic neurones.

Such a concept may, of course, be both oversimplified and inadequate. Indeed, recent work in this laboratory has shown that a discrete region of the cerebral cortex is intimately involved in the release of prolactin. By the use of a technique similar to that described by Tindal & Knaggs (1969) for stimulation of the brain stem it was found that electrical stimulation of the orbital region of the prefrontal cortex, in particular the area immediately dorsal and dorsolateral to the rhinal sulcus, caused the onset of lactogenesis in the pseudopregnant rabbit (Tindal & Knaggs, 1970*b*). The two top lactogenic ratings on the Chadwick (1963) scale were observed in such animals, which suggested that considerable quantities of prolactin had been released by the stimulation. This region of the prefrontal cortex projects, *inter alia*, to the lateral hypothalamus in the monkey (Nauta, 1962) and rat (Leonard, 1969). It is also closely associated with limbic structures in the forebrain, and although there is some overlap, the orbito-frontal region appears to be connected primarily to the amygdala, while the dorsal part of the prefrontal convexity is associated more with the hippocampus, in each case via the cortical region immediately associated with these structures (see Nauta, 1964). It is much too early to be able to do more than assert that the orbital region of the prefrontal cortex is involved in the control of prolactin secretion. The mechanism by which this is achieved must await further investigation. It may be that orbital cortex is the crucial structure which is activated by the suckling stimulus, itself acting on the limbic system to control release of prolactin, perhaps in the manner suggested by Tindal (1967). It may, of course, also be concerned with the release of prolactin in response to conditioned stimuli. The concept of cerebral cortical involvement in basic endocrine control mechanisms may appear unorthodox, yet it is in agreement with modern views. It has been suggested that prefrontal cortex can be regarded as the superstructure of limbic and visceral activity (Akert, 1964) and that it may supply the neural code to interpret the environment to the more basic mechanisms of the body (Nauta, 1964). Prolactin, therefore, may merely be the first of the anterior pituitary hormones whose release mechanism has been shown to be influenced by this little-understood region of the brain.

REFERENCES

Aberle, S. B. D. (1934). Growth of mammary gland in the rhesus monkey. *Proc. Soc. exp. Biol. Med.* **32**, 249–251.

Abolins, J. A. (1954). Das Stillen und die Temperatur der Brust. *Acta obstet. gynec. scand.* **33**, 60–68.

Adamiker, D. & Glawischnig, E. (1967). Elektronenmikroskopische Untersuchungen an der Schweinemilchdrüse. Befunde an Drüsen virgineller, gravider und laktierender Tiere. Diskussion der Befunde. *Wein tierärztl. Mschr.* **54**, 507–518, 575–583.

Adams, E. W. & Rickard, C. G. (1963). The antistreptococcic activity of bovine teat canal keratin. *Am. J. vet. Res.* **24**, 122–135.

Adams, E. W., Rickard, C. G. & Murphy, J. M. (1961). Some histological and histochemical observations on bovine teat epithelium. *Cornell Vet.* **51**, 124–154.

Ahmad, N., Lyons, W. R. & Ellis, S. (1969). Luteotrophic activity of rat hypophysial mammotrophin. *Endocrinology* **85**, 378–380.

Ahmed, M. M. U. & Kanagasuntheram, R. (1965). A note on the mammary glands in the lesser bush baby (*Galago senegalensis senegalensis*). *Acta anat.* **60**, 253–261.

Ahrén, K. (1959). Mammary gland development in hypophysectomized rats injected with anterior pituitary hormones and testosterone. *Acta endocr., Copenh.* **31**, 228–240.

Ahrén, K. & Etienne, M. (1957). The development of the mammary gland in normal and castrated male rats after the age of 21 days. *Acta physiol. scand.* **41**, 283–300.

— (1959). The effect of testosterone alone and combined with insulin on the mammary glands of castrated and hypophysectomized rats. *Acta endocr., Copenh.* **30**, 109–136.

Ahrén, K. & Hamberger, L. (1962). Direct action of testosterone propionate on the rat mammary gland. *Acta endocr., Copenh.* **40**, 265–276.

Akert, K. (1964). Discussion following Chap. 19. In *The Frontal Granular Cortex and Behavior*, edited by Warren, J. M. & Akert, K. New York: McGraw-Hill.

Albe-Fessard, D. (1967). Organization of central somatic projections. In *Contributions to Sensory Physiology*, edited by Neff, W. D., vol. 2, pp. 101–167. New York & London: Academic Press.

Amenomori, Y., Chen, C. L. & Meites, J. (1970). Serum prolactin levels in rats during different reproductive states. *Endocrinology* **86,** 506–510.

Amenomori, Y. & Nellor, J. E. (1969). Effect of suckling on serum prolactin levels in lactating rats. *Fedn Proc.* **28,** 505.

Aminov, S. A. (1961). Nature of the first phase of the reflex of milk ejection (mistranslated as milk 'secretion') *Sechenov physiol. J.* **47,** 496–501 [cover-to-cover translation of *Fiziol. Zh. SSSR im. I. M. Sechenova* **47,** 449–453.]

Amoroso, E. C. & Jewell, P. A. (1963). The exploitation of the milk-ejection reflex by primitive peoples. *Occasional paper No. 18 of the Royal Anthropological Institute,* 126–137.

Andersson, B. (1951*a*). Some observations on the neuro-hormonal regulation of milk-ejection. *Acta physiol. scand.* **23,** 1–7.

— (1951*b*). The effect and localization of electrical stimulation of certain parts of the brain stem in sheep and goats. *Acta physiol. scand.* **23,** 8–23.

Andrews, P. (1966). Molecular weights of prolactins and pituitary growth hormones estimated by gel filtration. *Nature, Lond.* **209,** 155–157.

— (1969). Molecular weight of human placental lactogen investigated by gel filtration. *Biochem. J.* **111,** 799–800.

Apostolakis, M. (1965). The extraction of prolactin from human pituitary glands. *Acta endocr., Copenh.* **49,** 1–16.

— (1968). Prolactin. In *Vitamins and Hormones,* edited by Harris, R. S., Wool, I. G. & Loraine, J. A., vol. 26, pp. 197–235. New York & London: Academic Press.

Apostolakis, M., Theile, L. & Berle, P. (1969). Darstellung eines albumin-freien, hypophysären, menschlichen Prolaktinpräparates. *Endokrinologie* **54,** 145–152.

Arai, Y. & Lee, T. H. (1967). A double-antibody radioimmunoassay procedure for ovine pituitary prolactin. *Endocrinology* **81,** 1041–1046.

Ardran, G. M., Cowie, A. T. & Kemp, F. H. (1957). A cineradiographic study of the teat sinus during suckling in the goat. *Vet. Rec.* **69,** 1100–1101.

— (1958). Further observations on the teat sinus of the goat during suckling. *Vet. Rec.* **70,** 808–809.

Ardran, G. M., Kemp, F. H. & Lind, J. (1958*a*). A cineradiographic study of bottle feeding. *Br. J. Radiol.* **31,** 11–22.

— (1958*b*). A cineradiographic study of breast feeding. *Br. J. Radiol.* **31,** 156–162.

Argonz, J. & del Castillo, E. B. (1953). A syndrome characterized by estrogenic insufficiency, galactorrhea and decreased urinary gonadotropin. *J. clin. Endocr. Metab.* **13,** 79–87.

Arimura, A., Saito, T., Müller, E. E., Bowers, C. Y., Sawano, S. & Schally, A. V. (1967). Absence of prolactin-release inhibiting activity in highly purified LH-releasing factor. *Endocrinology* **80,** 972–974.

Arizono, H. & Okamoto, S. (1957). Comparative neurologic study on the hypothalamo-hypophyseal neurosecretory system. *Med. J. Osaka Univ.* **8**, 195–228.

Arnold, J. (1905). Die Morphologie der Milch- und Colostrumsekretion sowie deren Beziehung zur Fettsynthese, Fettphagocytose, Fettsekretion und Fettdegeneration. *Beitr. path. Anat.* **38**, 422–449.

Arvy, L. (1961). Histoenzymologie de la glande mammaire chez la lapine en période de lactation *post-partum. C. r. hebd. Séanc. Acad. Sci., Paris* **253**, 2132–2134.

Aschaffenburg, R., Gregory, M. E., Kon, S. K., Rowland, S. J. & Thompson, S. Y. (1962). The composition of the milk of the reindeer. *J. Dairy Res.* **29**, 325–328.

Asling, C. W., Durbin, P. W., Johnson, M. E. & Parrott, M. W. (1959). Demonstration of the concentration of astatine-211 in the mammary tissue of the rat. *Endocrinology* **64**, 579–585.

Assenmacher, I. & Tixier-Vidal, A. (1964). Répercussions de la section des veines porte hypophysaires sur la préhypophyse du canard Pékin mâle, entier ou castré. *Archs Anat. microsc. Morph. exp.* **53**, 83–108.

Astrakhanskaya, N. A. (1955). Znachenie nervnoĭ sistemȳ dlya razvitiya i funktsii molochnoĭ zhelezȳ. Avtoreferat diss. Leningrad. Quoted by Zaks (1962).

Atkins, Sir Hedley (1968). Astley Cooper and diseases of the breast. *Guy's Hosp. Rep.* **117**, 199–206.

Aulsebrook, L. H. & Holland, R. C. (1965). Central inhibition of the neurohypophysial system. *Anat. Rec.* **151**, 319–320.

— (1969a). Central regulation of oxytocin release with and without vasopressin release. *Am. J. Physiol.* **216**, 818–829.

— (1969b). Central inhibition of oxytocin release. *Am. J. Physiol.* **216**, 830–842.

Averill, R. L. W. (1965). Restoration of lactation in rats with hypothalamic lesions which inhibit lactation. *J. Endocr.* **31**, 191–196.

Averill, R. L. W. & Purves, H. D. (1963). Differential effects of permanent hypothalamic lesions on reproduction and lactation in rats. *J. Endocr.* **26**, 463–477.

Bahn, R. C. & Bates, R. W. (1956). Histologic criteria for detection of prolactin: lack of prolactin in blood and urine of human subjects. *J. clin. Endocr. Metab.* **16**, 1337–1346.

Baker, B. L. (1970). Studies on hormone localization with emphasis on the hypophysis. *J. Histochem. Cytochem.* **18**, 1–8.

Baker, B. L. & Zanotti, D. B. (1966). Electrophoresis of pituitary proteins after treatment of rats with norethynodrel. *Endocrinology* **78**, 1037–1040.

Baker, E., Shaw, D. C. & Morgan, E. H. (1968). Isolation and characterization of rabbit serum and milk transferrins. Evidence for difference in sialic acid content only. *Biochemistry, N.Y.* **7**, 1371–1378.

Baldwin, R. L. (1969a). Development of milk synthesis. *J. Dairy Sci.* **52**, 729–736.

Baldwin, R. L. (1969*b*). Enzymic and metabolic changes in mammary tissue at lactogenesis. In *Lactogenesis: the initiation of milk secretion at parturition*, edited by Reynolds, M. & Folley, S. J., pp. 85–95. Philadelphia: University of Pennsylvania Press.

Baldwin, R. L. & Cheng, W. (1969). Metabolic changes associated with initiation and maintenance of lactation in rats and cows. *J. Dairy Sci.* **52**, 523–528.

Balinsky, B. I. (1950). On the prenatal growth of the mammary gland rudiment in the mouse. *J. Anat.* **84**, 227–235.

Ball, J. N. (1969). Prolactin (fish prolactin or paralactin) and growth hormone. In *Fish Physiology*, edited by Hoar, W. S. & Randall, D. J., vol. 2, chap. 3. New York & London: Academic Press.

Ballantyne, B. & Bunch, G. A. (1966). The neurohistology of quiescent mammary tissue in *Lepus albus*. *J. comp. Neurol.* **127**, 471–487.

Ban, T. & Omukai, F. (1959). Experimental studies on the fiber connections of the amygdaloid nuclei in the rabbit. *J. comp. Neurol.* **113**, 245–279.

Bangham, D. R., Mussett, M. V. & Stack-Dunne, M. P. (1963). The second international standard for prolactin. *Bull. Wld Hlth Org.* **29**, 721–728.

Barber, R. S., Braude, R. & Mitchell, K. G. (1955). Studies on milk production of Large White pigs. *J. agric. Sci., Camb.* **46**, 97–118.

Bargmann, W. (1964). Secretion and 'let-down' of milk. *Germ. med. Mon.* **9**, 309–313.

Bargmann, W., Fleischhauer, K. & Knoop, A. (1961). Über die Morphologie der Milchsekretion—II. Zugleich eine Kritik am Schema der Sekretionmorphologie. *Z. Zellforsch. mikrosk. Anat.* **53**, 545–568.

Bargmann, W. & Knoop, A. (1959). Über die Morphologie der Milchsekretion. Licht- und elekronenmikroskopische Studien an der Milchdrüse der Ratte. *Z. Zellforsch. mikrosk. Anat.* **49**, 344–388.

Bargmann, W. & Welsch, U. (1969). On the ultrastructure of the mammary gland. In *Lactogenesis: the Initiation of Milk Secretion at Parturition*, edited by Reynolds, M. & Folley, S. J., pp. 43–52. Philadelphia: University of Pennsylvania Press.

Barry, J. (1968). Recherches sur le rôle des monoamines infundibulaires au cours de l'allaitement chez la souris. *C. r. Séanc. Soc. Biol.* **162**, 1954–1955.

Bartke, A. & Lloyd, C. W. (1970). Influence of prolactin and pituitary isografts on spermatogenesis in dwarf mice and hypophysectomized rats. *J. Endocr.* **46**, 321–329.

Barȳshnikov, I. A. (1959). Reflex regulation of lactation. *Dairy Sci. Abstr.* **21**, 47–53. Translated from Russian: *Problemȳ fiziologii tsentral'noĭ nervnoĭ sistemȳ*, pp. 62–72 (1957). Moskva–Leningrad: Akademiya Nauk SSSR.

— (1965). Nervous control of mammary function. The reflex regulation of lactation. *Proc. 2nd Int. Congr. Endocr.* (*London, 1964*). Excerpta Medica International Congress Series No. 83, pp. 655–659.

Barȳshnikov, I. A., Borsuk, V. N., Zaks, M. G., Zotikova, I. N. Pavlov,

G. N. & Tolbukhin, V. I. (1953). K voprosu o nervnoĭ regulyatsii deyatel'nosti molochnoĭ zhelezȳ. *Zh. obshch. Biol.* **14,** 257–274. Quoted by Zaks (1962).

Barȳshnikov, I. A., Zaks, M. G., Zotikova, I. N., Levitskaya, E. S., Pavlov, G. N., Pavlov, E. F., Tverskoĭ, G. B., Tolbukhin, V. I. & Tsakhaev, G. A. (1951). O nervnoĭ regulyatsii dvigatel'noĭ funktsii molochnoĭ zhelezȳ. *Zh. obshch. Biol.* **12,** 423–439. Quoted by Zaks (1962).

Bässler, R. (1961). Elektronenmikroskopische Beobachtungen bei experimenteller Milchstauung. *Frank. Z. Path.* **71,** 398–422.

— (1963). Über die Enstehung des Eisenpigmentes in der Milchdrüse im elektronenmikroskopischen Bild. *Acta histochem.* suppl. III, 130–141.

— (1968). Neuere Aspekte der normalen und pathologischen Feinstruktur der Mamma. *Hippokrates* **7,** 237–244.

Bässler, R. & Brethfeld, V. (1968). Enzymhistochemische Studien an der Milchdrüse: Gravidität, Laktation, Involution und experimentelle Stauung mit besonderer Berücksichtigung myoepithelialer Zellen. *Histochemie* **15,** 270–286.

Bässler, R. & Flörchinger, J. (1966*a*). Histometrische Studien an der lactierenden Milchdrüse—I. Lactation und physiologische Involution. *Arch. Gynäk.* **203,** 366–399.

— (1966*b*). Histometrische Studien an der lactierenden Milchdrüse—II. Experimentelle Milchstauung und vermehrtes Flüssigkeitsangebot durch Periston-Infusionen. *Arch. Gynäk.* **203,** 400–422.

Bässler, R. & Forssmann, W. (1964). Experimenteller Strukturwandel der Drüsenzelle durch Hormonwirkung. *Verh. dt. Ges. Path.* **48,** 240–245.

Bässler, R. & Paek, S. (1968). Histochemisches Enzymmuster der Mamma unter dem experimentellen Einfluss von Geschlechtshormonen. *Histochemie* **13,** 29–44.

Bässler, R. & Schäfer, A. (1969*a*). Elektronenmikroskopische Zytomorphologie der männlichen Brustdrüse. *Z. Zellforsch. mikrosk. Anat.* **101,** 355–366.

— (1969*b*). Elektronenmikroskopische Cytomorphologie der Gynäkomastie. *Virchows Arch. path. Anat. Physiol.* **348,** 356–373.

Bässler, R., Schäfer, A. & Paek, S. (1967). Elektronenmikroskopische und histochemische Untersuchungen zur Morphologie und Funktion myoepithelialer Zellen. *Verh. dt. Ges. Path.* **51,** 301–307.

Bässler, R., Schulze, G. & Schriever, D. (1970). Histochemische Untersuchungen am Bindegewebe der hormonal stimulierten Mamma. *Beitr. path. Anat.* **140,** 212–236.

Bates, R. W., Garrison, M. M. & Cornfield, J. (1963). An improved bioassay for prolactin using adult pigeons. *Endocrinology* **73,** 217–223.

Baylis, E. M., Greenwood, F., James, V., Jenkins, J., Landon, J., Marks, V. & Samols, E. (1968). An examination of the control mechanisms postulated to control growth hormone secretion in man. In *Growth Hormone*, edited by Pecile, A. & Müller, E. E. *Excerpta Medica International Congress Series No. 158,* pp. 89–104.

Ben-David, M. (1967). A sensitive bioassay for prolactin based on H³-methyl-thymidine uptake by the pigeon-crop mucous epithelium. *Proc. Soc. exp. Biol. Med.* **125,** 705–708.

— (1968). Mechanism of induction of mammary differentiation in Sprague–Dawley female rats by perphenazine. *Endocrinology* **83,** 1217–1223.

Ben-David, M., Dikstein, S. & Sulman, F. G. (1964). Effect of different steroids on prolactin secretion in pituitary–hypothalamus organ co-culture. *Proc. Soc. exp. Biol. Med.* **117,** 511–513.

Ben-David, M., Roderig, H., Khazen, K. & Sulman, F. G. (1966). Effect of different steroids on lactating rats. *Proc. Soc. exp. Biol. Med.* **120,** 620–623.

Bengtsson, B. & Norgren, A. (1961). Interactions of oestrone and testosterone on mammary glands of male rabbits. *Acta endocr., Copenh.* **36,** 141–156.

Benoit, J. & DaLage, C. (1963) (Editors). *Cytologie de L'Adenohypophyse, Colloq. int. Cent. nat. Rech. sci.* No. 128.

Benson, G. K. & Cowie, A. T. (1956). Lactation in the rat after hypophysial posterior lobectomy. *J. Endocr.* **14,** 54–65.

Benson, G. K., Cowie, A. T., Cox, C. P., Folley, S. J. & Hosking, Z. D. (1965). Relative efficiency of hexoestrol and progesterone as oily solutions and as crystalline suspensions in inducing mammary growth and lactation in early and late ovariectomized goats. *J. Endocr.* **31,** 157–167.

Benson, G. K., Cowie, A. T., Cox, C. P. & Goldzveig, S. A. (1957). Effects of oestrone and progesterone on mammary development in the guinea-pig. *J. Endocr.* **15,** 126–144.

Benson, G. K. & Fitzpatrick, R. J. (1966). The neurohypophysis and the mammary gland. In *The Pituitary Gland*, edited by Harris, G. W. & Donovan, B. T., vol. 3, chap. 15. London: Butterworths.

Benson, G. K. & Folley, S. J. (1956). Oxytocin as stimulator for the release of prolactin from the anterior pituitary. *Nature, Lond.* **177,** 700.

— (1957). The effect of oxytocin on mammary gland involution in the rat. *J. Endocr.* **16,** 189–201.

Bergman, A. J. & Turner, C. W. (1940). The specificity of the lactogenic hormone in the initiation of lactation. *J. Dairy Sci.* **23,** 1229–1237.

Bern, H. A. (1967). Hormones and endocrine glands of fishes. *Science, N.Y.* **158,** 455–461.

Bern, H. A. & Nicoll, C. S. (1968). The comparative endocrinology of prolactin. *Recent Prog. Horm. Res.* **24,** 681–713.

Berson, S. A. & Yalow, R. S. (1962). Immunoassay of plasma insulin. *Ciba Fdn Colloq. Endocr.* **14,** 182–201.

— (1964). Immunoassay of protein hormones. In *The Hormones*, edited by Pincus, G., Thimann, K. V. & Astwood, E. B., vol. 4, chap. 11. New York & London: Academic Press.

Berswordt-Wallrabe, R. von, Moon, R. C. & Turner, C. W. (1960). Effect of lactogenic hormone, growth hormone and thyroxine in the lactating albino rat. *Proc. Soc. exp. Biol. Med.* **104,** 530–531.

Berswordt-Wallrabe, R. von, Steinbeck, H., Hahn, J. D. & Elger, W. (1969). Prolactin and the ventral prostate gland in juvenile rats. *Experientia* **25**, 533–534.

Berswordt-Wallrabe, R. von, & Turner, C. W. (1960). Successful replacement therapy in lactating thyro-parathyroidectomized rats. *Proc. Soc. exp. Biol. Med.* **104**, 113–116.

Bertkau, F. (1907). Ein Beitrag zur Anatomie und Physiologie der Milchdrüse. *Anat. Anz.* **30**, 161–180.

Bewley, T. A. & Li, C. H. (1970). Primary structures of human pituitary growth hormone and sheep pituitary lactogenic hormone compared. *Science, N.Y.* **168**, 1361–1362.

Beyer, C., Anguiano, L. G. & Mena, F. (1961). Oxytocin release in response to stimulation of cingulate gyrus. *Am. J. Physiol.* **200**, 625–627.

Beyer, C. & Mena, F. (1965a). Induction of milk secretion in the rabbit by removal of the telencephalon. *Am. J. Physiol.* **208**, 289–292.

— (1965b). Blockage of milk removal in the cat by periventricular diencephalic lesions. *Am. J. Physiol.* **208**, 585–588.

Beyer, C., Mena, F., Pacheco, P. & Alcaraz, M. (1962a). Effect of central nervous system lesions on lactation in the cat. *Fedn Proc.* **21**, 353.

— (1962b). Blockage of lactation by brain-stem lesions in the cat. *Am. J. Physiol.* **202**, 465–468.

Beyer, C., Tindal, J. S. & Sawyer, C. H. (1962). Electrophysiological study of projections from mesencephalic central grey matter to forebrain in the rabbit. *Expl Neurol.* **6**, 435–450.

Biborski, J. (1961). Badania nad rozwojem gruezołu mlecznego u płodów żeńskich bydła. *Roczn. Nauk roln.* (Ser B 3) **77**, 749–771.

Bílek, J., Janovský, M., Makoč, Z. & Kozlík, V. (1963). Hodnoty oxytocinu v krvi při ejekčním reflexu. *Živočišná Výroba* **8**, 41–46.

Bintarningsih, Lyons, W. R., Johnson, R. E. & Li, C. H. (1957). Hormonal requirements for lactation in the hypophysectomized rat. *Anat. Rec.* **127**, 266–267.

— (1958). Hormonally-induced lactation in hypophysectomized rats. *Endocrinology* **63**, 540–548.

Birge, C. A., Jacobs, L. S., Hammer, C. T. & Daughaday, W. H. (1970). Catecholamine inhibition of prolactin secretion by isolated rat adenohypophyses. *Endocrinology* **86**, 120–130.

Bisset, G. W. (1968). The milk-ejection reflex and the actions of oxytocin, vasopressin and synthetic analogues on the mammary gland. In *Handbook of Experimental Pharmacology*, Vol. 23, *Neurohypophysial Hormones and Similar Polypeptides*, edited by Berde, B., pp. 475–544. Berlin, Heidelberg, New York: Springer-Verlag.

Bisset, G. W., Clark, B. J. & Errington, M., (1970). The hypothalamic neurosecretory pathway for the release of oxytocin in the cat. *J. Physiol.* **207**, 21–22P.

Bisset, G. W., Clark, B. J. & Haldar, J. (1970). Blood levels of oxytocin and vasopressin during suckling in the rabbit and the problem of their independent release. *J. Physiol.* **206**, 711–722.

Bisset, G. W., Clark, B. J., Haldar, J., Harris, M. C., Lewis, G. P. & Rocha e Silva, M. (1967). The assay of milk-ejecting activity in the lactating rat. *Br. J. Pharmac. Chemother.* **31**, 537–549.

Bisset, G. W., Clark, B. J. & Lewis, G. P. (1967). The mechanism of the inhibitory action of adrenaline on the mammary gland. *Br. J. Pharmac. Chemother.* **31**, 550–559.

Bisset, G. W., Hilton, S. M. & Poisner, A. M. (1967). Hypothalamic pathways for independent release of vasopressin and oxytocin. *Proc. R. Soc.* B **166**, 422–442.

Bisset, G. W. & Lewis, G. P. (1962). A spectrum of pharmacological activity in some biologically active peptides. *Br. J. Pharmac. Chemother.* **19**, 168–182.

Bitensky, L. (1967). Histochemistry in experimental immunology. In *Handbook of Experimental Immunology*, edited by Weir, D. M., chap. 23. Oxford & Edinburgh: Blackwell Scientific Publications.

Blanc, B. & Isliker, H. (1963). Transfert de ^{59}Fe de ferriprotéines aux tissus et aux liquides biologiques (sérum et lait). *Helv. physiol. pharmac. Acta* **21**, 259–275.

Bland, E. P., Crawford, J. S., Docker, M. F. & Farr, R. F. (1969). Radio-active iodine uptake by thyroid of breast-fed infants after maternal blood-volume measurements. *Lancet* **ii**, 1039–1041.

Blaxter, K. L. (1961). Lactation and growth of the young. In *Milk: the Mammary Gland and its Secretion*, edited by Kon, S. K. & Cowie, A. T., vol. 2, chap. 19. New York & London: Academic Press.

Bogdashev, N. F. & Eliseev, A. P. (1951). *The Cow's Udder.* [In Russian.] Moscow, Leningrad: Sel'khozgiz. Quoted by Zaks (1962).

Boll, F. (1868). Ueber den Bau der Thränendrüse. *Arch. mikrosk. Anat. EntwMech.* **4**, 146–153.

Bonser, G. M., Dossett, J. A. & Jull, J. W. (1961). *Human and Experimental Breast Cancer.* London: Pitman Medical.

Boot, L. M. (1970). Prolactin and mammary gland carcinogenesis. The problem of human prolactin. *Int. J. Cancer* **5**, 167–175.

Bottomley, A. C. & Folley, S. J. (1938). The effect of androgenic substances on the growth of the teat and mammary gland in the immature male guinea-pig. *Proc. R. Soc.*, B, **126**, 224–240.

Bousquet, M., Fléchon, J. E. & Denamur, R. (1969). Aspects ultrastructuraux de la glande mammaire de lapine pendant la lactogénèse. *Z. Zellforsch. mikrosk. Anat.* **96**, 418–436.

Bradley, T. R. & Clarke, P. M. (1956). The response of rabbit mammary glands to locally administered prolactin. *J. Endocr.* **14**, 28–36.

Braude, R. (1954). Pig nutrition. In *Progress in the Physiology of Farm Animals*, edited by Hammond, J., vol. 1, chap. 2. London: Butterworths.

Braude, R. & Mitchell, K. G. (1950). 'Let-down' of milk in the sow. *Nature, Lond.* **165**, 937.

Breazile, J. E. & Kitchell, R. L. (1968a). Ventrolateral spinal cord afferents to the brain stem in the domestic pig. *J. comp. Neurol.* **133**, 363–372.

Breazile, J. E. & Kitchell, R. L. (1968*b*). A study of fiber systems within the spinal cord of the domestic pig that subserve pain. *J. comp. Neurol.* **133**, 373–382.

Bresciani, F. (1964). DNA synthesis in alveolar cells of the mammary gland: acceleration by ovarian hormones. *Science, N.Y.* **146**, 653–655.

Bresslau, E. (1920). *The Mammary Apparatus of the Mammalia in the Light of Ontogenesis and Phylogenesis.* London: Methuen.

Breuer, C. B. (1969). Stimulation of DNA synthesis in cartilage of hypophysectomized rats by native and modified placental lactogen and anabolic hormones. *Endocrinology* **85**, 989–999.

Brew, K. (1969). Secretion of α-lactalbumin into milk and its relevance to the organization and control of lactose synthetase. *Nature, Lond.* **223**, 671–672.

Brooks, C. McC., Ishikawa, T., Koizumi, K. & Lu, H-H. (1966). Activity of neurones in the paraventricular nucleus of the hypothalamus and its control. *J. Physiol.* **182**, 217–231.

Brown, D. & Snell, M. (1968). Inhibition of lactation with quinestrol. *Br. med. J.* **4**, 326–327.

Brown-Grant, K. (1957). The iodide concentrating mechanism of the mammary gland. *J. Physiol.* **135**, 644–654.

Browning, H. C., Larke, G. A. & Talamantes, F. (1968). Effect of norethynodrel-mestranol on the reproductive system and mammary glands of male BALB/c mice. *Proc. Soc. exp. Biol. Med.* **128**, 1199–1202.

Bruce, H. M. (1959). An exteroceptive block to pregnancy in the mouse. *Nature, Lond.* **184**, 105.

— (1960). A block to pregnancy in the mouse caused by proximity of strange males. *J. Reprod. Fert.* **1**, 96–103.

Bruce, H. M., Land, R. B. & Falconer, D. S. (1968). Inhibition of pregnancy block in mice by handling. *J. Reprod. Fert.* **15**, 289–294.

Brumby, H. I. & Forsyth, I. A. (1969). Bioassay of prolactin in the blood of goats at parturition. *J. Endocr.* **43**, xxiii–xxiv.

Bryant, G. D. & Greenwood, F. C. (1968). Radioimmunoassay for ovine, caprine and bovine prolactin in plasma and tissue extracts. *Biochem. J.* **109**, 831–840.

Bryant, G. D., Greenwood, F. C. & Linzell, J. L. (1968). Plasma prolactin levels in the goat: physiological and experimental modification. *J. Endocr.* **40**, iv–v.

Bryant, G. D., Linzell, J. L. & Greenwood, F. C. (1970). Plasma prolactin in goats measured by radioimmunoassay: the effects of teat stimulation, mating behavior, stress, fasting and of oxytocin, insulin and glucose injections. *Hormones* **1**, 26–35.

Buchanan, R. A., Eaton, C. J., Koeff, S. T. & Kinkel, A. W. (1968). Breast milk excretion of mefenamic acid. *Curr. ther. Res.* **10**, 592–596.

— (1969). The breast milk excretion of flufenamic acid. *Curr. ther. Res.* **11**, 533–588.

Buchheim, W. (1969). Über erste Erfahrungen mit der Gefrierätz-technik bei elektronenmikroskopischen Untersuchungen von Milch und Milchprodukten. *Milchwissenschaft* **24**, 6–11.

— (1970a). Der Verlauf der Fettkristallisation in den Fettkügelchen der Milch. Elektronenmikroskopische Untersuchungen mit Hilfe der Gefrierätztechnik. *Milchwissenschaft* **25**, 65–70.

— (1970b). Die molekulare Ordnung in doppelbrechenden Fettkugel-chen. *Milchwissenschaft* **25**, 223–227.

Bujard, E. (1966). La tétine et la peau aréolaire du cobaye gravide: activité de la glycéro-phosphatase alcaline. *Acta anat.* **64**, 263–281.

Bullis, D. D., Bush, L. J. & Barto, P. B. (1965). Effect of highly purified and commercial grade growth hormone preparations on milk pro-duction of dairy cows. *J. Dairy Sci.* **48**, 338–341.

Burns, J. H. (1947). Excretion of drugs in milk. *Br. med. Bull.* **5**, 190–192.

Buss, D. H. (1968). Gross composition and variation of the components of baboon milk during natural lactation. *J. Nutr.* **96**, 421–426.

Buss, D. H. & Kriewaldt, F. H. (1968). A machine for milking baboons. *Lab. Anim. Care* **18**, 644–647.

Caldeyro-Barcia, R. (1969). Milk ejection in women. In *Lactogenesis: the Initiation of Milk Secretion at Parturition*, edited by Reynolds, M. & Folley, S. J., pp. 229–243. Philadelphia: University of Pennsyl-vania Press.

Calma, I. (1965a). The activity of the posterior group of thalamic nuclei in the cat. *J. Physiol.* **180**, 350–370.

— (1965b). Thalamo-cortical relations in the sensory nuclei of the cat. *Nature, Lond.* **205**, 394–396.

Campbell, I. L., Davey, A. W. F., McDowall, F. H. Wilson, G. F. & Munford, R. E. (1964). The effect of adrenocorticotrophic hormone on the yield, composition and butterfat properties of cow's milk. *J. Dairy Res.* **31**, 71–79.

Capen, C. C. & Young, D. M. (1967). Thyrocalcitonin: evidence for release in a spontaneous hypocalcemic disorder. *Science, N.Y.* **157**, 205–206.

Cargill, D. I., Meli, A., Giannina, T. & Steinetz, B. G. (1969). Secretion of ethynylestradiol and its 3-cyclopentyl ether in the milk of lactating rats. *Proc. Soc. exp. Biol. Med.* **131**, 1362–1365.

Caruolo, E. V. & Mochrie, R. D. (1967). Ultrasonograms of lactating mammary glands. *J. Dairy Sci.* **50**, 225–230.

Cathcart, E. P., Gairns, F. W. & Garven, H. S. D. (1948). The innerva-tion of the human quiescent nipple, with notes on pigmentation, erection, and hyperneury. *Trans. Roy. Soc. Edinb.* **61**, 699–717.

Catt, K. & Moffat, B. (1967). Isolation of internally labeled rat prolactin by preparative disc electrophoresis. *Endocrinology* **80**, 324–328.

Catt, K. J., Moffat, B. & Niall, H. D. (1967). Human growth hormone and placental lactogen: structural similarity. *Science, N.Y.* **157**, 321.

Catt, K. J., Moffat, B., Niall, H. D. & Preston, B. N. (1967). Purification and physicochemical properties of human placental lactogen. *Biochem. J.* **102**, 27c–29c.

Catt, K. J. & Tregear, G. W. (1967). Solid-phase radioimmunoassay in antibody-coated tubes. *Science, N.Y.* **158**, 1570–1571.

— (1969). Solid-phase radioimmunoassay. In *Protein and Polypeptide Hormones*, edited by Margoulies, M., Excerpta Medica International Congress Series No. 161, pp. 45–48.

Ceriani, R. L. (1970a). Fetal mammary gland differentiation *in vitro* in response to hormones—I. Morphological findings. *Devl Biol.* **21**, 506–529.

— (1970b). Fetal mammary gland differentiation *in vitro* in response to hormones—II. Biochemical findings. *Devl Biol.* **21**, 530–546.

Cerruti, R. A. & Lyons, W. R. (1960). Mammogenic activities of the mid-gestational mouse placenta. *Endocrinology* **67**, 884–887.

Chadwick, A. (1963). Detection and assay of prolactin by the local lactogenic response in the rabbit. *J. Endocr.* **27**, 253–263.

Chadwick, A. & Folley, S. J. (1962). Lactogenesis in pseudopregnant rabbits treated with ACTH. *J. Endocr.* **24**, xi–xii.

Chan, W. Y. (1965). Mechanism of epinephrine inhibition of the milk ejecting response to oxytocin. *J. Pharmac. exp. Ther.* **147**, 48–53.

Chandler, R. L., Lepper, A. W. D. & Wilcox, J. (1969). Ultrastructural observations on the bovine teat duct. *J. comp. Path. Ther.* **79**, 315–319.

Chard, T., Forsling, M. L., James, M. A. R., Kitau, M. J. & Landon, J. (1970). The development of a radioimmunoassay for oxytocin: sensitivity of the assay in aqueous buffer solution, specificity and the dissociation of immunological and biological activity. *J. Endocr.* **46**, 533–542.

Chard, T., Forsling, M. L. & Kitau, M. J. (1969). Development of a radioimmunoassay for oxytocin. *J. Endocr.* **43**, lxi–lxii.

Chard, T., Kitau, M. J. & Landon, J. (1970). The development of a radioimmunoassay for oxytocin: radioiodination, antibody production and separation techniques. *J. Endocr.* **46**, 269–278.

Chatterton Jr, R. T., Chatterton, A. J. & Hellman, L. (1969). Metabolism of progesterone by the rabbit mammary gland. *Endocrinology* **85**, 16–24.

Chatwin, A. L., Linzell, J. L. & Setchell, B. P. (1969). Cardiovascular changes during lactation in the rat. *J. Endocr.* **44**, 247–254.

Cheever, E. V. & Lewis, U. J. (1969). Estimation of the molecular weights of the multiple components of growth hormone and prolactin. *Endocrinology* **85**, 465–473.

Cheever, E. V., Seavey, B. K. & Lewis, U. J. (1969). Prolactin of normal and dwarf mice. *Endocrinology* **85**, 698–703.

Chen, C. L., Bixler, E. J., Weber, A. I. & Meites, J. (1968). Hypothalamic stimulation of prolactin release from the pituitary of turkey hens and poults. *Gen. comp. Endocr.* **11**, 489–494.

Chen, C. L. & Meites, J. (1970). Effects of estrogen and progesterone on serum and pituitary prolactin levels in ovariectomized rats. *Endocrinology* **86**, 503–505.

Chen, C. L., Minaguchi, H. & Meites, J. (1967). Effects of transplanted pituitary tumors on host pituitary prolactin secretion. *Proc. Soc. exp. Biol. Med.* **126**, 317–320.

Chumakov, V. P. (1961). O. razvitii krovenosnȳkh kapillyarov v moloch-noĭ zheleze émbrionov korov. *Dokl. mosk. sel'.-khoz. Akad. K.A. Timiryazeva (Zootekh).* (69), 337–340.

Clark, M. J. (1967). Pregnancy in the lactating pigmy possum, *Cercartetus concinnus. Aust. J. Zool.* **15**, 673–683.

Clarke, P. M. & Folley, S. J. (1953). Some observations on prolactin assays by the pigeon crop-weight method. *Ciba Fdn Colloq. Endocr.* **5**, 90–103.

Clemens, J. A. & Meites, J. (1968). Inhibition by hypothalamic prolactin implants of prolactin secretion, mammary growth and luteal function. *Endocrinology* **82**, 878–881.

Clemens, J. A., Minaguchi, H., Storey, R., Voogt, J. L. & Meites, J. (1969). Induction of precocious puberty in female rats by prolactin. *Neuroendocrinology* **4**, 150–156.

Clemens, J. A., Sar, M. & Meites, J. (1969). Inhibition of lactation and luteal function in postpartum rats by hypothalamic implantation of prolactin. *Endocrinology* **84**, 868–872.

Cleverley, J. D. (1968a). The detection of oxytocin release in response to conditioned stimuli associated with machine milking in the cow. *J. Endocr.* **40**, ii-iii.

— (1968b). *Blood Levels of Oxytocin, with Special Reference to Lactation.* Ph.D. thesis, University of Reading.

Cleverley, J. D. & Folley, S. J. (1970). The blood levels of oxytocin during machine milking in cows with some observations on its half-life in the circulation. *J. Endocr.* **46**, 347–361.

Cleverley, J. D., Knaggs, G. S., Tindal, J. S. & Turvey, A. (1968). Blood milk-ejection activity after hypothalamic stimulation in the goat. *J. Endocr.* **42**, 609–610.

Clifton, K. H. & Furth, J. (1960). Ducto-alveolar growth in mammary glands of adreno-gonadectomized male rats bearing mammotropic pituitary tumors. *Endocrinology* **66**, 893–897.

Cobo, E., Bernal, M. M. de, Gaitan, E. & Quintero, C. A. (1967). Neuro-hypophyseal hormone release in the human—II. Experimental study during lactation. *Am. J. Obstet. Gynec.* **97**, 519–529.

Cobo, E. & Quintero, C. A. (1969). Milk-ejecting and antidiuretic activities under neurohypophyseal inhibition with alcohol and water overload. *Am. J. Obstet. Gynec.* **105**, 877–887.

Coch, J. A., Brovetto, J., Cabot, H. M., Fielitz, C. & Caldeyro-Barcia, R. (1965). Oxytocin equivalent activity in the plasma of women in labor and during the puerperium. *Am. J. Obstet. Gynec.* **91**, 10–17.

Coch, J. A., Fielitz, C., Brovetto, J., Cabot, H. M., Coda, H. & Fraga, A. (1968). Estimation of an oxytocin-like substance in highly purified extracts from the blood of puerperal women during suckling. *J. Endocr.* **40**, 137–144.

Cole, R. D. & Li, C. H. (1955). Studies on pituitary lactogenic hormone. XIV. A simplified procedure of isolation. *J. biol. Chem.* **213**, 197–201.

Convey, E. M. & Reece, R. P. (1969). Restoration of pituitary lactogen released in response to suckling. *Proc. Soc. exp. Biol. Med.* **131**, 543–546.

Cook, H. W. & Baker, B. E. (1969). Seal milk—I. Harp seal (*Pagophilus groenlandicus*) milk: composition and pesticide residue content. *Can. J. Zool.* **47**, 1129–1132.

Cook, H. W., Lentfer, J. W., Pearson, A. M. & Baker, B. E. (1970). Polar bear milk—IV. Gross composition, fatty acid, and mineral constitution. *Can. J. Zool.* **48**, 217–219.

Cook, H. W., Rausch, R. A. & Baker, B. E. (1970). Moose (*Alces alces*) milk. Gross composition, fatty acid, and mineral constitution. *Can. J. Zool.* **48**, 213–215.

Coombe, J. B., Wardrop, I. D. & Tribe, D. E. (1960). A study of milk production of the grazing ewe, with emphasis on the experimental technique employed. *J. agric. Sci., Camb.* **54**, 353–359.

Cooper, Sir Astley P. (1840). *On the Anatomy of the Breast.* London: Longman, Orme, Green, Brown, and Longman.

Courrier, R. (1945). *Endocrinologie de la Gestation.* Paris: Masson.

Cowie, A. T. (1949). The relative growth of the mammary gland in normal, gonadectomized and adrenalectomized rats. *J. Endocr.* **6**, 145–157.

— (1957). The maintenance of lactation in the rat after hypophysectomy. *J. Endocr.* **16**, 135–147.

— (1961). The hormonal control of milk secretion. In *Milk: the Mammary Gland and its Secretion*, edited by Kon, S. K. & Cowie, A. T., vol. 1, pp. 163–203. New York & London: Academic press.

— (1966). Anterior pituitary function in lactation. In *The Pituitary Gland*, edited by Harris, G. W. & Donovan, B. T., vol. 2, chap. 13. London: Butterworths.

— (1969a). Variations in the yield and composition of the milk during lactation in the rabbit and the galactopoietic effect of prolactin. *J. Endocr.* **44**, 437–450.

— (1969b). General hormonal factors involved in lactogenesis. In *Lactogenesis: the Initiation of Milk Secretion at Parturition*, edited by Reynolds, M. & Folley, S. J., pp. 157–169. Philadelphia: University of Pennsylvania Press.

— (1971). Influence of hormones on mammary growth and milk secretion. In *Lactation*, edited by Falconer, I. R., pp. 123–140. London: Butterworths.

Cowie, A. T., Cox, C. P., Folley, S. J., Hosking, Z. D., Naito, M. & Tindal, J. S. (1965). The effects of the duration of treatments with oestrogen and progesterone on the hormonal induction of mammary growth and lactation in the goat. *J. Endocr.* **32**, 129–139.

Cowie, A. T., Daniel, P. M., Knaggs, G. S., Prichard, M. M. L. & Tindal, J. S. (1964). Lactation in the goat after section of the pituitary stalk. *J. Endocr.* **28**, 253–265.

Cowie, A. T. & Folley, S. J. (1947a). The role of the adrenal cortex in mammary development and its relation to the mammogenic action of the anterior pituitary. *Endocrinology* **40**, 274–285.

— (1947b). The measurement of lactational performance in the rat in studies of the endocrine control of lactation. *J. Endocr.* **5**, 9–13.

— (1961). The mammary gland and lactation. In *Sex and Internal Secretions*, 3rd edn, edited by Young, W. C., vol. 1, chap. 10. Baltimore: Williams & Wilkins.

— (1970). The mammary gland and lactation. In *Scientific Foundations of Obstetrics and Gynaecology*, edited by Philipp, E. E., Barnes, J. & Newton, M., pp. 423–432. London: Heinemann Medical Books.

Cowie, A. T., Folley, S. J., Cross, B. A., Harris, G. W., Jacobsohn, D. & Richardson, K. C. (1951). Terminology for use in lactational physiology. *Nature, Lond.*, **168**, 421.

Cowie, A. T., Folley, S. J., Malpress, F. H. & Richardson, K. C. (1952). Studies on the hormonal induction of mammary growth and lactation in the goat. *J Endocr.* **8**, 64–88.

Cowie, A. T., Hartmann, P. E. & Turvey, A. (1969). The maintenance of lactation in the rabbit after hypophysectomy. *J. Endocr.* **43**, 651–662.

Cowie, A. T., Knaggs, G. S. & Tindal, J. S. (1964). Complete restoration of lactation in the goat after hypophysectomy. *J. Endocr.* **28**, 267–279.

Cowie, A. T., Knaggs, G. S., Tindal, J. S. & Turvey, A. (1968). The milking stimulus and mammary growth in the goat. *J. Endocr.* **40**, 243–252.

Cowie, A. T. & Tindal, J. S. (1957). Hormonal studies of lactation in the rat. *Rep. natn. Inst. Res. Dairy*, 55–56.

— (1961a). The maintenance of lactation in the rat after hypophysial anterior lobectomy during pregnancy. *J. Endocr.* **22**, 403–408.

— (1961b). The maintenance of lactation in the goat after hypophysectomy. *J. Endocr.* **23**, 79–96.

— (1965). Some aspects of the neuro-endocrine control of lactation. *Proc. 2nd Int. Congr. Endocr.* (*London* 1964). Excerpta Medica International Congress Series No. 83, pp. 646–654.

Cowie, A. T., Tindal, J. S. & Benson, G. K. (1960). Pituitary grafts and milk secretion in hypophysectomized rats. *J. Endocr.* **21**, 115–123.

Cowie, A. T., Tindal, J. S. & Yokoyama, A. (1966). The induction of mammary growth in the hypophysectomized goat. *J. Endocr.* **34**, 185–195.

Cowie, A. T. & Watson, S. C. (1966). The adrenal cortex and lactogenesis in the rabbit. *J. Endocr.* **35**, 213–214.

Cox, Jr. W. M. & Mueller, A. J. (1937). The composition of milk from stock rats and an apparatus for milking small laboratory animals. *J. Nutr.* **13**, 249–261.

Crosignani, P. G., Nakamura, R. M., Hovland, D. N. & Mishell, Jr. D. R. (1970). A method of solid phase radioimmunoassay utilizing polypropylene discs. *J. clin. Endocr. Metab.* **30**, 153–160.

Cross, B. A. (1952). Nursing behaviour and the milk-ejection reflex in rabbits. *J. Endocr.* **8**, xiii.

— (1954). Milk ejection resulting from mechanical stimulation of mammary myoepithelium in the rabbit. *Nature, Lond.* **173**, 450.

— (1955*a*). The hypothalamus and the mechanism of sympathetico-adrenal inhibition of milk ejection. *J. Endocr.* **12**, 15–28.

— (1955*b*). Neurohormonal mechanisms in emotional inhibition of milk ejection. *J. Endocr.* **12**, 29–37.

— (1961*a*). Neural control of oxytocin secretion. In *Oxytocin*, edited by Caldeyro-Barcia, R. & Heller, H., pp. 24–47. Oxford: Pergamon Press.

— (1961*b*). Neural control of lactation. In *Milk: the Mammary Gland and its Secretion*, edited by Kon, S. K. & Cowie, A. T., vol. 1, chap. 6. New York & London: Academic Press.

— (1966). Neural control of oxytocin secretion. In *Neuroendocrinology*, edited by Martini, L. & Ganong, F., vol. 1, chap. 7. New York & London: Academic Press.

Cross, B. A. & Findlay, A. L. R. (1969). Comparative and sensory aspects of milk ejection. In *Lactogenesis: the Initiation of Milk Secretion at Parturition*, edited by Reynolds, M. & Folley, S. J., pp. 245–252. Philadelphia: University of Pennsylvania Press.

Cross, B. A., Goodwin, R. F. W. & Silver, I. A. (1958). A histological and functional study of the mammary gland in normal and agalactic sows. *J. Endocr.* **17**, 63–74.

Cross, B. A. & Harris, G. W. (1950). Milk ejection following electrical stimulation of the pituitary stalk in rabbits. *Nature, Lond.* **166**, 994–995.

— (1951). The neurohypophysis and 'let down' of milk. *J. Physiol.* **113**, 35P.

— (1952). The role of the neurohypophysis in the milk-ejection reflex. *J. Endocr.* **8**, 148–161.

Cross, B. A., Novin, D. & Sundsten, J. W. (1969). Antidromic activation of neurones in the paraventricular nucleus by stimulation in the neural lobe of the pituitary. *J. Physiol.* **203**, 68–70P.

Cross, B. A. & Silver, I. A. (1956). Milk ejection and mammary engorgement. *Proc. R. Soc. Med.* **49**, 978–979.

— (1962). Mammary oxygen tension and the milk-ejection mechanism. *J. Endocr.* **23**, 375–384.

Cullen, G. A. (1966). Cells in milk. *Vet. Bull., Weybridge* **36**, 337–346.

Cupceancu, B., Neumann, F. & Ulloa, A. (1969). The influence of some progestogens on the mammary gland of the foetal mouse during the period of initial differentiation. *J. Endocr.* **44**, 475–480.

Curé, M. (1965). Étude histologique et caryométrique des vésicules Thyroïdiennes au cours de la gestation et de la lactation chez le hamster doré (*Mesocricetus auratus*, Waterh.). *C. r. Séanc. Soc. Biol.* **159**, 372–375.

Dabelow, A. (1934). Der Entfaltungsmechanismus der Mamma—I. Das Verhalten von Gefässsystem und Drüsenbaum während der Laktationsentwicklung der Mamma bei Maus, Ratte, Meerschweinchen und Kaninchen. *Gegenbaurs morph. Jb.* **73**, 69–99.

— (1941). Der Entfaltungsmechanismus der Mamma—II. Die postnatale Entwicklung der menschlichen Milchdrüse und ihre Korrelationen. (Hauptsächlich dargestellt an Färbungen im dicken Schnitt.) *Gegenbaurs morph. Jb.* **85**, 361–416.

— (1957). Die Milchdrüse In *Handbuch der mikroskopischen Anatomie des Menschen,* edited by von Möllendorff, W. & Bargmann, W., vol. 3, part 3, pp. 277–485. Berlin, Göttingen & Heidelberg: Springer-Verlag.

Dafny, N. & Feldman, S. (1968). Responsiveness of posterior hypothalamic neurons to striatal and peripheral stimuli. *Expl Neurol.* **21**, 397–412.

Daniel, C. W., DeOme, K. B., Young, J. T., Blair, P. B. & Faulkin, L. J. (1968). The *in vivo* life span of normal and preneoplastic mouse mammary glands: a serial transplantation study. *Proc. natn. Acad. Sci. U.S.A.* **61**, 53–60.

Daniel, D. G., Campbell, H. & Turnbull, A. C. (1967). Puerperal thrombo-embolism and suppression of lactation. *Lancet* **ii**, 287–289.

Daniel, P. M. & Prichard, M. M. L. (1958). The effects of pituitary stalk section in the goat. *Am. J. Path.* **34**, 433–469.

Danon, A., Dikstein, S. & Sulman, F. G. (1963). Stimulation of prolactin secretion by perphenazine in pituitary–hypothalamus organ culture. *Proc. Soc. exp. Biol. Med.* **114**, 366–368.

Davis, J. W. & Liu, T. M. Y. (1969). The adrenal gland and lactogenesis. *Endocrinology* **85**, 155–160.

Dawson, E. K. (1933). Carcinoma in the mammary lobule and its origin. *Edinb. med. J.* **40**, 57–82.

— (1934). A histological study of the normal mamma in relation to tumour growth—I. Early development to maturity. *Edinb. med. J.* **41**, 653–682.

— (1935). A histological study of the normal mamma in relation to tumour growth—II. The mature gland in pregnancy and lactation. *Edinb. med. J.* **42**, 569–660.

Debackere, M., Peeters, G. & Tuyttens, N. (1961). Reflex release of an oxytocic hormone by stimulation of genital organs in male and female sheep studied by a cross-circulation technique. *J. Endocr.* **22**, 321–334.

Deis, R. P. (1968). The effect of an exteroceptive stimulus on milk ejection in lactating rats. *J. Physiol.* **197**, 37–46.

De Jong, R. H. & Wagman, I. H. (1968). Block of afferent impulses in the dorsal horn of monkey. A possible mechanism of anesthesia. *Expl Neurol.* **20**, 352–358.

Dekker, A. (1968). Electron microscopic study of somatotropic and lactotropic pituitary cells of the Syrian hamster. *Anat. Rec.* **162**, 123–136.

Delost, P., Jean, Ch. & Jean, C. (1962). Production expérimentale de malformations mammaires chez le foetus de rat par injection d'oestradiol à la mère au 14ᵉ jour de la gestation. *C. r. Séanc. Soc. Biol.* **156**, 2048–2052.

Dempsey, E. W., Bunting, H. & Wislocki, G. B. (1947). Observations on the chemical cytology of the mammary gland. *Am. J. Anat.* **81**, 309–341.

Denamur, R. (1963). Les acides nucléiques de la glande mammaire pendant la gestation et la lactation de la lapine. *C. r. hebd. Séanc. Acad. Sci., Paris* **256**, 4748–4750.

— (1965*a*). Les acides nucléiques et les nucleotides libres de la glande mammaire pendant la lactogénèse et la galactopoièse. *Proc. 2nd Int. Congr. Endocr.* (*London*, 1964). Excerpta Medica International Congress Series No. 83, pp. 434–462.

— (1965*b*). The hypothalamo-neurohypophysial system and the milk-ejection reflex. *Dairy Sci. Abstr.* **27**, 193–224 & 263–280.

— (1969). Comparative aspects of hormonal control in lactogenesis. In *Progress in endocrinology*, edited by Gual, C. & Ebling, F. J. G., pp. 959–972. Amsterdam: Excerpta Medica Foundation.

— (1971). Hormonal control of lactogenesis. *J. Dairy Res.* **38**, 237–264.

Denamur, R. & Martinet, J. (1954). Enervation de la mamelle et lactation chez la brebis et la chèvre. *C. r. Séanc. Soc. Biol.* **148**, 833–836.

— (1959*a*). Les stimulus nerveux mammaires sont-ils nécessaires à l'entretien de la lactation chez la chèvre? *C. r. hebd. Séanc. Acad. Sci., Paris* **248**, 743–746.

— (1959*b*). Entretien de la lactation chez la chèvre après section de la moelle épinière et sympathectomie lombaire. *C. r. hebd. Séanc. Acad. Sci., Paris* **248**, 860–862.

— (1960). Physiological mechanisms concerned in the maintenance of lactation in the goat and sheep. *Nature, Lond.* **185**, 252–253.

Denamur, R., Stoliaroff, M. & Desclin, J. (1965). Effets de la traite sur l'activité corticotrope hypophysaire des petits ruminants en lactation. *C. r. hebd. Séanc. Acad. Sci., Paris* **260**, 3175–3178.

Denavit, M. (1968). *Zône Subthalamique Intervenant dans le Comportement de Veille et de Sommeil. Étude des Afférences Sensorielles qui l'activent.* Thèse Fac. Sci., Paris 158 pp. Quoted by Richard *et al.* (1970).

De Olmos, J. S. (1969). The stria terminalis: its projection field in the rat. *Anat. Rec.* **160**, 339–340.

Desclin, L. (1949). Effet de l'administration de thyroxine à des rats femelles en lactation sur la croissance des jeunes. *C. r. Séanc. Soc. Biol.* **143**, 1156–1158.

— (1952). Recherches sur le déterminisme des phénomènes de sécrétion dans la glande mammaire du rat. *Annls Endocr.* **13**, 120–136.

— (1962). Facteurs influencant la libération de la prolactine hypophysaire. *Proc. 22nd Int. Congr. Physiol. Sci., Leiden.* Excerpta Medica International Congress Series No. 47, pp. 715–739.

Desclin, L. & Flament-Durand, J. (1969). Effect of reserpine on the morphology of pituitaries grafted into the hypothalamus or under the kidney capsule in the rat. *J. Endocr.* **43**, lix–lx.

Desjardins, C., Kirton, K. T. & Hafs, H. D. (1967). Anterior pituitary levels of FSH, LH, ACTH and prolactin after mating in female rabbits. *Proc. Soc. exp. Biol. Med.* **126**, 23–26.

Desjardins, C., Paape, M. J. & Tucker, H. A. (1968). Contribution of pregnancy, fetuses, fetal placentas and deciduomas to mammary gland and uterine development. *Endocrinology* **83**, 907–910.

Desjardins, C., Sinha, Y. N., Hafs, H. D. & Tucker, H. A. (1965). Preservation of FSH, LH and prolactin activity. *J. Anim. Sci.* **24**, 915.

Deuben, R. R. & Meites, J. (1964). Stimulation of pituitary growth hormone releases by a hypothalamic extract *in vitro*. *Endocrinology* **74**, 408–414.

De Voe, W. F., Ramirez, V. D. & McCann, S. M. (1966). Induction of mammary secretion by hypothalamic lesions 'ı male rats. *Endocrinology* **78**, 158–164.

Dhariwal, A. P. S., Grosvenor, C. E., Antunes-Rodrigues, J. & McCann, S. M. (1968). Studies on the purification of ovine prolactin-inhibiting factor. *Endocrinology* **82**, 1236–1241.

Dickson, L. M. & Hewer, E. E. (1950). Structure of the breast. In *The Breast, Structure: Function: Disease*, edited by Saner, F. D., pp. 1–52. Bristol: John Wright.

Diczfalusy, E. (1969). Steroid metabolism in the foeto-placental unit. In *The Foeto-Placental Unit*, edited by Pecile, A. & Finzi, C., pp. 65–109. Amsterdam: Excerpta Medica Foundation.

Diczfalusy, E. & Mancuso, S. (1969). Oestrogen metabolism in pregnancy. In *Foetus and Placenta*, edited by Klopper, A. & Diczfalusy, E., pp. 191–248. Oxford & Edinburgh: Blackwell.

Dilley, W. G. & Nandi, S. (1968). Rat mammary gland differentiation *in vitro* in the absence of steroids. *Science, N.Y.* **161**, 59–60.

Dobson, W. J. & Deviney, G. T. (1967). The mammary system of the nutria, *Myocastor coypu*. *BioScience* **17**, 905.

Dodd, F. H. (1957). Factors affecting the rate of secretion of milk and lactation yields. In *Progress in the Physiology of Farm Animals*, edited by Hammond, J., vol. 3, chap. 20. London: Butterworths.

Domański, E., Traczyk, W. Z. & Lembowicz, K. (1967). Hypothalamic area in sheep associated with the lactation and secretion of prolactin. *Gen. comp. Endocr.* **9**, 446.

Domesick, V. B. (1969). Projections from the cingulate cortex in the rat. *Brain Res.* **12**, 296–320.

Donker, J. D., Koshi, J. H. & Petersen, W. E. (1954). The effect of exogenous oxytocin in blocking the normal relationship between endogenous oxytocic substance and the milk ejection phenomenon. *Science, N.Y.* **119**, 67–68.

Donovan, B. T. & van der Werff ten Bosch, J. J. (1957). The hypothalamus and lactation in the rabbit. *J. Physiol.* **137**, 410–420.

Dossett, J. A. (1960). The nature of breast secretion in infancy. *J. Path. Bact.* **80**, 93–99.

Dubois, M. P. & Herlant, M. (1968). Caractères cytologiques des cellules gonadotropes, thyréotropes, corticotropes, somatotropes, et des cellules a prolactine présentes dans le lobe antérieur de l'hypophyse des bovins. *Annls Biol. anim. Biochim. Biophys.* **8**, 5–26.

Dumont, J. N. (1965). Prolactin-induced cytologic changes in the mucosa of the pigeon crop during crop-'milk' formation. *Z. Zellforsch. mikrosk. Anat.* **68**, 755–782.

Duran-Jorda, F. (1944). Cell contents of milk. *Nature, Lond.* **154**, 704–705.

de Duve, C. (1969). The lysosome in retrospect. In *Lysosomes in Biology and Pathology*, edited by Dingle, J. T. & Fell, H. B., vol. 1, chap. 1. Amsterdam: North-Holland Publishing Co.

de Duve, C. & Wattiaux, R. (1966). Functions of lysosomes. *A. Rev. Physiol.* **28**, 436–492.

Eayrs, J. T. & Baddeley, R. M. (1956). Neural pathways in lactation. *J. Anat.* **90**, 161–171.

Eayrs, J. T. & Edwardson, J. A. (1965). Neuroendocrine interactions in the maintenance of lactation. *Acta endocr., Copenh.* Suppl. 100, 154.

Edwardson, J. A. & Eayrs, J. T. (1967). Neural factors in the maintenance of lactation in the rat. *J. Endocr.* **38**, 51–59.

Ehni, G. & Eckles, N. E. (1959). Interruption of the pituitary stalk in the patient with mammary cancer. *J. Neurosurg.* **16**, 628–652.

Ehrenbrand, F. (1962). Licht- und elektronenmikroskopische sowie chemohistologische Untersuchungen an der lactierenden Milchdrüse. *Fortschr. Med.* **80**, 711–716.

— (1964). Beiträge zur Orthologie der lactierenden Milchdrüse. (Lichtmikroskopische, elektronenoptische, polarisations- und fluoreszenzmikroskopische sowie chemohistologische Untersuchungen). *Acta histochem.* **18**, 1–5; **19**, 104–158.

El-Darwish, I. & Rivera, E. M. (1970). Temporal effects of hormones on DNA synthesis in mouse mammary gland *in vitro*. *J. exp. Zool.* **173**, 285–292.

Elger, W. & Neumann, F. (1966). The role of androgens in differentiation of the mammary gland in male mouse fetuses. *Proc. Soc. exp. Biol. Med.* **123**, 637–640.

Ellis, S. (1961). Studies on the serial extraction of pituitary proteins. *Endocrinology* **69**, 554–570.

Ellis, S., Grindeland, R. E., Nuenke, J. M. & Callahan, P. X. (1969). Purification and properties of rat prolactin. *Endocrinology* **85**, 886–894.

Ely, F. & Petersen, W. E. (1941). Factors involved in the ejection of milk. *J. Dairy Sci.* **24**, 211–223.

Emmart, E. W., Bates, R. W. & Turner, W. A. (1965). Localization of prolactin in rat pituitary and in a transplantable mammotropic pituitary tumor using fluorescent antibody. *J. Histochem. Cytochem.* **13**, 182–190.

Emmart, E. W., Spicer, S. S. & Bates, R. W. (1963). Localization of prolactin within the pituitary by specific fluorescent antiprolactin globulin. *J. Histochem. Cytochem.* **3**, 365–373.

Enders, R. K. (1966). Attachment, nursing and survival of young in some didelphids. *Symp. zool. Soc. Lond.* **15**, 195–203.

Erb, R. E., Estergreen Jr., V. L., Gomes, W. R., Plotka, E. D. & Frost, O. L. (1968). Progestin levels in corpora lutea and progesterone in ovarian venous and jugular vein blood plasma of the pregnant bovine. *J. Dairy Sci.* **51**, 401–410.

Ericsson, J. L. E., Trump, B. F. & Weibel, J. (1965). Electron microscopic studies of the proximal tubule of the rat kidney—II. Cytosegresomes and cytosomes: their relationship to each other and to the lysosome concept. *Lab. Invest.* **14**, 1341–1365.

Etkin, W. (1963). Metamorphosis-activating system of the frog. *Science, N.Y.* **139**, 810–814.

Etkin, W. & Lehrer, R. (1960). Excess growth in tadpoles after transplantation of the adenohypophysis. *Endocrinology* **67**, 457–466.

Evans, D. E. (1959). Milk composition of mammals whose milk is not normally used for human consumption. *Dairy Sci. Abstr.* **21**, 277–288.

Everett, J. W. (1954). Luteotrophic function of autografts of the rat hypophysis. *Endocrinology* **54**, 685–690.

— (1956). Functional corpora lutea maintained for months by autografts of rat hypophysis. *Endocrinology* **58**, 786–796.

— (1966). The control of the secretion of prolactin. In *The Pituitary Gland*, edited by Harris, G. W. & Donovan, B. T., vol. 2, chap. 5. London: Butterworths.

— (1969). Neuroendocrine aspects of mammalian reproduction. *A. Rev. Physiol.* **31**, 383–416.

Everett, J. W. & Quinn, D. L. (1966). Differential hypothalamic mechanisms inciting ovulation and pseudopregnancy in the rat. *Endocrinology* **78**, 141–150.

Everett, J. W. & Radford, H. M. (1961). Irritative deposits from stainless steel electrodes in the preoptic rat brain causing release of pituitary gonadotropin. *Proc. Soc. exp. Biol. Med.* **108**, 604–609.

Ewbank, R. (1964). Observations on the suckling habits of twin lambs. *Anim. Behav.* **12**, 34–37.

— (1967). Nursing and suckling behaviour amongst Clun Forest ewes and lambs. *Anim. Behav.* **15**, 251–258.

Ezekiel, E. (1965). The iron-binding proteins in milk and the secretion of iron by the mammary gland in the rat. *Biochim. biophys. Acta* **107**, 511–518.

Fabian, M., Forsling, M. L., Jones, J. J. & Lee, J. (1969). Comparison of two methods for the bioassay of oxytocin. *Endocrinology* **85**, 600–603.

Faulkin Jr., L. J. & DeOme, K. B. (1960). Regulation of growth and spacing of gland elements in the mammary fat pad of the C3H mouse. *J. natn. Cancer Inst.* **24**, 953–969.

Feasey, C. M., James, W. B. & Davison, M. (1970). A technique for breast thermography. *Br. J. Radiol.* **43**, 462–465.

Fegler, G. (1957). The reliability of the thermodilution method for determination of the cardiac output and the blood flow in central veins. *Q. Jl exp. Physiol.* **42**, 254–266.

Feldman, J. D. (1961). Fine structure of the cow's udder during gestation and lactation. *Lab. Invest.* **10**, 238–255.

Feller, W. F. & Boretos, J. (1967). Semiautomatic apparatus for milking mice. *J. natn. Cancer Inst.* **38**, 11–17.

Findlay, A. L. R. (1966). Sensory discharges from lactating mammary glands. *Nature, Lond.* **211**, 1183–1184.

— (1968). The effect of teat anaesthesia on the milk-ejection reflex in the rabbit. *J. Endocr.* **40**, 127–128.

— (1969). Nursing behavior and the condition of the mammary gland in the rabbit. *J. comp. physiol. Psychol.* **69**, 115–118.

Findlay, A. L. R. & Grosvenor, C. E. (1969). The role of mammary gland innervation in the control of the motor apparatus of the mammary gland: a review. *Dairy Sci. Abstr.* **31**, 109–116.

Findlay, A. L. R. & Roth, L. L. (1970). Long-term dissociation of nursing behavior and the condition of the mammary gland in the rabbit. *J. comp. physiol. Psychol.* **72**, 341–344.

Fink, R. P. & Heimer, L. (1967). Two methods for selective silver impregnation of degenerating axons and their synaptic endings in the central nervous system. *Brain Res.* **4**, 369–374.

Firth, P. S. (1969). Inhibition of lactation. *Br. med. J.* **1**, 254–255.

Fischer-Rasmussen, W. (1970). Plasma oestriol in normal human pregnancy. *J. Steroid Biochem.* **1**, 121–126.

Fiske, S., Courtecuisse, V. & Haguenau, F. (1966). Autoradiographie au microscope électronique de l'incorporation de leucine tritiée dans la glande mammaire de la souris en lactation. *C. r. hebd. Séanc. Acad. Sci., Paris* **262**, 126–129.

Fitzpatrick, R. J. (1961). The estimation of small amounts of oxytocin in blood. In *Oxytocin*, edited by Caldeyro-Barcia, R. & Heller, H., pp. 358–379. Oxford: Pergamon Press.

Fitzpatrick, R. J. & Bentley, P. J. (1968). The assay of neurohypophysial hormones in blood and other body fluids. In *Handbook of Experimental Pharmacology*, Vol. 23, *Neurohypophysial Hormones and Similar Polypeptides*, edited by Berde, B., pp. 190–285. Berlin, Heidelberg, New York: Springer-Verlag.

Flament-Durand, J. & Desclin, L. (1964). Observations concerning the hypothalamic control of pituitary luteotrophin secretion in the rat. *Endocrinology* **75**, 22–26.

Florini, J. R., Tonelli, G., Breuer, B., Coppola, J., Ringler, I. & Bell, P. H. (1966). Characterization and biological effects of purified placental protein (human). *Endocrinology* **79**, 692–708.

Flux, D. S. (1954*a*). Growth of the mammary duct system in intact and ovariectomized mice of the CHI strain. *J. Endocr.* **11**, 223–237.

Flux, D. S. (1954b). The effect of adrenal steroids on the growth of the mammary glands, uteri, thymus and adrenal glands of intact, ovariectomized and oestrone-treated ovariectomized mice. *J. Endocr.* **11**, 238–254.

Folley, S. J. (1947). The nervous system and lactation. *Br. med. Bull.* **5**, 142–148.

— (1949). Biochemical aspects of mammary gland function. *Biol. Rev.* **24**, 316–354.

— (1952). Lactation. In *Marshall's Physiology of Reproduction*. 3rd edn, edited by Parkes, A. S., vol. 2, chap. 20. London: Longmans, Green.

— (1956). *The Physiology and Biochemistry of Lactation*. Edinburgh & London: Oliver & Boyd.

— (1960). Disorders of mammary development and lactation. In *Clinical Endocrinology I*, edited by Astwood, E. B., chap. 8. New York: Grune & Stratton.

— (1963). Some observations on prolactin secretion. In *Advances in Neuroendocrinology*, edited by Nalbandov, A. V., pp. 277–282. Urbana: University of Illinois Press.

— (1969a). Symposium on lactogenesis: chairman's introduction. In *Lactogenesis: the Initiation of Milk Secretion at Parturition*, edited by Reynolds, M. & Folley, S. J., pp. 1–3. Philadelphia: University of Pennsylvania Press.

— (1969b). The milk-ejection reflex: a neuroendocrine theme in biology, myth and art. *J. Endocr.* **44**, x–xx.

Folley, S. J., Guthkelch, A. N. & Zuckerman, S. (1939). The mammary gland of the rhesus monkey under normal and experimental conditions. *Proc. R. Soc.* B **126**, 469–491.

Folley, S. J. & Knaggs, G. S. (1965a). Oxytocin levels in the blood of ruminants with special reference to the milking stimulus. In *Advances in Oxytocin Research*, edited by Pinkerton, J. H. M., pp. 37–49. Oxford: Pergamon Press.

— (1965b). Levels of oxytocin in the jugular vein blood of goats during parturition. *J. Endocr.* **33**, 301–315.

— (1966). Milk-ejection activity (oxytocin) in the external jugular vein blood of the cow, goat and sow, in relation to the stimulus of milking or suckling. *J. Endocr.* **34**, 197–214

Folley, S. J. & Malpress, F. H. (1948a). Hormonal control of mammary growth. In *The Hormones*, edited by Pincus, G. & Thimann, K. V., vol. 1, chap. 15. New York: Academic Press.

— (1948b). Hormonal control of lactation. In *The Hormones*, edited by Pincus, G. & Thimann, K. V., vol. 1, chap. 16. New York: Academic Press.

Folley, S. J., Scott Watson, H. M. & Bottomley, A. C. (1941). Studies on experimental teat and mammary development and lactation in the goat. *J. Dairy Res.* **12**, 241–264.

Folley, S. J. & Young, F. G. (1938). The effect of anterior pituitary extracts on established lactation in the cow. *Proc. R. Soc.* B **126**, 45–76.

Folley, S. J. & Young, F. G. (1940). Further experiments on the continued treatment of lactating cows with anterior pituitary extracts. *J. Endocr.* **2**, 226–236.

— (1941). Prolactin as a specific lactogenic hormone. *Lancet* **i**, 380–381.

Forbes, A. P., Henneman, P. H., Griswold, G. C. & Albright, F. (1954). Syndrome characterized by galactorrhea, amenorrhea and low urinary FSH: comparison with acromegaly and normal lactation. *J. clin. Endocr. Metab.* **14**, 265–271.

Forbes, J. M. & Rook, J. A. F. (1970). The effect of intravenous infusion of oestrogen on lactation in the goat. *J. Physiol.* **207**, 79–80P.

Forbes, T. R. (1950). Witch's milk and witches' marks. *Yale J. Biol. Med.* **22**, 219–225.

Ford, D. H. & Kantounis, S. (1957). The localization of neurosecretory structures and pathways in the male albino rabbit. *J. comp. Neurol.* **108**, 91–107.

Forsyth, I. A. (1967). Prolactin and placental lactogens. In *Hormones in Blood*, 2nd edn, edited by Gray, C. H. & Bacharach, A. L., vol. 1, chap. 11. London & New York: Academic Press.

— (1969). The role of primate prolactins and placental lactogens in lacto-genesis. In *Lactogenesis: the Initiation of Milk Secretion at Parturi-tion*, edited by Reynolds, M. & Folley, S. J., pp. 195–205. Phila-delphia: University of Pennsylvania Press.

— (1970). The detection of lactogenic activity in human blood by bioassay. *J. Endocr.* **46**, iv–v.

— (1971). Organ culture techniques and the study of hormone effects on the mammary gland. *J. Dairy Res.* **38**, 419–444.

Forsyth, I. A. & Folley, S. J. (1970). Prolactin and growth hormone in man and other mammals. In *Ovo-Implantation, Human Gonado-tropins and Prolactin*, edited by Hubinont, P. O., Leroy, F., Robyn, C. & Leleux, P., pp. 266–278. Basel & New York: Karger.

Forsyth, I. A., Folley, S. J. & Chadwick, A. (1965). Lactogenic and pigeon crop-stimulating activities of human pituitary growth hor-mone preparations. *J. Endocr.* **31**, 115–126.

Forsyth, I. A. & Hosking, Z. D. (1969). The design and precision of pigeon crop-sac assays for prolactin. *J. Endocr.* **44**, 545–555.

Fox, C. A. & Knaggs, G. S. (1969). Milk-ejection activity (oxytocin) in peripheral venous blood in man during lactation and in association with coitus. *J. Endocr.* **45**, 145–146.

Frank, R. T. & Unger, A. (1911). An experimental study of the causes which produce the growth of the mammary gland. *Archs int. Med.* **7**, 812–838.

Fredrikson, H. (1939). Endocrine factors involved in the development and function of the mammary glands of female rabbits. *Acta obstet. gynec. scand.* **19**, Suppl. 1.

Freud, J. & Uyldert, I. E. (1948). Mamma and lactation in rats and other species. *Archs int. Pharmacodyn. Thér.* **76**, 74–94.

Friedman, M. & Lehrman, D. S. (1968). Physiological conditions for the stimulation of prolactin secretion by external stimuli in the male ring dove. *Anim. Behav.* **16**, 233–237.

Friesen, H. G. (1968). Biosynthesis of placental proteins and placental lactogen. *Endocrinology* **83**, 744–753.

Friesen, H. G., Suwa, S. & Pare, P. (1969). Synthesis and secretion of placental lactogen and other proteins by the placenta. *Recent Prog. Horm. Res.* **25**, 161–205.

Fuchs, A-R. (1969). Ethanol and the inhibition of oxytocin release in lactating rats. *Acta endocr., Copenh.* **62**, 546–554.

Fuchs, A-R. & Wagner, G. (1963a). Quantitative aspects of release of oxytocin by suckling in unanaesthetized rabbits. *Acta endocr., Copenh.* **44**, 581–592.

— (1963b). The effect of ethyl alcohol on the release of oxytocin in rabbits. *Acta endocr., Copenh.* **44**, 593–605.

— (1963c). Effect of alcohol on release of oxytocin. *Nature, Lond.* **198**, 92–94.

Gachev, E. (1963). Rol' prolaktina v podderzhanii urovnya laktozȳ v moloke. *Zh. obshch. Biol.* **24**, 382–383.

— (1966). Einfluss des Hydrokortisons auf die Milchzuckersynthese in der Milchdrüse. *C. r. Acad. bulg. Sci.* **19**, 417–419.

— (1967). Inhibition of lactose synthesis by means of tri-iodothyronin. *C. r. Acad. bulg. Sci.* **20**, 369–371.

— (1968a). The lactation curve as a function of the peripheral stimulation. *C. r. Acad. bulg. Sci.* **21**, 577–579.

— (1968b). Duration of prolactin-induced lactose synthesis. *C. r. Acad. bulg. Sci.* **21**, 709–711.

Gadkari, S. V., Chapekar, T. N. & Ranadive, K. J. (1968). Response of mouse mammary glands to hormonal treatment *in vitro. Indian J. exp. Biol.* **6**, 75–79.

Gaines, W. L. (1915). A contribution to the physiology of lactation. *Am. J. Physiol.* **38**, 285–312.

Gala, R. R. & Reece, R. P. (1964). Influence of estrogen on anterior pituitary lactogen production *in vitro. Proc. Soc. exp. Biol. Med.* **115**, 1030–1035.

Gale, C. C. (1963). Non-essential role of prolactin in the hormonal restoration of lactation in goats with radio frequency hypothalamic lesions. *Acta physiol. scand.* **59**, 269–283.

Gale, C. C. & Larsson, B. (1963). Radiation induced 'hypophysectomy' and hypothalamic lesions in lactating goats. *Acta physiol. scand.* **59**, 299–318.

Gale, C. C., Taleisnik, S., Friedman, H. M. & McCann, S. M. (1961). Hormonal basis for impairments in milk synthesis and milk ejection following hypothalamic lesions. *J. Endocr.* **23**, 303–316.

Garn, S. M. (1952). Changes in areolar size during the steroid growth phase. *Child Dev.* **23**, 55–60.

Gerebtzoff, M. A. (1940). Les voies centrales de la sensibilité et du goût et leurs terminaisons thalamiques. *Cellule* **48**, 91–146.

Gershon-Cohen, J., Hermel, M. B. & Birsner, J. W. (1970). Advances in mammographic technique. *Am. J. Roentg.* **108,** 424–427.

Geschickter, C. F. (1945). *Diseases of the Breast: Diagnosis, Pathology, Treatment,* 2nd edn. Philadelphia, London, Montreal: Lippencott.

Geschwind, I. I. (1966). Species specificity of anterior pituitary hormones. In *The Pituitary Gland,* edited by Harris, G. W. & Donovan, B. T., vol. 2, chap. 21. London: Butterworths.

Gill, J. C. & Thompson, W. (1956). Observations on the behaviour of suckling pigs. *Br. J. Anim. Behav.* **4,** 46–51.

Gilliland, P. F. & Prout, T. E. (1965a) Immunologic studies of octapeptides—I. Radioiodination of oxytocin. *Metabolism* **14,** 912–917.

— (1965b). Immunologic studies of octapeptides—II. Production and detection of antibodies to oxytocin. *Metabolism* **14,** 918–923.

Girardie, J. (1967a). Localisation optique et ultrastructurale de l'activité phosphatasique alcaline dans l'epithélium mammaire. *C. r. hebd. Séanc. Acad. Sci., Sér. D, Paris* **264,** 2064–2067.

— (1967b). Fonction catabolique de l'epithélium mammaire. Étude histochimique et ultrastructurale. *Z. Zellforsch. mikrosk. Anat.* **80,** 385–412.

— (1968). Histo-cytomorphologie de la glande mammaire de la souris C3H et de trois autres rongeurs. *Z. Zellforsch. mikrosk. Anat.* **87,** 478–503.

Girardie, J., Gros, C. M., Le Gal, Y. & Porte, A. (1964). Sur la formation des corpuscules de Donné dans la mamelle de souris. Étude au microscope électronique. *C. r. Séanc. Soc. Biol.* **158,** 1940–1942.

Girardie, J. & Porte, A. (1965). Sur la variation de l'activité leucine amino-peptidasique dans la mamelle de souris. Sa relation avec certain aspects ultrastructuraux. *C. r. Séanc. Soc. Biol.* **159,** 748–750.

Girod, C. (1964). Quelques données sur la cytologie de la pars distalis de l'hypophyse chez les singes. *C. r. Ass. Anat.* **121,** 145–158.

Gitlin, D. & Biasucci, A. (1969). Ontogenesis of immunoreactive growth hormone, follicle-stimulating hormone, thyroid-stimulating hormone, luteinizing hormone, chorionic prolactin and chorionic gonadotropin in the human conceptus. *J. clin. Endocr. Metab.* **29,** 926–935.

Glass, R. L., Troolin, H. A. & Jenness, R. (1967). Comparative biochemical studies of milks—IV. Constituent fatty acids of milk fats. *Comp. Biochem. Physiol.* **22,** 415–425.

Glebina, E. I. (1940). Razvitie molochnoĭ zhelezẏ i ee sekretornogo protsessa. *Arkh. Anat. Gistol. Embriol.* **23,** 332–342.

Glick, S. M. Kumaresan, P., Kagan, A. & Wheeler, M. (1969). Radioimmunoassay of oxytocin. In *Protein and Polypeptide Hormones,* edited by Margoulies, M., pp. 81–83. Excerpta Medica International Congress Series No. 161.

Gofman, M. A. (1955). O reflektornoĭ regulyatsii molokootdachi. *Trudẏ Inst. Fiziol. I. P. Pavlova* **4,** 22–33.

Gold, J. J. & Cohen, M. R. (1959). Sex-steroid therapy for postpartum breast symptoms: a review. *Obstet. Gynec., N. Y.* **13,** 413–419.

Goluboff, L. G. & Ezrin, C. (1969). Effect of pregnancy on the somato-troph and the prolactin cell of the human adenohypophysis. *J. clin. Endocr. Metab.* **29**, 1533–1538.

Gomes, W. R. & Erb, R. E. (1965). Progesterone in bovine reproduction: a review. *J. Dairy Sci.* **48**, 314–330.

Gomez, E. T. (1939). The relation of the posterior hypophysis in the maintenance of lactation in hypophysectomized rats. *J. Dairy Sci.* **22**, 488.

Gorbunov, V. M. (1963). Voloknistȳe strukturȳ v strome molochnoĭ zhelezȳ u vzroslȳkh zhivotnȳkh i émbrionov krupnogo rogatogo skota. *Izv. Akad. Nauk SSSR (Ser. biol.)* No. 6, 892–898.

Gorman, G. M. & Swanson, E. W. (1968). Effects of oxytocin adminis-tered during the dry period on the succeeding lactation. *J. Dairy Sci.* **51**, 60–66.

Gorokhov, L. N. & Trofimov, Yu. N. (1965). Deĭstvie vnutrennikh i vneshnikh faktorov na oksitotsinovyĭ refleks u korov. *Dokl. vses. Akad. sel'.-khoz. Nauk* No. 7, 24–26.

Gourdji, D. & Tixier-Vidal, A. (1966). Mise en évidence d'un contrôle hypothalamique stimulant de la prolactine hypophysaire chez le canard. *C. r. hebd. Séanc. Acad. Sci., Sér. D, Paris* **263**, 162–165.

Grachev, I. I. (1949). O refleksakh s molochnoĭ zhelezȳ. *Zh. obshch. Biol.* **10**, 401–420.

— (1964). *Reflektornaya Regulyatsiya Laktatsii.* Izdatel'stvo Leningrad-skogo Universiteta.

Grachev, I. I. & Gostev, A. V. (1962). Materialȳ o reflektornom vliyanii s molochnoĭ zhelezȳ na limfootdelenie u koz. *Dokl. Akad. Nauk SSSR* **144**, 938–941.

Graf, G. C. & Lawson, D. M. (1968). Factors affecting intramammary pressures. *J. Dairy Sci.* **51**, 1672–1675.

Grant, D. B., Kaplan, S. L. & Grumbach, M. M. (1970). Studies on a monkey placental protein with immunochemical similarity to human growth hormone and human chorionic somatomammo-trophin. *Acta endocr., Copenh.* **63**, 736–746.

Greenbaum, A. L. & Darby, F. J. (1964). The effect of adrenalectomy on the metabolism of the mammary glands of lactating rats. *Biochem. J.* **91**, 307–317.

Greenbaum, A. L. & Slater, T. F. (1957). Studies on the particulate components of rat mammary gland. 2. Changes in the levels of the nucleic acids of the mammary glands of rats during pregnancy, lactation and mammary involution. *Biochem. J.* **66**, 155–161.

Greenwood, F. C. (1967*a*). Immunological procedures in the assay of protein hormones. In *Modern Trends in Endocrinology*, 3rd series, edited by Gardiner-Hill, H., chap. 14. London: Butterworths.

— (1967*b*). Growth hormone. In *Hormones in Blood*, 2nd edn, edited by Gray, C. H. & Bacharach, A. L., vol. 1, chap. 10. London & New York: Academic Press.

Grégoire, C. (1946). Factors involved in maintaining involution of the thymus during suckling. *J. Endocr.* **5**, 68–87.

Griffith, D. R., Williams, R. & Turner, C. W. (1963). Effects of orally administered progesterone-like compounds on mammary gland growth in rats. *Proc. Soc. exp. Biol. Med.* **113**, 401–403.

Griffiths, M. (1968). *Echidnas*. International series of monographs in pure and applied biology, Zoology Division, edited by Kerkut, G. A., vol. 38. Oxford: Pergamon Press.

Griffiths, M., McIntosh, D. L. & Coles, R. E. A. (1969). The mammary gland of the echidna, *Tachyglossus aculeatus*, with observations on the incubation of the egg and on the newly-hatched young. *J. Zool., Lond.* **158**, 371–386.

Grosvenor, C. E. (1961). Thyroid hormone secretion rate and milk yield in lactating rats. *Am. J. Physiol.* **200**, 483–485.

— (1964). Lactation in rat mammary glands after spinal cord section. *Endocrinology* **74**, 548–553.

— (1965*a*). Contraction of lactating rat mammary gland in response to direct mechanical stimulation. *Am. J. Physiol.* **208**, 214–218.

— (1965*b*). Evidence that exteroceptive stimuli can release prolactin from the pituitary gland of the lactating rat. *Endocrinology* **76**, 340–342.

— (1965*c*). Effect of nursing and stress upon prolactin-inhibiting activity of the rat hypothalamus. *Endocrinology* **77**, 1037–1042.

— (1969). General discussion III. In *Lactogenesis: the Initiation of Milk Secretion at Parturition*, edited by Reynolds, M. & Folley, S. J., p. 189. Philadelphia: University of Pennsylvania Press.

Grosvenor, C. E. & Findlay, A. L. R. (1968). Effect of denervation on fluid flow into rat mammary gland. *Am. J. Physiol.* **214**, 820–824.

Grosvenor, C. E., Krulich, L. & McCann, S. M. (1968). Depletion of pituitary concentration of growth hormone as a result of suckling in the lactating rat. *Endocrinology* **82**, 617–619.

Grosvenor, C. E., McCann, S. M. & Nallar, R. (1965). Inhibition of nursing-induced and stress-induced fall in pituitary prolactin concentration in lactating rats by injection of acid extracts of bovine hypothalamus. *Endocrinology* **76**, 883–889.

Grosvenor, C. E., Maiweg, H. & Mena, F. (1969*a*). Effect of SME extract and exogenous prolactin upon post-suckling reaccumulation of prolactin in the pituitary of the lactating rat. *Fedn Proc.* **28**, 437.

— (1969*b*). Observations on the development and retention during lactation of the mechanism for prolactin release by exteroceptive stimulation in the rat. In *Lactogenesis: the Initiation of Milk Secretion at Parturition*, edited by Reynolds, M. & Folley, S. J., pp. 181–188. Philadelphia: University of Pennsylvania Press.

— (1970). A study of factors involved in the development of the exteroceptive release of prolactin in the lactating rat. *Horm. Behav.* **1**, 111–120.

Grosvenor, C. E. & Mena, F. (1967). Effect of auditory, olfactory and optic stimuli upon milk ejection and suckling-induced release of prolactin in lactating rats. *Endocrinology* **80**, 840–846.

— (1969). Failure of self-licking of nipples to alter pituitary prolactin concentration in lactating rats. *Horm. Behav.* **1**, 85–91.

Grosvenor, C. E., Mena, F., Dhariwal, A. P. S. & McCann, S. M. (1967). Reduction of milk secretion by prolactin-inhibiting factor: further evidence that exteroceptive stimuli can release pituitary prolactin in rats. *Endocrinology* **81**, 1021–1028.

Grosvenor, C. E., Mena, F. & Schaefgen, D. A. (1967). Effect of non-suckling interval and duration of suckling on the suckling-induced fall in pituitary prolactin concentration in the rat. *Endocrinology* **81**, 449–453.

Grosvenor, C. E. & Turner, C. W. (1957a). Estimation of amount of oxytocin released as result of nursing stimuli in lactating rat. *Proc. Soc. exp. Biol. Med.* **95**, 131–133.

— (1957b). Release and restoration of pituitary lactogen in response to nursing stimuli in lactating rats. *Proc. Soc. exp. Biol. Med.* **96**, 723–725.

— (1958a). Assay of lactogenic hormone. *Endocrinology* **63**, 530–534·

— (1958b). Pituitary lactogenic hormone concentration and milk secretion in lactating rats. *Endocrinology* **63**, 535–539.

— (1959a). Effect of growth hormone and oxytocin upon milk yield in lactating rats. *Proc. Soc. exp. Biol. Med.* **100**, 158–161.

— (1959b). Thyroid hormone and lactation in the rat. *Proc. Soc. exp. Biol. Med.* **100**, 162–165.

— (1959c). Lactogenic hormone requirements for milk secretion in intact lactating rats. *Proc. Soc. exp. Biol. Med.* **101**, 699–703.

Grosz, H. J. & Rothballer, A. B. (1961). Hypothalamic control of lactogenic function in the cat. *Nature, Lond.* **190**, 349–350.

Grota, L. J. & Eik-Nes, K. B. (1967). Plasma progesterone concentrations during pregnancy and lactation in the rat. *J. Reprod. Fert.* **13**, 83–91.

Groves, W. E. & Sells, B. H. (1968). Purification of rat prolactin and growth hormone using preparative polyacrylamide gel electrophoresis. *Biochim. biophys. Acta* **168**, 113–121.

Grumbach, M. M. & Kaplan, S. L. (1964). On the placental origin and purification of chorionic 'growth hormone-prolactin' and its immunoassay in pregnancy. *Trans. N.Y. Acad. Sci.* Series II, **27**, 167–188.

Grumbach, M. M., Kaplan, S. L., Sciarra, J. J. & Burr, I. M. (1968). Chorionic growth hormone-prolactin (CGP): secretion, disposition, biologic activity in man, and postulated function as the 'growth hormone' of the second half of pregnancy. *Ann. N.Y. Acad. Sci.* **148**, 501–531.

Grünefeld, Y-F. (1964). Die Myoepithelzellen und die phosphatasehaltigen Strukturen der bovinen Milchdrüse. *Acta anat.* **58**, 317–332.

Gupta, B. N., Conner, G. H. & Langham, R. F. (1970). A device for collecting milk from guinea pigs. *Am. J. vet. Res.* **31**, 557–559.

Gusdon, J. P., Jr. (1967). An antibody to oxytocin. *Am. J. Obstet. Gynec.* **98**, 526–534.

Hadfield, G. & Young, S. (1958). The controlling influence of the pituitary on the growth of the normal breast. *Br. J. Surg.* **46**, 265–273.

Hahn, D. W. & Turner, C. W. (1966). Effect of corticosterone upon milk yield in the rat. *Proc. Soc. exp. Biol. Med.* **121**, 1056–1058.

Hakim, C. A., Elder, M. G. & Hawkins, D. F. (1969). Plasma factor IX levels in patients given hexoestrol or stilboestrol to suppress lactation. *Br. med. J.* **4**, 82–84.

Halász, B. (1968). The role of the hypothalamic hypophysiotrophic area in the control of growth hormone secretion. In *Growth Hormone*, edited by Pecile, A. & Müller, E. E., Excerpta Medica International Congress Series No. 158, pp. 204–210.

Halász, B., Pupp, L. & Uhlarik, S. (1962). Hypophysiotrophic area in the hypothalamus. *J. Endocr.* **25**, 147–154.

Hall, P. F. (1959). *Gynaecomastia*. Monographs of the Federal Council of the British Medical Association in Australia, No. 2.

Haller, A. von (1778). *Elementa Physiologiae Corporis Humani*, 2nd edn., tomus 7, pars 2, liber 28, sectio 1—Mammae. Lausanna: Societas Typographica (First edition was published in 1765).

Halsell, J. T., Smith, J. R., Bentlage, C. R., Park, O. K. & Humphreys, J. W., Jr. (1965). Lymphatic drainage of the breast demonstrated by vital dye staining and radiography. *Ann. Surg.* **162**, 221–226.

Hamberger, L. & Ahrén, K. (1964). Influence of the adrenal cortex on growth processes in the rat mammary gland. *J. Endocr.* **30**, 171–179.

Hampl, A. (1964). K otázce existence a morfologické úpravy TZV nadstrukových mízních uzlin mléčné žlázy skotu. *Sb. vys. Šk. zeměd. Brně, Řada B (Spisy Fak. Agron.)* No. 3, 569–577.

— (1965*a*). Lymphonodi intramammarii der Rindermilchdrüse—I. Makroskopisch-anatomische Verhältnisse. *Anat. Anz.* **116**, 281–298.

— (1965*b*). Lymphonodi intramammarii der Rindermilchdrüse—II. Mikroskopisch-anatomische Verhältnisse. *Anat. Anz.* **117**, 129–137.

— (1967). Die Lymphknoten der Rindermilchdrüse. *Anat. Anz.* **121**, 38–54.

— (1968). Příspěvek k otázce regionální příslušnosti intramamárních mízních uzlin a jejich vztahu k uzlinám supramamárním u skotu. *Sb. vys. Šk. zeměd. Brně, Řada A (Spisy Fak. Agron.)* **16**, 293–298.

Hampl, A., Bartoš, J. & Zedník, R. (1967). Lymphonodi supramammarii der Schafmilchdrüse. *Zentbl. VetMed.*, A. **14**, 570–577.

Hanrahan, J. P. & Eisen, E. J. (1970). A lactation curve for mice. *Lab. Anim. Care* **20**, 101–104.

Hansel, W. (1967). Studies on the formation and maintenance of the corpus luteum. In *Reproduction in the Female Mammal, Proc. 13th Easter Sch. agric. Sci. Univ. Nott., 1966*, edited by Lamming, G. E. & Amoroso, E. C., pp. 346–363. London: Butterworths.

Harris, G. W. & Jacobsohn, D. (1952). Functional grafts of the anterior pituitary gland. *Proc. R. Soc.* B **139**, 263–276.

Harrison, R. J. (1969). Reproduction and reproductive organs. In *The Biology of Marine Mammals*, edited by Andersen, H. T., chap. 8. New York & London: Academic Press.

Hartmann, P. E., Cowie, A. T. & Hosking, Z. D. (1970). Changes in enzymic activity, chemical composition and histology of the mammary glands and blood metabolites of lactating rabbits after hypophysectomy and replacement therapy with sheep prolactin, human growth hormone or bovine growth hormone. *J. Endocr.* **48**, 433–448.

Hartree, A. S., Kovačić, N. & Thomas, M. (1965). Growth-promoting and luteotrophic activities of human growth hormone. *J. Endocr.* **33**, 249–258.

Haun, C. K. & Sawyer, C. H. (1960). Initiation of lactation in rabbits following placement of hypothalamic lesions. *Endocrinology* **67**, 270–272.

— (1961). The role of the hypothalamus in initiation of milk secretion. *Acta endocr., Copenh.* **38**, 99–106.

Hawker, R. W. (1961). Oxytocin and an unidentified oxytocic substance in extracts of blood. In *Oxytocin*, edited by Caldeyro-Barcia, R. & Heller, H., pp. 425–436. Oxford: Pergamon Press.

Hawker, R. W. & Roberts, V. S. (1957). Oxytocin in lactating cows and goats. *Br. vet. J.* **113**, 459–464.

Hayashida, T. (1966). Immunological reactions of pituitary hormones. In *The Pituitary Gland*, edited by Harris, G. W. & Donovan, B. T., vol. 2, chap. 22. London: Butterworths.

Hayward, J. N. & Smith, W. K. (1964). Antidiuretic response to electrical stimulation in brain stem of the monkey. *Am. J. Physiol.* **206**, 15–20.

Heap, R. B. & Linzell, J. L. (1966). Arterial concentration, ovarian secretion and mammary uptake of progesterone in goats during the reproductive cycle. *J. Endocr.* **36**, 389–399.

Heap, R. B., Linzell, J. L. & Slotin, C. A. (1969). Quantitative measurement of progesterone metabolism in the mammary gland of the goat. *J. Physiol.* **200**, 38–40 P.

Hebb, C. O. & Linzell, J. L. (1951). Some conditions affecting the blood flow through the perfused mammary gland, with special reference to the action of adrenaline. *Q. Jl exp. Physiol.* **36**, 159–175.

— (1966). A histological study of the innervation of the mammary glands. *J. Physiol.* **186**, 82–83 P.

Heimer, L. & Nauta, W. J. H. (1969). The hypothalamic distribution of the stria terminalis in the rat. *Brain Res.* **13**, 284–297.

Hellig, H., Lefebvre, Y., Gattereau, D. & Bolté, E. (1969). Foetal progesterone synthesis in the human. In *The Foeto-Placental Unit*, edited by Pecile, A. & Finzi, C., pp. 152–161. Amsterdam: Excerpta Medica Foundation.

Helminen, H. J. & Ericsson, J. L. E. (1968*a*). Studies on mammary gland involution—I. On the ultrastructure of the lactating mammary gland. *J. Ultrastruct. Res.* **25**, 193–213.

— (1968*b*). Studies on mammary gland involution—II. Ultrastructural evidence for auto- and heterophagocytosis. *J. Ultrastruct. Res.* **25**, 214–227.

— (1968*c*). Studies on mammary gland involution—III. Alteration outside auto- and heterophagocytic pathways for cytoplasmic degradation. *J. Ultrastruct. Res.* **25**, 228–239.

Helminen, H. J. & Ericsson, J. L. E. (1970). Quantitation of lysosomal enzyme changes during enforced mammary gland involution. *Expl Cell Res.* **60**, 419–426.

Helminen, H. J., Ericsson, J. L. E. & Orrenius, S. (1968). Studies on mammary gland involution. IV. Histochemical and biochemical observations on alterations in lysosomes and lysosomal enzymes. *J. Ultrastruct. Res.* **25**, 240–252.

Herlant, M. (1960). Étude critique de deux techniques nouvelles destinées à mettre en évidence les différentes catégories cellulaires présentes dans la glande pituitaire. *Bull. Microsc. appl.* **10**, 37–44.

— (1965). Present state of knowledge concerning the cytology of the anterior lobe of the hypophysis. *Proc. 2nd Int. Congr. Endocr. (London, 1964).* Excerpta Medica International Congress Series No. 83, pp. 468–481.

Herlant, M. & Pasteels, J. (1967). Histophysiology of human anterior pituitary. In *Methods and Achievements in Experimental Pathology*, edited by Bajusz, E. & Jasmin, G., vol. 3, pp. 250–305. Basel & New York: Karger.

Herlyn, U., Jantzen, K., Flaskamp, D., Hoffmann, H. & Berswordt-Wallrabe, I. von (1969). A modification of the pigeon crop sac assay for lactotrophic hormone determinations by means of the addition of prednisolone. *Acta. endocr., Copenh.* **60**, 555–560.

Heyndrickx, G. V. (1959). Investigations on the lipids, proteins, lipo- and glycoproteins of udder lymph and plasma in cattle. *Q. Jl exp. Physiol.* **44**, 264–270.

— (1961). Further investigations on the lipids in udder lymph and plasma of cattle. *Q. Jl exp. Physiol.* **46**, 33–37.

Heyndrickx, G. V. & Peeters, G. (1958a). Investigations on the ionic balance of udder lymph among cattle. *Q. Jl exp. Physiol.* **43**, 174–179.

— (1958b). Investigations on the enzymes in udder lymph, plasma and milk of cattle. *Enzymologia* **20**, 161–166.

Hibbitt, K. G., Cole, C. B. & Reiter, B. (1969). Antimicrobial proteins isolated from the teat canal of the cow. *J. gen. Microbiol.* **56**, 365–371.

Higashi, K. (1961). Studies on the prolactin-like substance in human placenta III. *Endocr. jap.* **8**, 288–296.

— (1962). Studies on the prolactin-like substance in human placenta IV. *Endocr. jap.* **9**, 1–11.

Hirsch, P. F. & Munson, P. L. (1969). Thyrocalcitonin. *Physiol. Rev.* **49**, 548–622.

Hodges, D. R. & McShan, W. H. (1970). Electrophoretic separation of hormones associated with secretory granules from rat anterior pituitary glands. *Acta endocr., Copenh.* **63**, 378–384.

Holland, R. C., Aulsebrook, L. H. & Woods, W. H. (1963). Neurohypophyseal hormone release following electrical stimulation of the forebrain. *Fedn Proc.* **22**, 571.

Holland, R. C., Woods, W. H. & Aulsebrook, L. H. (1963). Brain stem afferents to paraventricular and supraoptic nuclei. *Anat. Rec.* **145**, 241.

L

Hollmann, K. H. (1959). L'ultrastructure de la glande mammaire normale de la souris en lactation. Étude au microscope électronique. *J. Ultrastruct. Res.* **2**, 423–443.

— (1966). Sur des aspects particuliers des protéines élaborées dans la glande mammaire. Étude au microscope électronique chez la lapine en lactation. *Z. Zellforsch. mikrosk. Anat.* **69**, 395–402.

— (1969). Quantitative electron microscopy of sub-cellular organization in mammary gland cells before and after parturition. In *Lactogenesis: the Initiation of Milk Secretion at Parturition*, edited by Reynolds, M. & Folley, S. J., pp. 27–41. Philadelphia: University of Pennsylvania Press.

Hollmann, K. H. & Verley, J. M. (1966). Individualisation au microscope optique des grains de proteine secretes par la glande mammaire. *Z. Zellforsch. mikrosk. Anat.* **75**, 601–604.

— (1967). La régression de la glande mammaire à l'arrét de la lactation—II. Étude au microscope électronique. *Z. Zellforsch. mikrosk. Anat.* **82**, 222–238.

— (1971). Morphology of secretion in mammary gland cells. In *Lactation*, edited by Falconer, I. R., pp. 31–40. London: Butterworths.

Holmes, R. L. (1956). Alkaline phosphatase in the rabbit mammary gland. *Nature, Lond.* **178**, 311–312.

Honour, A. J., Myant, N. B. & Rowlands, E. N. (1952). Secretion of radioiodine in digestive juices and milk in man. *Clin. Sci.* **11,** 447–462.

Horridge, G. A. (1968). *Interneurons.* London & San Francisco: Freeman.

Hoshino, K. (1964). Regeneration and growth of quantitatively transplanted mammary glands of normal female mice. *Anat. Rec.* **150**, 221–236.

— (1965). Development and function of mammary glands of mice prenatally exposed to testosterone propionate. *Endocrinology* **76**, 789–794.

— (1967). Transplantability of mammary gland in brown fat pads of mice. *Nature, Lond.* **213**, 194–195.

Houvenaghel, A. & Peeters, G. (1968). Influence de la bradykinine sur l'éjection du lait chez la brebis et la chèvre. *Archs int. Physiol. Biochim.* **76**, 647–657.

Houvenaghel, A., Peeters, G., Vandaele, G. & Djordjevic, N. (1968). Influence des kinines du plasma et des kallikréines sur l'éjection du lait chez les ruminants. *Archs int. Physiol. Biochim.* **76**, 658–679.

Howe, A., Richardson, K. C. & Birbeck, M. S. C. (1956). Quantitative observations on mitochondria from sections of guinea-pig mammary gland. *Expl Cell Res.* **10**, 194–213.

Hubben, K., Morse, G. E. & Mealey, M. M. (1966). Studies of bovine mastitis. Histochemical observations on the streak-canal epithelium. *Cornell Vet.* **56**, 648–658.

Huggins, C. & Mainzer, K. (1958). Hormone promotion and restraint of growth of experimental mammary tumours. In *Endocrine Aspects of Breast Cancer*, edited by Currie, A. R. & Illingworth, C. F. W., pp. 297–304. Edinburgh & London: Livingstone.

Hughes, E. S. R. (1950). The development of the mammary gland. *Ann. R. Coll. Surg.* **6**, 99–119.

Hughes, R. L. (1962). Reproduction in the macropod marsupial *Potorous tridactylus* (Kerr). *Aust. J. Zool.* **10**, 193–224.

Hunter, D. L., Erb, R. E., Randel, R. D., Garverick, H. A., Callahan, C. J. & Harrington, R. B. (1970). Reproductive steroids in the bovine—I. Relationships during late gestation. *J. Anim. Sci.* **30**, 47–59.

Hunter, W. M. (1967). The preparation of radioiodinated proteins of high activity, their reaction with antibody *in vitro*: the radioimmunoassay. In *Handbook of Experimental Immunology*, edited by Weir, D. M., chap. 18. Oxford & Edinburgh: Blackwell.

— (1969). Control of specificity in the radio-immunoassay. In *Protein and Polypeptide Hormones*, edited by Margoulies, M. Excerpta Medica International Congress Series No. 161, pp. 5–13.

Hutton, J. B. (1958). Oestrogen function in established lactation in the cow. *J. Endocr.* **17**, 121–133.

Huxley, J. S. (1932). *Problems of Relative Growth*. London: Methuen.

Huxley, J. S. & Teissier, G. (1936). Terminology of relative growth. *Nature, Lond.* **137**, 780–781.

Hymer, W. C., McShan, W. H. & Christiansen, R. G. (1961). Electron microscopic studies of anterior pituitary glands from lactating and estrogen-treated rats. *Endocrinology* **69**, 81–90.

Hytten, F. E. (1954). Clinical and chemical studies in human lactation—VI. The functional capacity of the breast. *Br. med. J.* **i**, 912–915.

Hytten, F. E. & Baird, D. (1958). The development of the nipple in pregnancy. *Lancet* **i**, 1201–1204.

Hytten, F. E. & Leitch, I. (1964). *The Physiology of Human Pregnancy*. Oxford: Blackwell.

Ichinose, R. R. & Nandi, S. (1966). Influence of hormones on lobulo-alveolar differentiation of mouse mammary glands *in vitro*. *J. Endocr.* **35**, 331–340.

Ingleby, H. & Gershon-Cohen, J. (1960). *Comparative Anatomy, Pathology and Roentgenology of the Breast*. Philadelphia: University of Pennsylvania Press.

Ishikawa, T., Koizumi, K. & Brooks, C. McC. (1966). Electrical activity recorded from the pituitary stalk of the cat. *Am. J. Physiol.* **210**, 427–431.

Ito, Y. & Higashi, K. (1961). Studies on the prolactin-like substance in human placenta II. *Endocr. jap.* **8**, 279–287.

Ivanov, N., Kichev, G., Gendzhev, Z. & Khristov, V. (1966). Oksitot-sinoviyat fon v krŭvta na kravi pri rŭchno i mashinno doene. *Zhivotn. Nauki, Sofia* **3**, 679–685.

Jacobsohn, D. (1948). On the mode of action of ovarian hormones on growth and development of the mammary gland. *Acta. physiol. scand.* **17**, Suppl. 57.

— (1958). Mammary gland growth in relation to hormones with metabolic actions. *Proc. R. Soc.* B **149**, 301–424.

Jacobsohn, D. (1962). Interactions of oestrogens and androgens on the mammary gland and growth of other tissues in hypophysectomized rats treated with insulin, cortisone and thyroxine. *Acta endocr., Copenh.* **41,** 287–300.

Jacobsohn, D. & Norgren, A. (1965). Estrogens and corticoids in relation to mammary gland growth in male rats. *Proc. Soc. exp. Biol. Med.* **118,** 1106–1109.

Jadassohn, W. & Fierz-David, H. E. (1943). Sexualhormonprobleme. Dir Wirkung von Sexualhormonen auf die Zitze und Brustdrüse des Meerschweinchens. *Vjschr. naturf. Ges., Zürich* **88,** 1–70.

Jadassohn, W., Uehlinger, E. & Margot, A. (1938). The nipple test. Studies in the local and systemic effects on topical application of various sex-hormones. *J. invest. Derm.* **1,** 31–43.

Jakovac, M. & Rapić, S. (1963). Mamografija u ovce. *Vet. Ark.* **33,** 115–120.

Jean, Ch. (1968a). Nature et fréquence des malformations mammaires du rat nouveau-né en fonction de la dose d'oestradiol injectée à la mère gravide. *C. r. Séanc. Soc. Biol.* **162,** 1144–1149.

— (1968b). Influence sur l'embryogenèse de la glande mammaire de l'hormone somatotrope injectée à la mère gravide on au foetus. *C. r. Séanc. Soc. Biol.* **162,** 1473–1477.

— (1969). Evolution post-natale de l'atrophie de la glande mammaire produite chez la souris nouveau-née par injection d'oestrogène à la mère gravide. *C. r. Séanc. Soc. Biol.* **163,** 1747–1754.

Jean, Ch. & Delost, P. (1965). Oestrogènes et malformations congénitales expérimentales de la morphogenèse mammaire. *C. r. Séanc. Soc. Biol.* **159,** 2357–2362.

Jean, Ch. & Jean, C. (1969). Action des androgènes sur la différenciation des ébauches mammaires du rat nouveau-né. *C. r. Séanc. Soc. Biol.* **163,** 1754–1758.

Jiang, N-S. & Wilhelmi, A. E. (1965). Preparation of bovine, ovine and porcine prolactin. *Endocrinology* **77,** 150–154.

Johke, T. (1969a). Prolactin release in response to milking stimulus in the cow and goat estimated by radioimmunoassay. *Endocr. jap.* **16,** 179–185.

— (1969b). Radioimmunoassay for bovine prolactin in plasma. *Endocr jap.* **16,** 581–589.

Jones, A. E., Fisher, J. N., Lewis, U. J. & Vanderlaan, W. P. (1965). Electrophoretic comparison of pituitary glands from male and female rats. *Endocrinology* **76,** 578–583.

Jones, E. A. (1967). Changes in the enzyme pattern of the mammary gland of the lactating rat after hypophysectomy and weaning. *Biochem. J.* **103,** 420–427.

— (1968). The relationship between milk accumulation and enzyme activities in the involuting rat mammary gland. *Biochim. biophys. Acta* **177,** 158–160.

— (1969). Recent developments in the biochemistry of the mammary gland. *J. Dairy Res.* **36,** 145–167.

Jordan, S. M. & Morgan, E. H. (1969). The serum and milk whey proteins of the echidna. *Comp. Biochem. Physiol.* **29**, 383–391.

Joshi, U. M. & Rao, S. S. (1968). Effect of an oral contraceptive agent on lactation—differential response in three species of animals. *J. Reprod. Fert.* **16**, 15–19.

Josimovich, J. B. & MacLaren, J. A. (1962). Presence in the human placenta and term serum of a highly lactogenic substance immunologically related to pituitary growth hormone. *Endocrinology* **71**, 209–220.

Jouvet, M. (1969). Biogenic amines and the states of sleep. *Science, N.Y.* **163**, 32–41.

Jull, J. W. & Dossett, J. A. (1964). Hormone excretion studies of gynaecomastia of puberty. *Br. med. J.* **ii**, 795–797.

Kaern, T. (1967). Effect of an oral contraceptive immediately post partum on initiation of lactation. *Br. med. J.* **3**, 644–645.

Kahler, H. (1942). Apparatus for milking mice. *J. natn. Cancer Inst.* **2**, 457–458.

Kahn, R. H. & Baker, B. L. (1964). Effect of norethynodrel alone or combined with mestranol on the mammary glands of the adult female rat. *Endocrinology* **75**, 818–821.

— (1969). Effect of long-term treatment with norethynodrel on A/J and C3H/HeJ mice. *Endocrinology* **84**, 661–668.

Kahn, R. H., Baker, B. L. & Zanotti, D. B. (1965). Factors modifying the stimulatory action of norethynodrel on the mammary gland. *Endocrinology* **77**, 162–168.

Kanematsu, S. & Sawyer, C. H. (1963*a*). Effects of intrahypothalamic and intrahypophysial estrogen implants on pituitary prolactin and lactation in the rabbit. *Endocrinology* **72**, 243–252.

— (1963*b*). Effects of hypothalamic estrogen implants on pituitary LH and prolactin in rabbits. *Am. J. Physiol.* **205**, 1073–1076.

— (1963*c*). Effects of intrahypothalamic implants of reserpine on lactation and pituitary prolactin content in the rabbit. *Proc. Soc. exp. Biol. Med.* **113**, 967–969.

Kaplan, S. L. & Grumbach, M. M. (1964). Studies of a human and simian placental hormone with growth hormone-like and prolactin-like activities. *J. clin. Endocr. Metab.* **24**, 80–100.

Karg, H., Hoffmann, B. & Schams, D. (1969). Verlauf der Blutspiegal an Progesteron, Luteinisierungshormon und Prolaktin während des Zyklus bei einer Kuh. *Zuchthygiene* **4**, 149–153.

Katz, H. P., Grumbach, M. M. & Kaplan, S. L. (1969). Diminished growth hormone response to arginine in the puerperium. *J. clin. Endocr. Metab.* **29**, 1414–1419.

Kaveshnikova, K. I., Chudnovskiĭ, L. A. & Shenger, I. F. (1969). Vliyanie razdrazheniya supraopticheskikh yader gipotalamusa na oksitoticheskuyu aktivnost' krovi laktiruyushchikh krol' chikh. *Dokl. Akad. Nauk SSSR* **187**, 949–951.

Kawakami, M., Seto, K. & Yoshida, K. (1968). Influence of corticosterone implantation in limbic structure upon biosynthesis of adrenocortical steroid. *Neuroendocrinology* **3**, 349–354.

Keenan, T. W., Morré, D. J., Olson, D. E., Yunghans, W. N. & Patton, S. (1970). Biochemical and morphological comparison of plasma membrane and milk fat globule membrane from bovine mammary gland. *J. Cell Biol.* **44**, 80–93.

Kendall, J. W., Grimm, Y. & Shimshak, G. (1969). Relation of cerebrospinal fluid circulation to the ACTH-suppressing effects of corticosteroid implants in the rat brain. *Endocrinology* **85**, 200–208.

Kett, K., Varga, G. & Lukács, L. (1970). Direct lymphography of the breast. *Lymphology* **3**, 3–12.

Khazan, N., Primo, C., Danon, A., Assael, M., Sulman, F. G. & Winnik, H. Z. (1962). The mammotropic effect of tranquillizing drugs. *Archs int. Pharmacodyn. Thér.* **141**, 291–305.

Kilpatrick, R., Armstrong, D. T. & Greep, R. O. (1962). Maintenance of the corpus luteum. *Lancet* **ii**, 462.

— (1964). Maintenance of the corpus luteum by gonadotrophins in the hypophysectomized rabbit. *Endocrinology* **74**, 453– 461.

Kinzey, W. G. (1968). Hormonal activity of the rat placenta in the absence of dietary protein. *Endocrinology* **82**, 266–270.

Kjaersgaard, P. (1968*a*). Determination of udder weight in live cows. *Acta vet. scand.* **9**, 177–179.

— (1968*b*). Mammary blood flow ante and post partum in cows. *Acta vet. scand.* **9**, 180–181.

Klein, M-J., Porte, A. & Stutinsky, F. (1968). Contacts synaptiques axo-axoniques dans les noyaux supra-optiques et paraventriculaires du rat et de la souris. *C. r. hebd. Séanc. Acad. Sci., Sér. D, Paris* **267**, 1007–1009.

Knaggs, G. S. (1963). Blood oxytocin levels in the cow during milking and in the parturient goat. *J. Endocr.* **26**, xxiv–xxv.

— (1966). *Blood Oxytocin Levels in Relation to Lactation and Reproduction.* Ph. D. thesis, University of Reading.

Knaggs, G. S., Tindal, J. S. & Turvey, A. (1971). Paraventricular-hypophysial neurosecretory pathways in the guinea-pig. *J. Endocr.* **50**, 153–162.

Knowles, J. A. (1965). Excretion of drugs in milk—a review. *J. Pediat.* **66**, 1068–1082.

Kobayashi, H., Nagai, J. & Naito, M. (1963). Breeding of mice with spontaneous alveolar formation in the mammary gland—II. Relation between the spontaneous alveolar formation and estrous cycle. *Endocr. jap.* **10**, 169–174.

Koch, B. (1969). Liaisons de la corticostérone aux protéines plasmatiques et régulation du niveau du stéroide libre au cours de la gestation et de la lactation chez la ratte. *Hormone metab. Res.* **1**, 129–135.

Kohmoto, K. & Bern, H. A. (1970). Demonstration of mammotrophic activity of the mouse placenta in organ culture and by transplantation. *J. Endocr.* **48**, 99–107.

Kolessnikow, N. (1877). Die Histologie der Milchdrüse der Kuh und die pathologisch- anatomischen Veränderungen derselken bei der Perlsucht. *Virchows Arch. path. Anat. Physiol.* **70**, 531–546.

Kora, S. J. (1969). Effect of oral contraceptives on lactation. *Fert. Steril.* **20**, 419–423.

Kottman, J., Hampl, A. & Pravda, D. (1970). The collection of lymph from efferent vessel of supramammary lymphatic gland of the cow in a long-term experiment. *Acta vet. Brno* **39**, 197–203.

Kovačić, N. (1962). Prolongation of dioestrus in the mouse as a quantitative assay of luteotrophic activity of prolactin. *J. Endocr.* **24**, 227–231.

— (1963). The deciduoma assay: a method for measuring prolactin. *J. Endocr.* **28**, 45–58.

— (1965). Prolactin assay by the decidual reaction in the mouse. *J. Endocr.* **33**, 295–299.

— (1968). Mouse hyperaemic corpora lutea assay of prolactin. *J. Reprod. Fert.* **15**, 259–266.

Kragt, C. L. (1966). *Studies on the Neuroendocrine Control of Prolactin Release in Mammals and Birds.* Ph. D. thesis, Michigan State University, East Lansing, Mich. (quoted by Meites, 1967).

Kragt, C. L. & Meites, J. (1965). Stimulation of pigeon pituitary prolactin release by pigeon hypothalamic extract *in vitro. Endocrinology* **76**, 1169–1176.

— (1967). Dose–response relationships between hypothalamic PIF and prolactin release by rat pituitary tissue *in vitro. Endocrinology* **80**, 1170–1173.

Kratochwil, K. (1969). Organ specificity in mesenchymal induction demonstrated in the embryonic development of the mammary gland of the mouse. *Dev. Biol.* **20**, 46–71.

Kronfeld, D. S. (1969). Biosynthesis of milk constituents at lactogenesis. In *Lactogenesis: the Initiation of Milk Secretion at Parturition*, edited by Reynolds, M. & Folley, S. J., pp. 109–120. Philadelphia: University of Pennsylvania Press.

Kronfeld, D. S., Mayer, G. P., Robertson, J. McD. & Raggi, F. (1963). Depression of milk secretion during insulin administration. *J. Dairy Sci.* **46**, 559–563.

Krulich, L., Dhariwal, A. P. S. & McCann, S. M. (1968). Stimulatory and inhibitory effects of purified hypothalamic extracts on growth hormone release from rat pituitary *in vitro. Endocrinology* **83**, 783–790.

Kudryavtsev, P. N. & Glebina, E. I. (1941). Massazh vymeni remontnȳkh svineĭ do perovogo pokrytiya i ikh produktivnost'. *Vest. sel'.-khoz. Nauki, Mosk. Zhivotn. 1941*, No. 2, 136–150.

Kuhn, N. J. (1969*a*). Progesterone withdrawal as the lactogenic trigger in the rat. *J. Endocr.* **44**, 39–54.

— (1969*b*). Specificity of progesterone inhibition of lactogenesis. *J. Endocr.* **45**, 615–616.

— (1971). Control of lactogenesis and lactose biosynthesis. In *Lactation*, edited by Falconer, I. R., pp. 161–176. London: Butterworths.

Kuhn, N. J. & Briley, M. S. (1970). The roles of pregn-5-ene-3β, 20α-diol and 20α-hydroxy steroid dehydrogenase in the control of progesterone synthesis preceding parturition and lactogenesis in the rat. *Biochem. J.* **117**, 193–201.

Kuhn, N. J. & Linzell, J. L. (1970). Measurement of the quantity of lactose passing into mammary venous plasma and lymph in goats and a cow. *J. Dairy Res.* **37**, 203–208.

Kumaresan, P , Anderson, R. R. & Turner, C. W. (1967). Effect of litter size upon milk yield and litter weight gains in rats. *Proc. Soc. exp. Biol. Med.* **126**, 41–45.

Kumaresan, P. & Turner, C. W. (1965a). Effect of graded levels of insulin on lactation in the rat. *Proc. Soc. exp. Biol. Med.* **119**, 415–416.

— (1965b). Effect of alloxan on lactation and replacement therapy with insulin in the rat. *Proc. Soc. exp. Biol. Med.* **119**, 1133–1135.

— (1966). Effect of oxytocin upon litter weight gain in rats. *Proc. Soc. exp. Biol. Med.* **123**, 70–72.

Kuosaïte, B. A. (1965). Kompensatornaya gipertrofiya molochnoĭ zhelezȳ morskoĭ svinki posle udaleniya parnogo organa. *Byull. éksp. Biol. Med.* **59**, (3) 97–100.

Kurcz, M. (1966). Specificity of the micro-test of the pigeon's crop-sac for prolactin determination. *Annls Univ. Scient. bpest. Rolando Eötvös, Sect. Biol.* **8**, 149–154.

Kurcz, M., Nagy, I. & Baranyai, P. (1969). New biochemical micro-method for the determination of prolactin in rat adenohypophysis. *Acta biochim. biophys. hung.* **4**, 287–295.

Kurcz, M., Nagy, I., Kiss, C. & Halmy, L. (1969a). Estimation of the blood prolactin level. *Acta physiol. hung.* **35**, 153–166.

— (1969b). Ergebnisse der prolactinbestimmung in Blut. *Arch. Gynäk.* **208**, 19–32.

Kurosaki, M. (1961). Prolactin-like substance of human placenta. *Tohuku J. exp. Med.* **75**, 122–136.

Kurosumi, K., Kobayashi, Y. & Baba, N. (1968). The fine structure of mammary glands of lactating rats, with special reference to the apocrine secretion. *Expl Cell Res.* **50**, 177–192.

Kwa, H. G., Bent, E. M. van der, & Prop, F. S. A. (1967). Studies on hormones from the anterior pituitary gland—II: Identification and isolation of prolactin from the 'granular' fraction of transplanted rat pituitary tumours. *Biochim. biophys. Acta* **133**, 301–318.

Kwa, H. G., Gugten, A. A. van der & Verhofstad, F. (1969). Radio-immunoassay of rat prolactin. Comparison of rat prolactin preparations isolated from the granular fraction of pituitary tumour transplants and from normal pituitary glands. *Eur. J. Cancer* **5**, 559–569.

Kwa, H. G. & Verhofstad, F. (1967). Radioimmunoassay of rat prolactin. *Biochim. biophys. Acta* **133**, 186–188.

Kwa, H. G., Verhofstad, F. & Bent, E. M. van der (1967). Radioimmunoassay of mouse prolactin based upon a protein isolated from prolactin-producing pituitary tumours. *Acta physiol. pharmac. néerl.* **14**, 514–518.

Labussière, J. (1966). Relation entre le niveau de production laitière des brebis et leur aptitude à la traite. *Proc. 17th Int. Dairy Congr., Munich*, Section A:1, pp. 43–51.

Labussière, J. & Martinet, J. (1964). Description de deux appareils permettant le controle automatique des débits de lait au cours de la traite a la machine premiers résultats obtenus chez la brebis. *Annls Zootech.* **13**, 199–212.

Labussière, J., Martinet, J. & Denamur, R. (1969). The influence of the milk-ejection reflex on the flow rate during the milking of ewes. *J. Dairy Res.* **36**, 191–201.

Lacroix, E. (1894). De l'existence de 'cellules en pamiers' dans l'acinus et les conduits excréteurs de la glande mammaire. *C. r. hebd. Séanc. Acad. Sci., Paris* **119**, 748–751.

Lane, G. T., Dill, C. W., Armstrong, B. C. & Switzer, L. A. (1970). Influence of repeated oxytocin injections on composition of dairy cows' milk. *J. Dairy Sci.* **53**, 427–429.

Langer, E. & Huhn, S. (1958). Der submikroskopische Bau der Myoepithelzelle. *Z. Zellforsch. mikrosk. Anat.* **47**, 507–516.

Langhans, T. (1873). Zur pathologischen Histologie der weiblichen Brüstdrüse. *Virchows Arch. path. Anat. Physiol.* **58**, 132–160.

Lansing, A. I. & Opdyke, D. L. (1950). Histological and histochemical studies of the nipples of estrogen treated guinea pigs with special reference to keratohyalin granules. *Anat. Rec.* **107**, 379–397.

Lascelles, A. K. (1962). The absorption of serum albumin and casein from the mammary gland of the merino ewe. *Q. Jl exp. Physiol.* **47**, 48–56.

Lascelles, A. K., Cowie, A. T., Hartmann, P. E. & Edwards, M. J. (1964). The flow and composition of lymph from the mammary gland of lactating and dry cows. *Res. vet. Sci.* **5**, 190–201.

Lascelles, A. K., Gurner, B. W. & Coombs, R. R. A. (1969). Some properties of human colostral cells. *Aust. J. exp. Biol. med. Sci.* **47**, 349–360.

Lascelles, A. K. & Morris, B. (1961). Surgical techniques for the collection of lymph from unanaesthetized sheep. *Q. Jl exp. Physiol.* **44**, 199–205.

Lasfargues, E. Y. & Murray, M. R. (1959). Hormonal influences on the differentiation and growth of embryonic mouse mammary glands in organ culture. *Devl Biol.* **1**, 413–435.

Lauer, B. H. & Baker, B. E. (1969). Whale milk—I. Fin whale (*Balaenoptera physalus*) and beluga whale (*Delphinapterus leucas*) milk: gross composition and fatty acid constitution. *Can. J. Zool.* **47**, 95–97.

Lawson, D. M. & Graf, G. C. (1968). Plasma oxytocic activity and intramammary pressure in lactating dairy cows. *J. Dairy Sci.* **51**, 1676–1679.

Lawson, W., Stroud, S. W. & Williams, P. C. (1944). Oestrogen excretion in milk from oestrogenized cattle. *J. Endocr.* **4**, 83–89.

Lawton, A. R., Asofsky, R. & Mage, R. G. (1970). Synthesis of secretory IgA in the rabbit. *J. Immun.* **104**, 388–396, 397–408.

Leake, N. H. & Burt, R. L. (1969). Solid-phase radioimmunoassay of human placental lactogen. *Obstet. Gynec.*, *N.Y.* **34**, 471–477.

Lee, C. S. & Lascelles, A. K. (1969a). The histological changes in involuting mammary glands of ewes in relation to the local allergic response. *Aust. J. exp. Biol. med. Sci.* **47**, 613–623.

—— (1969b). Distribution of lymphatic vessels in mammary glands of ewes. *Am. J. Anat.* **126**, 489–495.

Lee, C. S., McDowell, G. H. & Lascelles, A. K. (1969). The importance of macrophages in the removal of fat from the involuting mammary gland. *Res. vet. Sci.* **10**, 34–38.

Lehrman, D. S. (1961). Hormonal regulation of parental behavior in birds and infrahuman mammals. In *Sex and Internal Secretions*, 3rd edn, edited by Young, W. C., vol. 2, chap. 21. Baltimore: Williams & Wilkins.

—— (1965). Interaction between internal and external environments in the regulation of the reproductive cycle of the ring dove. In *Sex and Behavior*, edited by Beach, F. A., chap. 15. New York: John Wiley.

—— (1967). Reproductive behavior. In *McGraw-Hill Encyclopedia Science and Technology*, pp. 454–462. New York & London: McGraw-Hill.

Lelong, M., Giraud, P., Roche, J., Liardet, J. & Coignet, J. (1950). Sur l'action galactogène des proteines iodées chez la femme. Essais thérapeutiques. *Archs fr. Pédiat.* **7**, 1–13.

Lemon, M. & Bailey, L. F. (1966). A specific protein difference in the milk from two mammary glands of a red kangaroo. *Aust. J. exp. Biol. med. Sci.* **44**, 705–708.

Lemon, M. & Poole, W. E. (1969). Specific proteins in the whey from milk of the grey kangaroo. *Aust. J. exp. Biol. med. Sci.* **47**, 283–285.

Lengemann, F. W. (1970). Metabolism of radioiodide by lactating goats given iodine-131 for extended periods. *J. Dairy Sci.* **53**, 165–170.

Lennep, E. W. van & Utrecht, W. L. van (1953). Preliminary report on the study of the mammary glands of whales. *Norsk Hvalfangst-Tidende* (5), 249–259.

Leonard, C. M. (1969). The prefrontal cortex of the rat—I. Cortical projections of the mediodorsal nucleus. II. Efferent connections. *Brain Res.* **12**, 321–343.

Levine, M. D., Reisch, M. L. & Thurlbeck, W. M. (1970). Automated measurement of the internal surface area of the human lung. *IEEE Transactions on biomedical Engineering* **17**, 254–262.

Levitskaya, E. S. (1955). Prizhiznennoe issledovanie raboty̆ vy̆vodnogo apparata molochnoǐ zhelezy̆ beloǐ my̆shi. *Trudy̆ Inst. Fiziol. I. P. Pavlova* **4**, 58–62.

Levy, H. R. (1964). The effects of weaning and milk on mammary fatty acid synthesis. *Biochim. biophys. Acta* **84**, 229–238.

Lewis U. J. & Cheever, E. V. (1967). Effect of toluene on bovine growth hormone and prolactin in pituitary extracts. *Endocrinology* **81**, 1338–1348.

Lewis, U. J., Cheever, E. V. & Seavey, B. K. (1969). Aggregate-free human growth hormone—I. Isolation by ultrafiltration. *Endocrinology* **84**, 325–331.

Lewis, U. J., Cheever, E. V. & VanderLaan, W. P. (1965). Alteration of the proteins of the pituitary gland of the rat by estradiol and cortisol. *Endocrinology* **76**, 362–368.

Lewis, U. J., Litteria, M. & Cheever, E. V. (1969). Growth hormone and prolactin components of disc electrophoretic patterns: quantitative determination of the amount of protein in a stained band. *Endocrinology* **85**, 690–697.

Lewis, U. J., Parker, D. C., Okerlund, M. D., Boyar, R. M., Litteria, M. & VanderLaan, W. P. (1969). Aggregate-free human growth hormone—II. Physicochemical and biological properties. *Endocrinology* **84**, 332–339.

Li, C. H. (1961). Biochemistry of prolactin. In *Milk: the Mammary Gland and its Secretion*, edited by Kon, S. K. & Cowie, A. T., vol. 1, chap. 5. New York & London: Academic Press.

— (1968). The chemistry of human pituitary growth hormone: 1956–1966. In *Growth Hormone*, edited by Pecile, A. & Müller, E. E., Excerpta Medica International Congress Series No. 158, pp. 3–28.

Li, C. H., Dixon, J. S. & Liu, W-K. (1969). Human pituitary growth hormone—XIX. The primary structure of the hormone. *Arch Biochem. Biophys.* **133**, 70–91.

Li, C. H., Dixon, J. S., Lo, T-B., Pankov, Y. A. & Schmidt, K. D. (1969). Amino-acid sequence of ovine lactogenic hormone. *Nature, Lond.* **244**, 695–696.

Li, C. H., Grumbach, M. M., Kaplan, S. L., Josimovich, J. B., Friesen, H. & Catt, K. J. (1968). Human chorionic somato-mammotropin (HCS), proposed terminology for designation of a placental hormone. *Experientia* **24**, 1288.

Ling, E. R., Kon, S. K. & Porter, J. W. G. (1961). The composition of milk and the nutritive value of its components. In *Milk: the Mammary Gland and its Secretion*, edited by Kon, S. K. & Cowie, A. T., vol. 2, chap. 17. New York & London: Academic Press.

Linnerud, A. C., Caruolo, E. V., Miller, G. E., Marx, G. D. & Donker J. D. (1966). Lactation studies—X. Total daily production as affected by number of times milked, number of times stimulated, and method of stimulation. *J. Dairy Sci.* **49**, 1529–1532

Linzell, J. L. (1952). The silver staining of myoepithelial cells, particularly in the mammary gland, and their relation to the ejection of milk. *J. Anat.* **86**, 49–57.

— (1953). The blood and nerve supply to the mammary glands of the cat, and other laboratory animals. *Br. vet. J.* **109**, 427–433.

— (1955). Some observations on the contractile tissue of the mammary glands. *J. Physiol.* **130**, 257–267.

— (1959a). The innervation of the mammary glands in the sheep and goat with some observations on the lumbo-sacral autonomic fibres. *Q. Jl. exp. Physiol.* **44**, 160–176.

Linzell, J. L. (1959*b*). Physiology of the mammary glands. *Physiol. Rev.* **39**, 534–576.

— (1960*a*). Valvular incompetence in the venous drainage of the udder. *J. Physiol.* **153**, 481–491.

— (1960*b*). The flow and composition of mammary gland lymph. *J. Physiol.* **153**, 510–521.

— (1961). Recent advances in the physiology of the udder. *Vet. A.* **3**, 44–53.

— (1963). Some effects of denervating and transplanting mammary glands. *Q. Jl exp. Physiol.* **48**, 34–60.

— (1966*a*). Measurement of venous flow by continuous thermodilution and its application to measurement of mammary blood flow in the goat. *Circulation Res.* **18**, 745–754.

— (1966*b*). Measurement of udder volume in live goats as an index of mammary growth and function. *J. Dairy Sci.* **49**, 307–311.

— (1967). The effect of very frequent milking and of oxytocin on the yield and composition of milk in fed and fasted goats. *J. Physiol.* **190**, 333–346.

— (1971). Mammary blood vessels, lymphatics and nerves. In *Lactation*, edited by Falconer, I. R., pp. 41–50. London: Butterworths.

Lippmann, W., Leonardi, R., Ball, J. & Coppola, J. A. (1967). Relationship between hypothalamic catecholamines and gonadotrophin synthesis in rats. *J. Pharmac. exp. Ther.* **156**, 258–266.

Lombardo, N. (1955). Rilievi radiografica sulla mammella della capra. *Clinica vet., Milano* **78**, 104–110.

Long, C. A. (1969). The origin and evolution of mammary glands. *BioScience* **19**, 519–523.

Lukášová, J. & Lukáš, Z. (1965). Cholinesterázová aktivita a inervace mléčné žlázy. *Vet. Med., Praha* **10**, 293–297.

Lundahl, W. S., Meites, J. & Wolterink, L. F. (1950). A technique for whole mount autoradiographs of rabbit mammary glands. *Science, N.Y.* **112**, 599–600.

Lyne, A. G., Pilton, P. E. & Sharman, G B. (1959). Oestrous cycle, gestation period and parturition in the marsupial *Trichosurus vulpecula*. *Nature, Lond.* **183**, 622–623.

Lyons, W. R. (1942). The direct mammotrophic action of lactogenic hormone. *Proc. Soc. exp. Biol. Med.* **51**, 308–311.

— (1958). Hormonal synergism in mammary growth. *Proc. R. Soc. B* **149**, 303–325.

— (1962). Tests for investigation of endocrine effects on the mammary gland. In *Laboratory Tests in Diagnosis and Investigation of Endocrine Functions*, edited by Escamilla, R. F., chap. 35. Oxford: Blackwell.

— (1969). Human hypophysial mammotrophin distinct from somatotrophin. In *Lactogenesis: the Initiation of Milk Secretion at Parturition*, edited by Reynolds, M. & Folley, S. J., pp. 223–228. Philadelphia: University of Pennsylvania Press.

Lyons, W. R., & Dixon, J. S. (1966). The physiology and chemistry of the mammotrophic hormone. In *The Pituitary Gland*, edited by Harris, G. W. & Donovan, B. T., vol. 1, pp. 527–581. London: Butterworths.

Lyons, W. R., Gutiérrez, J., Cervantes, A. & Rice-Wray, E. (1968). Intentos para incrementar la lactación en mujeres con mamosomatotrofina hipofisiaria humana. *Revta mex. Pediat.* **37**, 111–121.

Lyons, W. R., Li, C. H., Ahmad, N. & Rice-Wray, E. (1968). Mammotrophic effects of human hypophysial growth hormone preparations in animals and man. In *Growth Hormone*, edited by Pecile, A. & Müller, E. E., Excerpta Medica International Congress Series No. 158, pp. 349–363.

Lyons, W. R., Li, C. H. & Johnson, R. E. (1958). The hormonal control of mammary growth. *Recent Prog. Horm. Res.* **14**, 219–248.

— (1960). Mammary-stimulating activities of human pituitary hormones. *Proc. 1st Int. Congr. Endocr. (Copenhagen)*, edited by Fuchs, F., p. 1145. Copenhagen: Periodica.

Lyons, W. R. & Page, E. (1935). Detection of mammotropin in the urine of lactating women. *Proc. Soc. exp. Biol. Med.* **32**, 1049–1050.

McBride, G. (1963). The 'teat order' and communication in young pigs. *Anim. Behav.* **11**, 53–56.

McBride, A. F. & Kritzler, H. (1951). Observations on pregnancy, parturition, and postnatal behavior in the bottlenose dolphin. *J. Mammal.* **32**, 251–266.

McBurney, J. J., Meier, H. & Hoag, W. G. (1964). Device for milking mice. *J. Lab. Clin. Med.* **64**, 485–487.

McCann, S. M., Dhariwal, A. P. S. & Porter, J. C. (1967). Regulation of the adenohypophysis. *A. Rev. Physiol.* **30**, 589–640.

McCann, S. M., Mack R. & Gale, C. (1959). The possible role of oxytocin in stimulating the release of prolactin. *Endocrinology* **64**, 870–889.

McCann, S. M. & Porter, J. C. (1969). Hypothalamic pituitary stimulating and inhibiting hormones. *Physiol. Rev.* **49**, 240–284.

McCullagh, K. G. & Widdowson, E. M. (1970). The milk of the African elephant. *Br. J. Nutr.* **24**, 109–117.

McDonald, J. S. (1968). Radiographic method for anatomic study of the teat canal: observations on 22 lactating dairy cows. *Am. J. vet. Res.* **29**, 1315–1319.

Mackenzie, D. D. S. (1968). Studies on the transfer of protein across the glandular epithelium of the mammary gland during involution. *Aust. J. exp. Biol. med. Sci.* **46**, 273–283.

McKerrow, M. J. (1954). The lactation cycle of *Elephantulus myurnus jamesoni* (Chubb). *Phil. Trans. R. Soc.* Ser. B **238**, 62–98.

MacLean, P. D. (1966). The limbic and visual cortex in phylogeny: further insights from anatomic and microelectrode studies. In *Evolution of the Forebrain*, edited by Hassler, R. & Stephen H., pp. 443–453. Stuttgart: Georg Thieme.

MacLeod, R. M. (1969). Influence of norepinephrine and catecholamine-depleting agents on the synthesis and release of prolactin and growth hormone. *Endocrinology* **85**, 916–923.

326 *The physiology of lactation*

MacLeod, R. M., Smith, M. C. & DeWitt, G. W. (1966). Hormonal properties of transplanted pituitary tumors and their relation to the pituitary gland. *Endocrinology* **79**, 1149–1156.

McNeilly, J. R. (1971). A solid phase radioimmunoassay for ovine prolactin. *J. Endocr.* **49**, 141–149.

McShan, W. H. (1956). Ultrastructure and function of the anterior pituitary gland. *Proc. 2nd Int. Congr. Endocr. (London, 1964)*. Excerpta Medica International Congress Series No. 83, pp. 382–391.

Ma, R. C. S. & Nalbandov, A. V. (1963). In *Advances in Neuroendocrinology*, edited by Nalbandov, A. V., discussion of chap. 9, pp. 306–311. Urbana: University of Illinois Press.

Maanen, J. H. van & Smelik, P. G. (1967). Depletion of monoamines in the hypothalamus and prolactin secretion. *Acta physiol. pharmac. néerl.* **14**, 519–520.

— (1968). Induction of pseudopregnancy in rats following local depletion of monoamines in the median eminence of the hypothalamus. *Neuroendocrinology* **3**, 177–186.

Macy, J. G. & Kelly, H. J. (1961). Human milk and cow's milk in infant nutrition. In *Milk: the Mammary Gland and its Secretion*, edited by Kon, S. K. & Cowie, A. T., vol. 2, chap. 18. New York & London: Academic Press.

Marcum, R. G. & Wellings, S. R. (1969). Subgross pathology of the human breast: method and initial observations. *J. natn Cancer Inst.* **42**, 115–121.

Margoulies, M. (editor) (1969). *Protein and polypeptide hormones*. Excerpta Medica International Congress Series 161.

Marshall, F. H. A. (1910). *The Physiology of Reproduction*, chap. 13. Lactation, pp. 553–585. London, New York, Bombay & Calcutta: Longmans, Green.

Martin, R. D. (1966). Tree shrews: unique reproductive mechanism of systematic importance. *Science, N.Y.* **152**, 1402–1404.

Martinet, L. (1962) Embryologie de la mamelle chez le mouton. *Annls Biol. anim. Biochim. Biophys.* **2**, 175–184.

Martini, L., Fraschini, F. & Motta, M. (1968). Neural control of anterior pituitary functions. *Recent Prog. Horm. Res.* **24**, 439–485.

Marx, G. D. & Caruolo, E. V. (1963). Method of biopsy of the mammary gland of cows and goats. *J. Dairy Sci.* **46**, 576–579.

Masson, P. L., Heremans, J. F. & Ferin, J. (1968). Presence of an iron-binding protein (lactoferrin) in the genital tract of the human female—I. Its immunohistochemical localization in the endometrium. *Fert. Steril.* **19**, 679–689.

Masson, P. L., Heremans, J. F., Prignot, J. J. & Wauters, G. (1966). Immunohistochemical localization and bacteriostatic properties of an iron-binding protein from bronchial mucus. *Thorax* **21**, 538–544.

Masson, P. L. Heremans, J. F., Schonne, E. & Crabbé, P. A. (1969). New data on lactoferrin, the iron-binding protein of secretions. *Protides biol. Fluids* **16**, 633–638.

Matthies, D. L. (1967). Studies of the luteotropic and mammotropic factor found in trophoblast and maternal peripheral blood of the rat at mid-pregnancy. *Anat. Rec.* **159,** 55–67.

— (1968). A rapid assay for the lactogenic activity of rat chorionic mammotropin. *Proc. Soc. exp. Biol. Med.* **127,** 1126–1129.

Mayberry, H. E. (1964). Macrophages in post-secretory mammary involution in mice. *Anat. Rec.* **149,** 99–112.

Mayer, G. & Duluc, A-J. (1967). Stérilisation des petits par administration à la mère de stilboestrol au cours de la lactation. *C. r. hebd. Séanc. Acad. Sci., Sér. D, Paris* **264,** 2043–2044.

Mayer, G. & Klein, M. (1949). Physiologie de la lactation. Les facteurs de l'activité fonctionnelle du parenchyme mammaire. *Annls. Nutr. Aliment.* **3,** 667–747.

— (1961). Histology and cytology of the mammary gland. In *Milk: the Mammary Gland and its Secretion*, edited by Kon, S. K. & Cowie, A. T., vol. 1, chap. 2. New York & London: Academic Press.

Mehler, W. R., Feferman, M. E. & Nauta, W. J. H. (1960). Ascending axon degeneration following anterolateral cordotomy. An experimental study in the monkey. *Brain* **83,** 718–750.

Meier, A. H., Farner, D. S. & King J. R. (1965). A possible endocrine basis for migratory behaviour in the white-crowned sparrow, *Zonotrichia leucophrys gambelii. Anim. Behav.* **13,** 453–465.

Meites, J. (1961). Farm animals: hormonal induction of lactation and galactopoiesis. In *Milk: the Mammary Gland and its Secretion*, edited by Kon, S. K. & Cowie, A. T., vol. 1, chap. 8. New York & London: Academic Press.

— (1966). Control of mammary growth and lactation. In *Neuroendocrinology*, edited by Martini, L. & Ganong, W. F., vol. 1, chap. 16. New York & London: Academic Press.

— (1967). Control of prolactin secretion. *Archs Anat. microsc. Morph. exp.* **56,** Suppl. to No. 3–4, 516–529.

Meites, J. & Hopkins, T. F. (1960). Induction of lactation and mammary growth by pituitary grafts in intact and hypophysectomized rats. *Proc. Soc. exp. Biol. Med.* **104,** 263–266.

— (1961). Mechanism of action of oxytocin in retarding mammary involution: study in hypophysectomized rats. *J. Endocr.* **22,** 207–213.

Meites, J., Kahn, R. H. & Nicoll, C. S. (1961). Prolactin production by rat pituitary *in vitro. Proc. Soc. exp. Biol. Med.* **108,** 440–443.

Meites, J. & Nicoll, C. S. (1966). Adenohypophysis: prolactin. *A. Rev. Physiol.* **28,** 57–88.

Meites, J., Nicoll, C. S. & Talwalker, P. K. (1963). The central nervous system and the secretion and release of prolactin. In *Advances in Neuroendocrinology*, edited by Nalbandov, A. V., chap. 8. Urbana: University of Illinois Press.

Meites, J., Talwalker, P. K. & Nicoll, C. S. (1960). Initiation of lactation in rats with hypothalamic or cerebral tissue. *Proc. Soc. exp. Biol. Med.* **103,** 298–300.

Meites, J. & Turner, C. W. (1947). The induction of lactation during pregnancy in rabbits and the specificity of the lactogenic hormone. *Am. J. Physiol.* **150**, 394–399.

Melampy, R. M., Gurland, J. & Rakes, J. M. (1959). Estrogen excretion by cows after oral administration of diethylstilboestrol. *J. Anim. Sci.* **18**, 178–186.

Mellin, T. N. & Erb, R. E. (1965). Estrogens in the bovine—a review. *J. Dairy Sci.* **48**, 687–700.

Melzack, R. & Wall, P.D. (1965). Pain mechanisms: a new theory. *Science, N. Y.* **150**, 971–979.

Mena, F. & Beyer, C. (1963). Effect of high spinal section on established lactation in the rabbit. *Am. J. Physiol.* **205**, 313–316.

— (1968*a*). Effect of spinal cord lesions on milk ejection in the rabbit. *Endocrinology* **83**, 615–617.

— (1968*b*). Induction of milk secretion in the rabbit by lesions in the temporal lobe. *Endocrinology* **83**, 618–620.

Mena, F & Grosvenor, C. E. (1968). Effect of number of pups upon suckling-induced fall in pituitary prolactin concentration and milk-ejection in the rat. *Endocrinology* **82**, 623–626.

Mena, F., Maiweg, H. & Grosvenor, C. E. (1968). Effect of ectopic pituitary glands upon prolactin concentration by the *in situ* pituitary of the lactating rat. *Endocrinology* **83**, 1359–1362.

Mendell, L. M. (1966). Physiological properties of unmyelinated fiber projection to the spinal cord. *Expl Neurol.* **16**, 316–332.

Merchant, J. C. & Sharman, G. B. (1966). Observations on the attachment of marsupial pouch young to the teats and on the rearing of pouch young by foster-mothers of the same or different species. *Aust. J. Zool.* **14**, 593–609.

Mielke, H. & Brabant, W. (1963). Laktogenese und Galactopoese beim Rind ohne Saug-, Melk-oder andere exogene, zur Milcheejektion führende Euterreize. *Arch. exp. Vet.-Med.* **16**, 909–919.

Miller, M. R. & Kasahara, M. (1959). The cutaneous innervation of the human female breast. *Anat. Rec.* **135**, 153–167.

Miller, M. R., Ralston, H. J. III & Kasahara, M. (1958). The pattern of cutaneous innervation of the human hand, *Am. J. Anat.* **102**, 183–217.

Milligan, J. V. & Kraicer, J. (1970). Adenohypophysial transmembrane potentials: polarity reversal by elevated external potassium ion concentration. *Science, N.Y.* **167**, 182–184.

Mills, E. & Wang, S. C. (1964). Liberation of antidiuretic hormone: location of ascending pathways. *Am. J. Physiol.* **207**, 1399–1404.

Mills, E. S. & Topper, Y. J. (1970). Some ultrastructural effects of insulin, hydrocortisone, and prolactin on mammary gland explants. *J. Cell Biol.* **44**, 310–328.

Mills, J. B., Ashworth, R. B., Wilhelmi, A. E. & Hartree, A. S. (1969) Improved method for the extraction and purification of human growth hormone. *J. clin. Endocr. Metab.* **29**, 1456–1459.

Minaguchi, H. & Meites, J. (1967). Effects of suckling on hypothalamic LH-releasing factor and prolactin-inhibiting factor, and on pituitary LH and prolactin. *Endocrinology* **80**, 603–607.

Mishkinsky, J., Dikstein, S., Ben-David, M., Azeroual, J. & Sulman, F. G. (1967). A sensitive *in vitro* method for prolactin determination. *Proc. Soc. exp. Biol. Med.* **125**, 360–363.

Mishkinsky, J., Khazen, K. & Sulman, F. G. (1968). Prolactin-releasing activity of the hypothalamus in post-partum rats. *Endocrinology* **82**, 611–613.

Mishkinsky, J., Lajtos, Z. K. & Sulman, F. G. (1966). Initiation of lactation by hypothalamic implantation of perphenazine. *Endocrinology* **78**, 919–922.

Mishkinsky, J., Nir, I. & Sulman, F. G. (1969). Internal feedback of prolactin in the rat. *Neuroendocrinology* **5**, 48–52.

Miyawaki, H. (1965). Histochemistry and electron microscopy of iron-containing granules, lysosomes, and lipofuscin in mouse mammary glands. *J. natn. Cancer Inst.* **34**, 601–623.

Mizuno, H. (1961). The changes of nucleic acids content in the mouse mammary glands in the course of involution and the effects of pregnancy, prolactin or progesterone on them. *Endocr. jap.* **8**, 27–34.

Mizuno, H. & Satoh, K. (1970). Further studies on inhibition of milk ejection by administration of oxytocin to the mouse. *Endocr. jap.* **17**, 15–22.

Mizuno, H. & Shiiba, N. (1969). Inhibitory effect of oxytocin administration on lactation in mice. *Endocr. jap.* **16**, 547–553.

Mizuno, H., Talwalker, P. K. & Meites, J. (1967). Central inhibition by serotonin of reflex release of oxytocin in response to suckling stimulus in the rat. *Neuroendocrinology* **2**, 222–231.

Molen, H. J. van der & Aakvaag, A. (1969). Progesterone. In *Hormones in Blood*, 2nd edn., edited by Gray, C. H. & Bacharach, A. L , vol. 2, chap. 6. London & New York: Academic Press.

Molen, H. J. van der, Hart, P. G. & Wijmenga, H. G. (1969). Studies with 4-^{14}C-lynestrol in normal and lactating women. *Acta endocr., Copenh.* **61**, 255–274.

Moltz, H., Levin, R. & Leon, M. (1969). Prolactin in the postpartum rat: synthesis and release in the absence of suckling stimulation. *Science, N. Y.* **163**, 1083–1084.

Moon, R. C. (1965). Mammary growth in rats treated with somatotropin during pregnancy and/or lactation. *Proc. Soc. exp. Biol. Med.* **118**, 181–183.

— (1969). Mammary growth and milk yield as related to litter size. *Proc. Soc. exp. Biol. Med.* **130**, 1126–1128.

Morag, M. (1968*a*). A galactopoietic effect from oxytocin administered between milkings in the cow. *Annls Biol. anim. Biochim. Biophys.* **8**, 27–43.

— (1968*b*). The effect of regular intravenous injections of oxytocin at milking time on the proportion of the yield obtained as residue in the ewe. *J. Dairy Res.* **35**, 377–381.

Morag, M. (1969). The relation between the passage of time and the secretion of milk in the ewe. *Aust. J. agric. Res.* **20**, 941–951.

Morag, M. & Brick, D. (1969). The stimulation and inhibition of milk secretion by oxytocin in the rat. *Life Sci.* **8**, 143–150.

Morag, M. & Fox, S. (1966). Galactokinetic responses to oxytocin in the ewe. *Annls Biol. anim. Biochim. Biophys.* **6**, 467–478.

Motta, M., Fraschini, F. & Martini, L. (1969). 'Short' feedback mechanisms in the control of anterior pituitary function. In *Frontiers in Neuroendocrinology*, 1969, edited by Ganong, W. F. & Martini, L., chap. 6, pp. 211–253. Oxford: Oxford University Press.

Mueller, A. J. (1939). A modified apparatus for milking small laboratory animals. *J. Lab. clin. Med.* **24**, 426–427.

Munford, R. E. (1963a). Changes in the mammary glands of rats and mice during pregnancy, lactation and involution—1. Histological structure. *J. Endocr.* **28**, 1–15.

— (1963b). Changes in the mammary glands of rats and mice during pregnancy, lactation and involution—2. Levels of deoxyribonucleic acid, and alkaline phosphatases. *J. Endocr.* **28**, 17–34.

— (1963c). Changes in the mammary glands of rats and mice during pregnancy, lactation and involution—3. Relation of structural and biochemical changes. *J. Endocr.* **28**, 35–44.

— (1964). A review of anatomical and biochemical changes in the mammary gland with particular reference to quantitative methods of assessing mammary development. *Dairy Sci. Abstr.* **26**, 293–304.

Munro, J. (1956). Observations on the suckling behaviour of young lambs. *Br. J. Anim. Behav.* **4**, 34–36.

Murad, T. M. (1970). Ultrastructural study of rat mammary gland during pregnancy. *Anat. Rec.* **167**, 17–36.

Murakawa, S. & Raben, M. S. (1968). Effect of growth hormone and placental lactogen on DNA synthesis in rat costal cartilage and adipose tissue. *Endocrinology* **83**, 645–650.

Murillo, G. J. & Goldman, A. S. (1970). The cells of human colostrum— II. Synthesis of IgA and β1C. *Pediat. Res.* **4**, 71–75.

Nagai, J. (1962). Breeding of mice with spontaneous alveolar formation in the mammary gland. 1. Frequency of spontaneous alveolar formation and sexual cycle in mouse strains. *Jap. J. zootech. Sci.* **33**, 256–264.

Nagai, J. & Yamada J. (1957). Establishment of mice strains with special reference to mammary growth responses. 1. Comparison of several measuring methods of mammary duct areas in immature mice treated with estrogen. *Endocr. jap.* **4**, 179–183.

Nagasawa, H., Iwahashi, H., Kanzawa, F., Fujimoto, M. & Kuretani, K. (1967). A comparative study on the normal mammary gland development in a high and low mammary tumor strains of virgin mice. *Gann* **58**, 45–53.

Nagasawa, H. & Naito, M. (1962). Effects of growth hormone and/or prolactin on the function of the mammary glands of guinea-pigs in the declining phase of lactation (I). *Jap. J. zootech. Sci.* **33**, 165–173.

Nagasawa, H. & Naito, M. (1963). Effects of growth hormone and/or pro-lactin on the function of the mammary glands of guinea-pigs in the declining phase of lactation (II). *Jap. J. zootech. Sci.* **34,** 174–179.

Nagasawa, H., Tôzaki, T., Shôda, Y. & Naito, M. (1960). Lactation curve of guinea-pig. *Jap. J. zootech. Sci.* **31,** 195–199.

Nakane, P. K. (1970). Classifications of anterior pituitary cell types with immunoenzyme histochemistry. *J. Histochem. Cytochem.* **18,** 9–20.

Nakane, P. K. & Pierce Jr., G. B. (1967). Enzyme-labeled antibodies for the light and electron microscopic localization of tissue antigens. *J. Cell Biol.* **33,** 307–318.

Nandi, S. (1959). Hormonal control of mammogenesis and lactogenesis in the C3H/He Crgl mouse. *Univ. Calif. Publs Zool.* **65,** 1–128.

Nandi, S. & Bern, H. A. (1961). The hormones responsible for lacto-genesis in BALB/cCrgl mice. *Gen. comp. Endocr.* **1,** 195–210.

Nauta, W. J. H. (1960). Some neural pathways related to the limbic system. In *Electrical Studies on the Unanesthetized Brain*, edited by Ramey, E. R. & O'Doherty, D. S., chap. 1. New York: Hoeber.

— (1962). Neural associations of the amygdaloid complex in the monkey. *Brain* **85,** 505–520.

— (1964). Some efferent connections of the prefrontal cortex in the monkey. In *The Frontal Granular Cortex and Behavior*, edited by Warren, J. M. & Akert, K., chap. 19. New York: McGraw-Hill.

Nayak, R., McGarry, E. E. & Beck, J. C. (1968). Site of prolactin in the pituitary gland, as studied by immunofluorescence *Endocrinology* **83,** 731–736.

Neill, J. D. & Reichert, L. E. (1970). Radioimmunoassay of rat prolactin. *Fedn Proc.* **29,** Abstr. 1865.

Nelson. W. L., Kaye, A., Moore, M., Williams, H. H. & Herrington, B. L. (1951). Milking techniques and the composition of guinea-pig milk. *J. Nutr.* **44,** 585–594.

Neuenschwander, J. & Talmage, R. V. (1963). Influence of the para-thyroids on composition of rat milk. *Proc. Soc. exp. Biol. Med.* **112,** 297–299.

Neumann, F. & Elger, W. (1966). The effect of the anti-androgen 1,2α-methylene-6-chloro-$\Delta^{4,6}$-pregnadiene-17α-ol-3,20-dione-17α-acetate (cyproterone acetate) on the development of the mammary glands of male foetal rats. *J. Endocr.* **36,** 347–352.

— (1967). Steroidal stimulation of mammary glands in prenatally feminized male rats. *Eur. J. Pharm.* **1,** 120–123.

Neumann, F., Elger, W. & Berswordt-Wallrabe, R. von (1966). The structure of the mammary glands and lactogenesis in feminized male rats. *J. Endocr.* **36,** 353–356.

Newton, M. (1961). Human lactation. In *Milk: the Mammary Gland and its Secretion*, edited by Kon, S. K. & Cowie, A. T., vol. 1, chap. 7. New York & London: Academic Press.

Newton, M. & Egli, G. E. (1958). The effect of intranasal administration of oxytocin on the let-down of milk in lactating women. *Am. J. Obstet. Gynec.* **76,** 103–107.

Newton, N. & Newton, M. (1967). Psychologic aspects of lactation. *New Engl. J. Med.* **277**, 1179–1188.

Nicholson, P. M. (1970). Physiological variations in prolactin content of the mouse pituitary gland examined by disc electrophoresis and bioassay. *J. Endocr.* **47**, 403–409.

Nicoll, C. S. (1965a). Growth autoregulation and the mammary gland. *J. natn. Cancer Inst.* **34**, 131–140.

— (1965b). Neural regulation of adenohypophysial prolactin secretion in tetrapods: indications from *in vitro* studies. *J. exp. Zool.* **158**, 203–210.

— (1967). Bioassay of prolactin: analysis of the pigeon crop-sac response to local prolactin injection by an objective and quantitative method. *Endocrinology* **80**, 641–655.

— (1969). Bioassay of prolactin. *Acta endocr., Copenh.* **60**, 91–100.

Nicoll, C. S. & Bern, H. A. (1968). Further analysis of the occurrence of pigeon crop-sac-stimulating activity (prolactin) in the vertebrate adenohypophysis. *Gen. comp. Endocr.* **11**, 5–20.

Nicoll, C. S. & Meites, J. (1962a). Estrogen stimulation of prolactin production by rat adenohypophysis *in vitro*. *Endocrinology* **70**, 272–277.

— (1962b). Prolactin secretion *in vitro*: comparative aspects. *Nature, Lond.* **195**, 606–607.

— (1963). Prolactin secretion *in vitro*: effects of thyroid hormones and insulin. *Endocrinology* **72**, 544–551.

Nicoll, C. S., Parsons, J. A., Fiorindo, R. P. & Nichols Jr. C. W. (1969). Estimation of prolactin and growth hormone levels by polyacrylamide disc electrophoresis. *J. Endocr.* **45**, 183–196.

Nicoll, C. S., Parsons, J. A., Fiorindo, R. P., Nichols, Jr., C. W. & Sakuma, M. (1970). Evidence of independent secretion of prolactin and growth hormone *in vitro* by adenohypophyses of rhesus monkeys. *J. clin. Endocr. Metab.* **30**, 512–519.

Nicoll, C. S., Talwalker, P. K. & Meites, J. (1960). Initiation of lactation in rats by nonspecific stresses. *Am. J. Physiol.* **198**, 1103–1106.

Nicoll, C. S. & Tucker, H. A. (1965). Estimates of parenchymal, stromal, and lymph node deoxyribonucleic acid in mammary glands of C3H/Crgl/2 mice. *Life Sci.* **4**, 993–1001.

Niswender, G. D., Chen, C. L., Midgeley Jr., A. R., Meites, J. & Ellis, S. (1969). Radioimmunoassay for rat prolactin. *Proc. Soc. exp. Biol. Med.* **130**, 793–797.

Norgren, A. (1966). Effects of different doses of oestrone and progesterone on mammary glands of gonadectomized rabbits. *Acta Univ. lund.* Sectio II, No. 31, p. 24.

— (1968). Modifications of mammary development of rabbits injected with ovarian hormones. *Acta Univ. lund.* Sectio II, No. 4, p. 41.

O'Donnell, V. J. & Preedy, J. R. K. (1967). The oestrogens. In *Hormones in Blood*, 2nd edn, edited by Gray, C. H. & Bacharach, A. L., vol. 2, chap. 4. London & New York: Academic Press.

Okada, M. (1956a). Histology of the mammary gland—I. Cytological and cytochemical studies of colostrum bodies appearing in mammary gland of pregnant, lactating and post-weaning mice. *Tohoku J. agric. Res.* **7,** 35–45.

— (1956b). Histology of the mammary gland—II. Effects of stagnant milk on the colostrum bodies in the mammary glands of rats. *Tohoku J. agric. Res.* **7,** 115–129.

— (1957). Histology of the mammary gland—III. Wandering cells in mammary tissues at the farrowing and weaning stage and their relation to circulating blood leucocytes in mice. *Tohoku J. agric. Res.* **8,** 121–127.

— (1958a). Histology of the mammary gland—IV. Comparative morphology of the degenerative lymphoid cells in the mammary tissues, lymphoid organs and gut of mice. *Tohoku J. agric. Res.* **9,** 1–21.

— (1958b). Histology of the mammary gland—V. Effect of ACTH on the lymphoid cell counts in the mammary glands of lactating mice and rats. *Tohoku J. agric. Res.* **9,** 23–35.

— (1959). Histology of the mammary gland—VI. Effects of ACTH on the cell count in milk and in various organs of milking goats. *Tohoku J. agric. Res.* **10,** 369–381.

— (1960). Histology of the mammary gland—VII. Histological and histo-chemical studies of cells in the milk of domestic animals. *Tohoku J. agric. Res.* **11,** 31–51.

Oram, J. D. & Reiter, B. (1968). Inhibition of bacteria by lactoferrin and other iron-chelating agents. *Biochim. biophys. Acta* **170,** 351–365.

Oshima, M. & Goto, T. (1955). A study of involution of the mammary gland after weaning in the albino rat. *Bull. natn. Inst. agric. Sci., Chiba,* Ser. G. No. 11, 81–86.

Ôta, K. (1964). Mammary involution and engorgement after arrest of suckling in lactating rats indicated by the contents of nucleic acids and milk protein of the gland. *Endocr. jap.* **11,** 146–152.

Ôta, K. & Yokoyama, A. (1967). Body weight and food consumption of lactating rats nursing various sizes of litters. *J. Endocr.* **38,** 263–268.

Ott, I. & Scott, J. C. (1910). The action of infundibulin upon the mammary secretion. *Proc. Soc. exp. Biol. Med.* **8,** 48–49.

Ozzello, L. & Speer, F. D. (1958). The mucopolysaccharides in the normal and diseased breast. *Am. J. Path.* **34,** 993–1009.

Paape, M. J. & Guidry, A. J. (1969). Effect of milking on leucocytes in the subcutaneous abdominal vein of the cow. *J. Dairy Sci.* **52,** 998–1002.

Paape, M. J. & Tucker, H. A. (1966). Somatic cell content variation in fraction-collected milk. *J. Dairy Sci.* **49,** 265–267.

— (1969a). Mammary nucleic acid, hydroxyproline, and hexosamine of pregnant rats during lactation and post-lactational involution. *J. Dairy Sci.* **52,** 380–385.

— (1969b). Influence of length of dry period on subsequent lactation in the rat. *J. Dairy Sci.* **52,** 518–522.

Palić, D. (1954). Vaskularizatsiya vimena ovtse. *Acta vet., Beogr.* **4**, 85–97.

Palmiter, R. D. (1969a). Hormonal induction and regulation of lactose synthetase in mouse mammary gland. *Biochem. J.* **113**, 409–417.

— (1969b). Early macromolecular syntheses in cultured mammary tissue from midpregnant mice. *Endocrinology* **85**, 747–751.

Parcells, A. J., Dahlgren, D. A. & Evans, J. S. (1969). A comparison of the effects of chemical and enzymatic degradations of human growth hormone (HGH) and human placental lactogen (HPL). In *3rd International Congress of Endocrinology—free communications*, International Congress Series No. 157, p. 74, abstract 184. Amsterdam: Excerpta Medica Foundation.

Parkes, A. S. & Bruce, H. M. (1961). Olfactory stimuli in mammalian reproduction. *Science, N.Y.* **134**, 1049–1054.

Parlow, A. F., Wilhelmi, A. E. & Reichert, Jr., L. E. (1965). Further studies on the fractionation of human pituitary glands. *Endocrinology* **77**, 1126–1134.

Parsons, J. A. (1969). Calcium ion requirement for prolactin secretion by rat adenohypophyses *in vitro*. *Am. J. Physiol.* **217**, 1599–1603.

Pasteels, J. L. (1961a). Sécrétion de prolactine par l'hypophyse en culture de tissus. *C. r. hebd. Séanc. Acad. Sci., Paris* **253**, 2140–2142.

— (1961b). Premiers résultats de culture combinée *in vitro* d'hypophyse et d'hypothalamus dans le but d'en apprecier la sécrétion de prolactine. *C. r. hebd. Séanc. Acad. Sci., Paris*, **253**, 3074–3075.

— (1963). Recherches morphologiques et expérimentales sur la sécrétion de prolactine. *Archs Biol., Liège* **74**, 439–553.

— (1967). Contrôle de la sécrétion de prolactine par le système nerveux. *Archs Anat. microsc. Morph. exp.* **56**, Suppl. to No. 3–4, 530–544.

— (1969). Lactation in the human: hypothalamic control of prolactin secretion. In *Lactogenesis: the Initiation of Milk Secretion at Parturition*, edited by Reynolds, M. & Folley, S. J., pp. 207–216. Philadelphia: University of Pennsylvania Press.

Pasteels, J. L. & Herlant, M. (1962). Notions nouvelles sur la cytologie de l'antehypophyse chez le rat. *Z. Zellforsch. mikrosk. Anat.* **56**, 20–39.

Patton, S. & Fowkes, F. M. (1967). The role of the plasma membrane in the secretion of milk fat. *J. theor. Biol.* **15**, 274–281.

Pavlov, G. N. (1955). Analiz refleksa molokootdachi u koz s pomosch'yu lokal'nogo okhazhdeniya spinnogo mozga. *Trudȳ Inst. Fiziol. I. P. Pavlova* **4**, 17–21.

Payne, J. M. & Chamings, J. (1964). The effect of thyro-parathyroidectomy in the goat with particular respect to clinical effects and changes in the concentrations of plasma calcium inorganic phosphorus and magnesium. *J. Endocr.* **29**, 19–28.

Peake, G. T., McKeel, D. W., Jarett, L. & Daughaday, W. H. (1969). Ultrastructural, histologic and hormonal characterization of a prolactin-rich human pituitary tumor. *J. clin. Endocr. Metab.* **29**, 1383–1399.

Pecile, A. & Müller, E. E. (1966). Control of growth hormone secretion. In *Neuroendocrinology*, edited by Martini, L. & Ganong, W. F., vol. 1, chap. 13. New York & London: Academic Press.

—— (Editors) (1968). *Growth Hormone*. Excerpta Medica Int. Congr. Series No. 158.

Peckham, W. D. (1967). The preparation of homogeneous monkey and human pituitary growth hormones. *J. biol Chem.* **242**, 190–196.

Peckham, W. D., Hotchkiss, J., Knobil, E. & Nicoll, C. S. (1968). Prolactin activity of homogeneous primate growth hormone preparations. *Endocrinology* **82**, 1247–1248.

Peeters, G., Cocquyt, G. & De Moor, A. (1963). L'écoulement de la lymphe de la glande mammaire chez la vache laitière. *Annls Endocr.* **24**, 717–718.

—— (1964). Het kollekteren van lymfe van de uier bij de lacterende koe. *Vlaams diergeneesk. Tijdschr.* **33**, 97–102.

Peeters, G., Coussens, R. & Oyaert, W. (1949). Physiology of the cistern of the bovine mammary gland. *Archs int. Pharmacodyn. Thér.* **79**, 113–122.

Peeters, G., Coussens, R. & Sierens, G. (1949). Physiology of the nerves in the bovine mammary gland. *Archs int. Pharmacodyn. Thér.* **79**, 75–82.

Peeters, G., Massart, L. & Coussens, R. (1947). L'éjection du lait chez les bovides. *Archs int. Pharmacodyn. Thér.* **75**, 85–89.

Peeters, G., Sierens, G. & Silver, M. (1952). Expulsion of milk in the isolated perfused udder of the cow. *Archs int. Pharmacodyn. Thér.* **88**, 413–424.

Peeters, G., Stormorken, H. & Vanschoubroek, F. (1960). The effect of different stimuli on milk ejection and diuresis in the lactating cow. *J Endocr.* **20**, 163–172.

Perl, E. R. & Whitlock, D. G. (1961). Somatic stimuli exciting spinothalamic projections to thalamic neurons in cat and monkey. *Expl Neurol.* **3**, 256–296.

Peruzy, A. D., Amoruso, M. R. & Pavoni, P. (1963). Nuova tecnica di dosaggio della prolattina mediante radiofosforo. *Folia endocr.* **16**, 670–678.

Petersen, W. E. & Ludwick, T. M. (1942). The humoral nature of the factor causing the let-down of milk. *Fedn Proc.* **1**, 66–67.

Pickford, M. (1960). Factors affecting milk release in the dog and the quantity of oxytocin liberated by suckling. *J. Physiol.* **152**, 515–526.

Pickford, G. E. & Phillips, J. G. (1959). Prolactin, a factor in promoting survival of hypophysectomized killifish in fresh water. *Science, N.Y.* **130**, 454–455.

Pickford, G. E., Robertson, E. E. & Sawyer, W. H. (1965). Hypophysectomy, replacement therapy, and the tolerance of the euryhaline killifish, *Fundulus heteroclitus*, to hypotonic media. *Gen. comp. Endocr.* **5**, 160–180.

Pincus, G. (1965). *The Control of Fertility*. New York & London: Academic Press.

Pitelka, D. R., Kerkof, P. R., Gagné, H. T., Smith, S. & Abraham, S. (1969). Characteristics of cells dissociated from mouse mammary glands—I. Method of separation and morphology of parenchymal cells from lactating glands. *Expl Cell Res.* **57**, 43–62.

Plotka, E. D., Erb, R. E., Callahan, C. J. & Gomes, W. R. (1967). Levels of progesterone in peripheral blood plasma during the estrous cycle of the bovine. *J. Dairy Sci.* **50**, 1158–1160.

Poggio, G. F. & Mountcastle, V. B. (1960). A study of the functional contributions of the lemniscal and spinothalamic systems to somatic sensibility. *Bull. Johns Hopkins Hosp.* **106**, 266–316.

Pope, G. S., Gupta, S. K. & Munro, I. B. (1969). Progesterone levels in the systemic plasma of pregnant, cycling and ovariectomized cows. *J. Reprod. Fert.* **20**, 369–381.

Pope, G. S., Jones, H. E. H. & Waynforth, H. B. (1965). Oestrogens in the blood of the cow. *J. Endocr.* **33**, 385–395.

Pope, G. S. & Waynforth, H. B. (1970). Secretion of oestrogen into the ovarian venous blood of pregnant rats. *J. Endocr.* **48**, i–ii.

Popovici, D. G. (1963). Recherches neurophysiologiques sur le réflexe d'évacuation du lait. *Rev. Biol., Bucarest* **8**, 75–81.

Porter, R. M., Conrad, H. R. & Gilmore, L. D. (1966). Milk secretion rate as related to milk yield and frequency of milking. *J. Dairy Sci.* **49**, 1064–1067.

Pounden, W. D. & Grossman, J. D. (1950). Wall structure and closing mechanism of the bovine teat. *Am. J. vet. Res.* **11**, 349–354.

Prentice, J. H. (1969). The milk fat globule membrane, 1955–1968. *Dairy Sci. Abstr.* **31**, 353–356.

Prop, F. J. A. (1963). Hypophyseal hormones and mammary glands in organ cultures. *Acta physiol. pharmac. néerl.* **12**, 172–176.

Propper, A. & Gomot, L. (1967). Interactions tissulaires au cours de l'organogenèse de la glande mammaire de l'embryon de lapin. *C. r. hebd. Séanc. Acad. Sci., Sér. D, Paris* **264**, 2573–2575.

Prusty, J. N. (1958). Distribution of the elastic tissue in the mammary gland of a cow. *Br. vet. J.* **114**, 411–413.

Puca, G. A. & Bresciani, F. (1969). Interactions of 6,7-^{3}H-17β-estradiol with mammary gland and other organs of the C3H mouse *in vivo*. *Endocrinology* **85**, 1–10.

Purves, H. D. (1966). Cytology of the adenohypophysis. In *The Pituitary Gland*, edited by Harris, G. W. & Donovan, B. T., vol. 1, chap. 4. London: Butterworths.

Quabbe, H-J. (1969). Sources of error in the immunoprecipitation system of radioimmunoassays. In *Protein and Polypeptide Hormones*, edited by Margoulies, M. Excerpta Medica International Congress Series No. 161, pp. 21–25.

Raben, M. S. (1959). Human growth hormone. *Recent Prog. Horm. Res.* **15**, 71–105.

Racadot, J. (1957). La thyroïde de la chatte durant la gestation et la lactation. *C. r. Séanc. Soc. Biol.* **151**, 1005–1007.

Ramirez, V. D. & McCann, S. M. (1964). Induction of prolactin secretion by implants of estrogen into the hypothalamo-hypophysial region of female rats. *Endocrinology* **75**, 206–214.

Rao, G. S., Breazile, J. E. & Kitchell, R. L. (1969). Distribution and termination of spinoreticular afferents in the brain stem of sheep. *J. comp. Neurol.* **137**, 185–196.

Rao, P. M., Robertson, M. C., Winnick, M. & Winnick, T. (1967). Biosynthesis of prolactin and growth hormone in slices of bovine anterior pituitary tissue. *Endocrinology* **80**, 1111–1119.

Rasmussen, F. (1963). The mammary blood flow in the goat as measured by antipyrine absorption. *Acta vet. scand.* **4**, 271–280.

— (1965). The mammary blood flow in the cow as measured by the antipyrine absorption method. *Acta vet. scand.* **6**, 135–149.

— (1966). *Studies on the Excretion and Absorption of Drugs.* Thesis. Copenhagen: Mortensen.

Ratner, A. & Meites, J. (1964). Depletion of prolactin-inhibiting activity of rat hypothalamus by estradiol or suckling stimulus. *Endocrinology* **75**, 377–382.

Ratner, A., Talwalker, P. K. & Meites, J. (1963). Effect of estrogen administration *in vivo* on prolactin release by rat pituitary *in vitro*. *Proc. Soc. exp. Biol. Med.* **112**, 12–15.

— (1965). Effect of reserpine on prolactin-inhibiting activity of rat hypothalamus. *Endocrinology* **77**, 315–319.

Rawlinson, H. E. & Pierce, G. B. (1950). Iron content as a quantitative measurement of the effect of previous pregnancies on the mammary glands of mice. *Endocrinology* **46**, 426–433.

Raynaud, A. (1961). Morphogenesis of the mammary gland. In *Milk: the Mammary Gland and its Secretion*, edited by Kon, S. K. & Cowie, A. T., vol. 1, chap. 1. New York & London: Academic Press.

— (1969). Mamelles. In *Traité de Zoologie*, edited by Grassé, P-P., vol. 16, fascicule 6, pp. 1–147. Paris: Masson, Libraires de l'Académie de Médecine.

— (1971). Foetal development of the mammary gland and hormonal effects on its morphogenesis. In *Lactation*, edited by Falconer, I. R., pp. 3–30. London: Butterworths.

Read, C. H., Eash, S. A. & Najjar, S. (1962). Experiences with the haemagglutination method of human growth hormone assay. *Ciba Fdn Colloq. Endocr.* **14**, 45–61.

Reddy, R. R. & Donker, J. D. (1964). Lactation studies—V. Effect of litter size and number of lactation upon milk yields in Sprague–Dawley rats with observations on rates of gains of young in litters of various sizes. *J. Dairy Sci.* **47**, 1096–1098.

Relkin, R. (1967). Neurologic pathways involved in lactation. *Dis. nerv. Syst.* **28**, 94–97.

Reynaert, H., Peeters, G., Verbeke, R. & Houvenaghel, A. (1968). Further studies of the physiology of plasma kinins and kallikreins in the udder of ruminants. *Archs int. Pharmacodyn. Thér.* **176**, 473–475.

Reynolds, M. (1962). Composition of mammary lymph in lactating goats. *J. Dairy Sci.* **45**, 742–746.

— (1964). Use of nitrous oxide to measure mammary blood flow in anesthetized lactating goats. *Am. J. Physiol.* **206**, 183–188.

— (1965). Udder blood flow in unanesthetized, lactating goats measured with nitrous oxide. *Am. J. Physiol.* **209**, 669–672.

— (1969). Relationship of mammary circulation and oxygen consumption to lactogenesis. In *Lactogenesis: the Initiation of Milk Secretion at Parturition*, edited by Reynolds, M. & Folley, S. J., pp. 145–151. Philadelphia: University of Pennsylvania Press.

Reynolds, M., Linzell, J. L. & Rasmussen, F. (1968). Comparison of four methods for measuring mammary blood flow in conscious goats. *Am. J. Physiol.* **214**, 1415–1424.

Richard, P. (1970). An electrophysiological study in the ewe of the tracts which transmit impulses from the mammary glands to the pituitary stalk. *J. Endocr.* **47**, 37–44.

Richard, P. & Urban, I. (1969). Mise en evidence du faisceau spino-cervico-thalamique chez le mouton. *C. r. hebd. Séanc. Acad. Sci., Sér. D, Paris* **268**, 115–117.

Richard, P., Urban, I. & Denamur, R. (1970). The role of the dorsal tracts of the spinal cord and of the mesencephalic and thalamic lemniscal system in the milk-ejection reflex during milking in the ewe. *J. Endocr.* **47**, 45–53.

Richards, R. C. & Benson, G. K. (1969). Ultrastructural changes associated with hormonally induced inhibition of mammary involution. *Acta endocr., Copenh.* Suppl. 138, 257.

Richardson, K. C. (1947). Some structural features of the mammary tissues. *Br. med. Bull.* **5**, 123–129.

— (1949). Contractile tissues in the mammary gland, with special reference to myoepithelium in the goat. *Proc. R. Soc.* B **136**, 30–45.

— (1951). Structural investigation of the contractile tissues in the mammary gland. *Colloq. int. Cent. natn. Rech. scient.* **32**, 167–169.

— (1953). Measurement of the total area of secretory epithelium in the lactating mammary gland of the goat. *J. Endocr.* **9**, 170–184.

Riddle, O. (1963). Prolactin or progesterone as key to parental behaviour: a review. *Anim. Behav.* **11**, 419–432.

Riddle, O., Bates, R. W. & Dykshorn, S. W. (1933). The preparation, identification and assay of prolactin—a hormone of the anterior pituitary. *Am. J. Physiol.* **105**, 191–216.

Ringler, I. (1968). The biological characterization of purified placental protein (human). In *Pharmacology of Hormonal Polypeptides and Proteins*, edited by Back, N., Martini, L. & Paoletti, R., pp. 473–482. New York: Plenum Press.

Rivera, E. M. (1964*a*). Maintenance and development of whole mammary glands of mice in organ culture. *J. Endocr.* **30**, 33–39.

— (1964*b*). Differential responsiveness to hormones of C3H and A mouse mammary tissues in organ culture. *Endocrinology* **74**, 853–864.

Rivera, E. M., Forsyth, I. A. & Folley, S. J. (1967). Lactogenic activity of mammalian growth hormones *in vitro*. *Proc. Soc. exp. Biol. Med.* **124**, 859–865.

Rivera, E. M. & Kahn, R. H. (1970). Endocrine secretion *in vitro*: prolactin. In *In Vitro Advances in Tissue Culture*, edited by Waymouth, C., vol. 5, pp. 28–39. Baltimore: Williams & Wilkins.

Robinson, J. J., Foster, W. H. & Forbes, T. J. (1969). The estimation of the milk yield of a ewe from body weight data on the suckling lamb. *J. agric. Sci., Camb.* **72**, 103–107.

Robinson, M. (1947). Clinical treatment of hypogalactia by hormonal methods. *Br. med. Bull.* **5**, 164–166.

Rook, J. A. F. & Hopwood, J. B. (1970). The effects of intravenous infusions of insulin and of sodium succinate on milk secretion in the goat. *J. Dairy Res.* **37**, 193–198.

Rook, J. A. F., Storry, J. E. & Wheelock, J. V. (1965). Plasma glucose and acetate and milk secretion in the ruminant. *J. Dairy Sci.* **48**, 745–747.

Rook, J. A. F. & Wheelock, J. V. (1967). Reviews of the progress of dairy science. Dairy chemistry. The secretion of water and of water-soluble constituents in milk. *J. Dairy Res.* **34**, 273–287.

Roth, J., Glick, S. M., Yalow, R. S. & Berson, S. A. (1963*a*). Hypoglycemia: a potent stimulus to secretion of growth hormone. *Science, N.Y.* **140**, 987–988.

— (1963*b*). Secretion of human growth hormone: physiological and experimental modification. *Metabolism* **12**, 577–579.

Roth, L. L. & Rosenblatt, J. S. (1966). Mammary glands of pregnant rats; development stimulated by licking. *Science, N.Y.* **151**, 1403–1404.

— (1968). Self-licking and mammary development during pregnancy in the rat. *J. Endocr.* **42**, 363–378.

Rothballer, A. B. (1966). Pathways of secretion and regulation of posterior pituitary factors. *Res. Publs. Ass. Res. nerv. ment. Dis.* **43**, 86–131.

Rothschild, H. de (1901). *Bibliographia Lactaria. Bibliographie Générale des Travaux parus sur le Lait et sur l'Allaitement.* Paris: Octave Doin. Premier supplément (année 1900) (1901). Deuxième supplément (année 1901) (1902).

Saji, M. A. (1967). An immunological estimation of prolactin in sheep blood. In *Reproduction in the Female Mammal*, edited by Lamming, G. E. & Amoroso, E. C., pp. 157–172. London: Butterworths.

Saji, M. A. & Crighton, D. B. (1968). A study of the antihormonal activity of an antiserum to ovine prolactin using the local lactogenic response in the rabbit. *J. Endocr.* **41**, 555–561.

Salter J. & Best, C. H. (1953). Insulin as a growth hormone. *Br. med. J.* **ii**, 353–359.

Sander, S. (1968). The uptake of 17β-oestradiol in breast tissue of female rats. *Acta endocr., Copenh.* **58**, 49–56.

Sar, M. & Meites, J. (1967). Changes in pituitary prolactin release and hypothalamic PIF content during the estrous cycle of rats. *Proc. Soc. exp. Biol. Med.* **125**, 1018–1021.

Sar, M. & Meites, J. (1969). Effects of suckling on pituitary release of prolactin, GH, and TSH in postpartum lactating rats. *Neuroendocrinology* **4**, 25–31.

Sas, M., Viski, S. & Gellén, J. (1969). Der Steroidgehalt der Frauenmilch. *Arch. Gynäk.* **207**, 452–459.

Saunders, F. J. (1967). Effects of norethynodrel combined with mestranol on the offspring when administered during pregnancy and lactation in rats. *Endocrinology* **80**, 447–452.

Sawyer, W. H. (1966). Biological assays for neurohypophysial principles in tissues and in blood. In *The Pituitary Gland*, edited by Harris, G. W. & Donovan, B. T., vol. 3, chap. 10. London: Butterworths.

Schade, A. L., Pallavicini, C. & Wiesman, U. (1969). Ekkrinosiderophilin of human milk. *Protides biol. Fluids* **16**, 619–625.

Schally, A. V., Meites, J., Bowers, C. Y. & Ratner, A. (1964). Identity of prolactin inhibiting factor (PIF) and luteinizing hormone-releasing factor (LRF). *Proc. Soc. exp. Biol. Med.* **117**, 252–254.

Schams, D. & Karg, H. (1969). Radioimmunologische Bestimmung von Prolaktin im Blutserum vom Rind. *Milchwissenschaft* **24**, 263–265.

— (1970). Untersuchungen über Prolaktin im Rinderblut mit einer radioimmunologischen Bestimmungsmethode. *Zentbl. VetMed.*, A **17**, 193–212.

Scheibel, M. E. & Scheibel, A. B. (1966). Patterns of organization in specific and nonspecific thalamic fields. In *The Thalamus*, edited by Purpura, D. P. & Yahr, M., pp. 13–46. New York: Columbia University Press.

— (1967). Structural organization of non-specific thalamic nuclei and their projection toward cortex. *Brain Res.* **6**, 60–94.

Schmidt, G. H. (1966). Effect of insulin on yield and composition of milk of dairy cows. *J. Dairy Sci.* **49**, 381–385.

Schmidt, G. H., Chatterton Jr., R. T. & Hansel, W. (1962). Histological changes during involution of the mammary glands of ovariectomized and intact lactating goats. *J. Dairy Sci.* **45**, 1380–1382.

Schmidt, G. H. & Moger, W. H. (1967). Effect of thyroactive materials upon mammary gland growth and lactation in rats. *Endocrinology* **81**, 14–18.

Schoefl, G. I. & French, J. E. (1968). Vascular permeability to particulate fat: morphological observations on vessels of lactating mammary gland and of lung. *Proc. R. Soc. B*, **169**, 153–165.

Sciarra, J. J., Kaplan, S. L. & Grumbach, M. M. (1963). Localization of anti-human growth hormone serum within the human placenta: evidence for a human chorionic 'growth hormone-prolactin'. *Nature, Lond.* **199**, 1005–1006.

Scott, D. G. & Daniel, C. W. (1970). Filaments in the division furrow of mouse mammary cells. *J. Cell. Biol.* **45**, 461–466.

Sekhri, K. K. & Faulkin Jr., L. J. (1967). Ultrastructure studies on the dog mammary gland during various physiological conditions. *J. Ultrastruct. Res.* **21**, 161.

Sekhri, K. K., Pitelka, D. R. & DeOme, K. B. (1967a). Studies of mouse mammary glands—I. Cytomorphology of the normal mammary gland. *J. natn. Cancer Inst.* **39**, 459–490.

— (1967b). Studies of mouse mammary glands—II. Cytomorphology of mammary transplants in inguinal fat pads, nipple-excised host glands, and whole mammary-gland transplants. *J. natn. Cancer Inst.* **39**, 491–527.

Selye, H. (1934). On the nervous control of lactation. *Am. J. Physiol.* **107**, 535–538.

Sgouris, J. T. & Meites, J. (1953). Differential inactivation of prolactin by mammary tissue from pregnant and parturient rats. *Am. J. Physiol.* **175**, 319–321.

Shani (Mishkinsky), J., Zanbelman, L., Khazen, K. & Sulman, F. G. (1970). Mammotrophic and prolactin-like effects of rat and human placentae and amniotic fluid. *J. Endocr.* **46**, 15–20.

Sharman, G. B. (1962). The initiation and maintenance of lactation in the marsupial, *Trichosurus vulpecula*. *J. Endocr.* **25**, 375–385.

— (1970). Reproductive physiology of marsupials. *Science, N.Y.* **167**, 1221–1228.

Sharman, G. B. & Pilton, P. E. (1964). The life history and reproduction of the red kangaroo (*Megaleia rufa*). *Proc. zool. Soc. Lond.* **142**, 29–48.

Sherry, W. E. & Nicoll, C. S. (1967). RNA and protein synthesis in the response of pigeon crop-sac to prolactin. *Proc. Soc. exp. Biol. Med.* **126**, 824–829.

Sherwood, L. M. (1967). Similarities in the chemical structure of human placental lactogen and pituitary growth hormone. *Proc. natn. Acad. Sci. U.S.A.* **58**, 2307–2314.

Shino, M. & Rennels, E. G. (1966). Cellular localizations of prolactin and growth hormone in the anterior pituitary glands of the rat and rabbit. *Tex. Rep. Biol. Med.* **24**, 659–673.

Short, R. H. D. (1950). Alveolar epithelium in relation to growth of the lung. *Phil. Trans. R. Soc. Ser. B* **235**, 35–86.

Sica-Blanco, Y., Mendez-Bauer, C., Sala, N., Cabot, H. & Caldeyro-Barcia, R. (1959). Nuevo metodo para el estudio de la funcionalidad mamaria en la mujer. *Archos. urug. Ginec. Obstet.* **17**, 63–72.

Silver, I. A. (1954). Myoepithelial cells in the mammary and parotid glands. *J. Physiol.* **125**, 8–9 P.

— (1956). Vascular changes in the mammary gland during engorgement with milk. *J. Physiol.* **133**, 65–66 P.

Silver, M. (1953a). A quantitative analysis of the role of oestrogen in mammary development in the rat. *J. Endocr.* **10**, 17–34.

— (1953b). The onset of allometric mammary growth in the female hooded Norway rat. *J. Endocr.* **10**, 35–45.

Simkin, B. & Goodart, D. (1960). Preliminary observations on prolactin activity in human blood. *J. clin. Endocr. Metab.* **20**, 1095–1106.

Simon, C. (1968). *Sur l'Histoire de la Physiologie Mammaire* (1800–1928). Thèse, Faculté de Médecine de Strasbourg, No. 67.

Simpson, A. A. & Schmidt, G. H. (1970). Lactate dehydrogenase in the rat mammary gland. *Proc. Soc. exp. Biol. Med.* **133,** 897–900.

Sinha, Y. N. & Tucker, H. A. (1966). Mammary gland growth of rats between 10 and 100 days of age. *Am. J. Physiol.* **210,** 601–605.

— (1968). Pituitary prolactin content and mammary development after chronic administration of prolactin. *Proc. Soc. exp. Biol. Med.* **128,** 84–88.

— (1969). Mammary development and pituitary prolactin level of heifers from birth through puberty and during the estrous cycle. *J. Dairy Sci.* **52,** 507–512.

Sisodia, C. S. & Stowe, C. M. (1964). The mechanism of drug secretion into bovine milk. *Ann. N.Y. Acad. Sci.* **111,** 650–661.

Slater, T. F. (1962). Studies on mammary involution—I. Chemical changes. *Archs int. Physiol. Biochim.* **70,** 167–178.

Slater, T. F., Greenbaum, A. L. & Wang, D. Y. (1963). Lysosomal changes during liver injury and mammary involution. In *Ciba Foundation Symposium: Lysosomes,* edited by Reuck, A. V. S. de & Cameron, M. P., pp. 311–334. London: J. & A. Churchill.

Slijper, E. J. (1962). *Whales.* London: Hutchinson.

— (1966). Functional morphology of the reproductive system in cetacea. In *Whales, Dolphins and Porpoises,* edited by Norris, K. S., chap. 15. Berkeley & Los Angeles: University of California Press.

Slotin, C. A., Heap, R. B., Christiansen, J. M. & Linzell, J. L. (1970). Synthesis of progesterone by the mammary gland of the goat. *Nature, Lond.* **225,** 385–386.

Smith, A., Wheelock, J. V. & Dodd, F. H. (1966). Effect of milking throughout pregnancy on milk yield in the succeeding lactation. *J. Dairy Sci.* **49,** 895–896.

Smith, C. W. & Goldman, A. S. (1968). The cells of human colostrum— I. *In vitro* studies of morphology and functions. *Pediat. Res.* **2,** 103–109.

Smithells, R. W. & Morgan, D. M. (1970). Transmission of drugs by the placenta and the breasts. *Practitioner* **204,** 14–19.

Sod-Moriah, U. A. & Schmidt, G. H. (1968). Deoxyribonucleic acid content and proliferative activity of rabbit mammary gland epithelial cells. *Expl Cell. Res.* **49,** 584–597.

Soemarwoto, I. N. & Bern, H. A. (1958). The effect of hormones on the vascular pattern of the mouse mammary gland. *Am. J. Anat.* **103,** 403–435.

Soloveĭ, M. Ya. & Ēktov, V. A. (1961). Razvitie molochnoĭ zhelezȳ chistoporodnȳkh u pomesnȳkh svineĭ v protsesse ikh individual'nogo razvitiya. *Dokl. mosk. sel'.-khoz. Akad. K. A. Timiryazeva,* No. 70, 317–323.

Speert, H. (1948). The normal and experimental development of the mammary gland of the rhesus monkey, with some pathological correlations. *Contr. Embryol.* **32,** 9–65.

Spellacy, W. N. & Buhi, W. C. (1969). Pituitary growth hormone and placental lactogen levels measured in normal term pregnancy and at the early and late postpartum periods. *Am. J. Obstet. Gynec.* **105,** 888–896.

Stabenfeldt, G. H., Ewing, L. L. & McDonald, L. E. (1969). Peripheral plasma progesterone levels during the bovine oestrous cycle. *J. Reprod. Fert.* **19,** 433–442.

Stabenfeldt, G. H., Osburn, B. I. & Ewing, L. L. (1970). Peripheral plasma progesterone levels in the cow during pregnancy and parturition. *Am. J. Physiol.* **218,** 571–575.

Steele, S. J. (1968). Inhibition of lactation by oestrogens. *Br. med. J.* **4,** 578.

Stein, O. & Stein, Y. (1967). Lipid synthesis, intracellular transport, and secretion—II. Electron microscopic radioautographic study of the mouse lactating mammary gland. *J. Cell Biol.* **34,** 251–263.

Steiner, F. A., Ruf, K. & Akert, K. (1969). Steroid-sensitive neurones in rat brain: anatomical localization and responses to neurohumours and ACTH. *Brain Res.* **12,** 74–85.

Stephenson, F. A. & Greenwood, F. C. (1969). A new hormone of lactation or an artefact of radioimmunoassay. In *Protein and Polypeptide Hormones,* edited by Margoulies, M. Excerpta Medica International Congress Series No. 161, p. 28.

Stewart, K. S., Kerridge, D. F. & Dennis, K. J. (1969). Suppression of lactation. *Br. med. J.* **2,** 249.

Sticker, A. (1899). Zur Histologie der Milchdrüse. *Arch. mikrosk. Anat. Entwges.* **54,** 1–23.

Stockinger, L. & Zarzicki, J. (1962). Elektronenmikroskopische Untersuchungen der Milchdrüse des laktierenden Meerschweinchens mit Berücksichtigung des Saugaktes. *Z. Zellforsch. mikrosk. Anat.* **57,** 106–123.

Stodart, E. (1966). Management and behaviour of breeding groups of the marsupial *Perameles nasuta* Geoffroy in captivity. *Aust. J. Zool.* **14,** 611–623.

Stokes, H. & Boda, J. M. (1968). Immunofluorescent localization of growth hormone and prolactin in the adenohypophysis of fetal sheep. *Endocrinology* **83,** 1362–1366.

Storry, J. E. (1970). Ruminant metabolism in relation to the synthesis and secretion of milk fat. *J. Dairy Res.* **37,** 139–164.

Stott, G. H. & Smith, V. R. (1964). Histology, cytology, and size of the parathyroid in bovine related to age and function. *J. Dairy Sci.* **47,** 426–432.

Stricker, P. (1951). Comment fut découverte l'existence d'une hormone lactogène dans le lobe antérieur de l'hypophyse. *Colloq. int. Cent. nat. Rech. sci.* **32,** 15–17.

Stricker, P. & Grueter, F. (1928). Action du lobe antérieur de l'hypophyse sur la montée laiteuse. *C. r. Séanc. Soc. Biol.* **99,** 1978–1980.

— (1929). Recherches expérimentales sur les fonctions du lobe antérieur sur l'appareil génital de la lapine et sur la montée laiteuse. *Presse méd.* **37,** 1268–1271.

Stürmer, E. (1968). Bioassay procedures for neurohypophysial hormones and similar polypeptides. In *Handbook of Experimental Pharmacology*, vol. 23, *Neurohypophysial hormones and similar polypeptides*, edited by Berde, B., pp. 130–189. Berlin, Heidelberg, New York: Springer-Verlag.

Stutinsky, F. & Guerne, Y. (1967). Effets des lésions croisées de l'hypothalamus postérieur et de l'amygdale sur l'allaitement chez la Ratte. *J. Physiol., Paris* **59**, 505–506.

Stutinsky, F. & Terminn, Y. (1964*a*). Effets des lésions hypothalamiques postérieures sur le réflexe d'éjection de lait chez la Ratte. *C. r. Séanc. Soc. Biol.* **158**, 833–835.

— (1964*b*). Les voies nerveuses du réflexe d'éjection du lait chez la Ratte. *J. Physiol., Paris* **56**, 443–444.

— (1965). Effets des lésions du complexe amygdalien sur le réflexe d'éjection de lait chez la Ratte. *J. Physiol., Paris* **57**, 279–280.

Sud, S. C., Tucker, H. A. & Meites, J. (1968). Estrogen–progesterone requirements for udder development in ovariectomized heifers. *J. Dairy Sci.* **51**, 210–214.

Sulman, F. G. (1956). Chromatophorotropic activity of human blood: review of 1,200 cases. *J. clin. Endocr. Metab.* **16**, 755–774.

Sundaram, K. & Sonenberg, M. (1969). Immunochemical studies of human growth hormone, ovine prolactin, bovine growth hormone and a tryptic digest of bovine growth hormone. *J. Endocr.* **44**, 517–522.

Suwa, S. & Friesen, H. (1969*a*). Biosynthesis of human placental proteins and human placental lactogen (HPL) *in vitro*—I. Identification of ^{3}H-labeled HPL. *Endocrinology* **85**, 1028–1036.

— (1969*b*). Biosynthesis of human placental proteins and human placental lactogen (HPL) *in vitro*—II. Dynamic studies of normal term placentas. *Endocrinology* **85**, 1037–1045.

Suzuki, H. & Kato, H. (1969). Neurons with visual properties in the posterior group of the thalamic nuclei. *Expl Neurol.* **23**, 353–365.

Swanson, E. W. (1965). Comparing continuous milking with sixty-day dry periods in successive lactations. *J. Dairy Sci.* **48**, 1205–1209.

Swanson, E. W., Pardue, F. E. & Longmire, D. B. (1967). Effect of gestation and dry period on deoxyribonucleic acid and alveolar characteristics of bovine mammary glands. *J. Dairy Sci.* **50**, 1288–1292.

Swanson, E. W. & Turner, C. W. (1941). Evidence for the presence of smooth muscle elements surrounding the alveoli of the mammary gland. *J. Dairy Sci.* **24**, 635–638.

Swett, W. W. & Matthews, C. A. (1949). Some studies of the circulatory system of the cow's udder. *Tech. Bull. U.S. Dep. Agric.* No. 982, 36 pp.

Talanti, S. & Hopsu, V. K. (1961). Leucine aminopeptidase in the mammary gland of the cow and rat. *Nature, Lond.* **191**, 86–87.

Taleisnik, S. & Deis, R. P. (1964). Influence of cerebral cortex in inhibition of oxytocin release induced by stressful stimuli. *Am. J. Physiol.* **207**, 1394–1398.

Taleisnik, S. & Orías, R. (1966). Pituitary melanocyte-stimulating hormone (MSH) after suckling stimulus. *Endocrinology* **78**, 522–526.

Talwalker, P. K. & Meites, J. (1961). Mammary lobulo-alveolar growth induced by anterior pituitary hormones in adreno-ovariectomized and adreno-ovariectomized-hypophysectomized rats. *Proc. Soc. exp. Biol. Med.* **107**, 880–883.

— (1964). Mammary lobulo-alveolar growth in adreno-ovariectomized rats following transplant of 'mammotropic' pituitary tumor. *Proc. Soc. exp. Biol. Med.* **117**, 121–124.

Talwalker, P. K., Meites, J. & Nicoll, C. S. (1960). Effects of hydrocortisone, prolactin and oxytocin on lactational performance of rats. *Am. J. Physiol.* **199**, 1070–1072.

Talwalker, P. K., Nicoll, C. S. & Meites, J. (1961). Induction of mammary secretion in pregnant rats and rabbits by hydrocortisone acetate. *Endocrinology* **69**, 802–808.

Talwalker, P. K., Ratner, A. & Meites, J. (1963). *In vitro* inhibition of pituitary prolactin synthesis and release by hypothalamic extract. *Am. J. Physiol.* **205**, 213–218.

Tanaka, Y. & Oota, K. (1970). A stereomicroscopic study of the mastopathic human breast—I. Three-dimensional structures of abnormal duct evolution and their histologic entity. *Virchows Arch. path. Anat. Physiol.* A **349**, 195–214.

Tashjian Jr., A. H. (1969). Animal cell cultures as a source of hormones. *Biotechnol. Bioengng* **9**, 109–126.

Temple, P. L. & Kon, S. K. (1937). A simple apparatus for milking small laboratory animals. *Biochem. J.* **31**, 2197–2198.

Tenen, S. S. (1968). Antagonism of the analgesic effect of morphine and other drugs by *p*-chlorophenyl-alanine, a serotonin depletor. *Psychopharmacologia, Berl.* **12**, 278–285.

Thatcher, W. W. & Tucker, H. A. (1970). Lactational performance of rats injected with oxytocin, cortisol-21-acetate, prolactin and growth hormone during prolonged lactation. *Endocrinology* **86**, 237–240.

Tillson, S. A., Erb, R. E. & Niswender, G. D. (1970). Comparison of luteinizing hormone and progesterone in blood and metabolites of progesterone in urine of domestic sows during the estrous cycle and early pregnancy. *J. Anim. Sci.* **30**, 795–805.

Tindal, J. S. (1967). Studies on the neuroendocrine control of lactation. In *Reproduction in the Female Mammal, Proc. 13th Easter Sch. agric. Sci. Univ. Nott., 1966*, edited by Lamming, G. E. & Amoroso, E. C., pp. 79–109. London: Butterworths.

Tindal, J. S., Beyer, C. & Sawyer, C. H. (1963). Milk-ejection reflex and maintenance of lactation in the rabbit. *Endocrinology* **72**, 720–724.

Tindal, J. S. & Knaggs, G. S. (1966). Lactogenesis in the pseudopregnant rabbit after the local placement of oestrogen in the brain. *J. Endocr.* **34**, ii–iii.

— (1969). An ascending pathway for release of prolactin in the brain of the rabbit. *J. Endocr.* **45**, 111–120.

Tindal, J. S. & Knaggs, G. S. (1970*a*). Environmental stimuli and the mammary gland. *Mem. Soc. Endocr.* **18**, 239–258.

— (1970*b*). Release of prolactin in the rabbit after electrical stimulation of the forebrain. *J. Endocr.* **48**, xxxii–xxxiii.

— (1971). Determination of the detailed hypothalamic route of the milk-ejection reflex in the guinea-pig. *J. Endocr.* **50**, 135–152.

Tindal, J. S., Knaggs, G. S. & Turvey, A. (1967*a*). Studies on the ascending path of the milk-ejection reflex in the brain of the guinea-pig. *J. Endocr.* **37**, xli.

— (1967*b*). Central nervous control of prolactin secretion in the rabbit: effect of local oestrogen implants in the amygdaloid complex. *J. Endocr.* **37**, 279–287.

— (1967*c*). The afferent path of the milk-ejection reflex in the brain of the guinea-pig. *J. Endocr.* **38**, 337–349.

— (1968). Preferential release of oxytocin from the neuropophysis after electrical stimulation of the afferent path of the milk-ejection reflex in the brain of the guinea-pig. *J. Endocr.* **40**, 205–214.

— (1969). The afferent path of the milk-ejection reflex in the brain of the rabbit. *J. Endocr.* **43**, 663–671.

Tindal, J. S. & Yokoyama, A. (1960). Bioassay of milk-ejection hormone (oxytocin) in body fluids in relation to the milk-ejection reflex. *Rep. natn. Inst. Res. Dairy.* pp. 52–53.

— (1962). Assay of oxytocin by the milk-ejection response in the anaesthetized lactating guinea-pig. *Endocrinology* **71**, 196–202.

Toaff, R., Ashkenazi, H., Schwartz, A. & Herzberg, M. (1969). Effects of oestrogen and progesterone on the composition of human milk. *J. Reprod. Fert.* **19**, 475–482.

Toaff, R. & Jewelewicz, R. (1963). Inhibition of lactogenesis by combined oral progestogens and oestrogens. *Lancet* **ii**, 322–324.

Toker, C. (1967). Observations on the ultrastructure of a mammary ductule. *J. Ultrastruct. Res.* **21**, 9–25.

Topper, Y. J. (1968). Multiple hormone interactions related to the growth and differentiation of mammary gland *in vitro*. *Trans. N.Y. Acad. Sci.*, Ser. II, **30**, 869–874.

— (1970). Multiple hormone interactions in the development of mammary gland *in vitro*. *Recent Prog. Horm. Res.* **26**, 207–308.

Traurig, H. H. (1967*a*). Cell proliferation in the mammary gland during late pregnancy and lactation. *Anat. Rec.* **157**, 489–504.

— (1967*b*). A radioautographic study of cell proliferation in the mammary gland of the pregnant mouse. *Anat. Rec.* **159**, 239–248.

Tsakhaev, G. A. (1953*a*). O prirode afferentnȳkh puteĭ refleksa molokootdachi. *Dokl. Akad. Nauk SSSR* **93**, 941–944.

— (1953*b*). Ob izmenenii sekretornoĭ i dvigatel'noĭ funktsiĭ vȳmeni u koz v usloviyakh ego polovinnoĭ denervatsii. *Dokl. Akad. Nauk SSSR* **93**, 1131–1133.

Tsubokawa, T. & Sutin, J. (1963). Mesencephalic influence upon the hypothalamic ventromedial nucleus. *Electroenceph. clin. Neurophysiol.* **15**, 804–810.

Tucker, H. A. & Reece, R. P. (1963). Nucleic acid content of rat mammary glands during post-lactational involution. *Proc. Soc. exp. Biol. Med.* **112**, 1002–1004.

— (1964). Nucleic acid content of suckled and non-suckled mammary glands within lactating rats. *Proc. Soc. exp. Biol. Med.* **115**, 887–890.

Tucker, H. A. & Thatcher, W. W. (1968). Pituitary growth hormone and luteinizing hormone content after various nursing intensities. *Proc. Soc. exp. Biol. Med.* **129**, 578–580.

Turkington, R. W. (1968). Hormone-dependent differentiation of mammary gland *in vitro*. *Curr. Topics dev. Biol.* **3**, 199–218.

— (1969*a*). The role of epithelial growth factor in mammary gland development *in vitro*. *Expl Cell Res.* **57**, 79–85.

— (1969*b*). Homogeneous differentiation of mammary alveolar cells. *Expl Cell Res.* **58**, 296–302.

Turkington, R. W. & Hill, R. L. (1969). Lactose sythetase: progesterone inhibition of the induction of α-lactalbumin. *Science, N.Y.* **163**, 1458–1460.

Turner, C. W. (1939). *The Comparative Anatomy of the Mammary Glands*. Columbia, Missouri: University Cooperative Store.

— (1952). *The Mammary Gland. 1. The Anatomy of the Udder of Cattle and Domestic Animals*. Columbia, Missouri: Lucas Brothers.

Turner, C. W. & Gomez, E. T. (1933). The normal development of the mammary gland of the male and female albino mouse. *Res. Bull. Mo. agric. Exp. Stn* No. 182.

Turner, C. W. & Slaughter, I. S. (1930). The physiological effect of pituitary extract (posterior lobe) on the lactating mammary gland. *J. Dairy Sci.* **13**, 8–24.

Tverskoĭ, G. B. (1953). O prirode chuvstvitelnȳkh stimulov s vȳmeni, uchastvuyushchikh v reflektornoĭ regulyatsii sekretsii moloka. *Zh. obshch. Biol.* **14**, 349–359.

— (1957). O roli chuvstvitel'noĭ innervatsii molochnoĭ zhelezȳ v reflektornoĭ regulyatsii sekretsii moloka i molochnogo zhira. *Zh. obshch. Biol.* **18**, 169–184.

— (1958). Sekretsiya moloka u koz posle polnoĭ pererezki spinnogo mozga. *Dokl. Akad. Nauk SSSR* **123**, 1137–1139.

— (1960). Influence of cervical sympathectomy and pituitary stalk secretion upon milk secretion in goats. *Nature, Lond.* **186**, 782–784.

— (1962). Rol' éfferentnoĭ innervatsii molochnoĭ zhelezȳ v regulatsii sekretsii molochnogo zhira u koz. *Dokl. Akad. Nauk SSSR* **142**, 728–731.

Valenstein, E. S. & Nauta, W. J. H. (1959). A comparison of the distribution of the fornix system in the rat, guinea pig, cat, and monkey. *J. comp. neurol.* **113**, 337–363.

Van Dongen, C. G. & Hays, R. L. (1966). A sensitive *in vitro* assay for oxytocin. *Endocrinology* **78**, 1–6.

Van Dongen, C. G. & Marshall, J. M. (1967). Effect of various hormones on the milk ejection response of tissue isolated from the rat mammary gland. *Nature, Lond.* **213**, 632–633.

Verbeke, R. & Peeters, G. (1965). Uptake of free plasma amino acids by the lactating cow's udder and amino-acid composition of udder lymph. *Biochem. J.* **94**, 183–189.

Verhaart, W. J. C. (1960). Comparative aspects of the medial lemniscus. In *Structure and Function of the Cerebral Cortex*. Proceedings 2nd International Meeting of Neurobiologists (Amsterdam, 1959), edited by Tower, D. B. & Schadé, J. P., pp. 150–158. Amsterdam: Elsevier.

Verley, J. M. & Hollmann, K. H. (1966). Synthèse et réabsorption des protéines dans la glande mammaire en stase, étude autoradiographique au microscope électronique. *Z. Zellforsch. mikrosk. Anat.* **75**, 605–610.

— (1967). La régression de la glande mammaire a l'arrêt de la lactation— I. Étude au microscope optique. *Z. Zellforsch. mikrosk. Anat.* **82**, 212–221.

du Vigneaud, V. (1956). Hormones of the posterior pituitary gland: oxytocin and vasopressin. *Harvey Lect.*, Series L, pp. 1–26.

Vogt, M. (1965). Effect of drugs on metabolism of catecholamines in the brain. *Br. med. Bull.* **21**, 57–61.

— (1969). Release from brain tissue of compounds with possible transmitter function: interaction of drugs with these substances. *Br. J. Pharmac. Chemother.* **37**, 325–337.

Voogt, J. L., Clemens, J. A. & Meites, J. (1969). Stimulation of pituitary FSH release in immature female rats by prolactin implant in median eminence. *Neuroendocrinology* **4**, 157–163.

Voogt, J. L., Sar, M. & Meites, J. (1969). Influence of cycling, pregnancy, labor, and suckling on corticosterone-ACTH levels. *Am. J. Physiol.* **216**, 655–658.

Voytovich, A. E., Owens, I. S. and Topper, Y. J. (1969). A novel action of insulin on phosphoprotein formation by mammary gland explants. *Proc. natn. Acad. Sci., U.S.A.* **63**, 213–217.

Vuorenkoski, V., Wasz-Höckert, O., Koivisto, E. & Lind, J. (1969). The effect of cry stimulation on the temperature of the lactating breast of primapara. A thermographic study. *Experientia* **25**, 1286–1287.

Wagner, G. & Fuchs, A-R. (1968). Effect of ethanol on uterine activity during suckling in post-partum women. *Acta endocr., Copenh.* **58**, 133–141.

Wakabayashi, K., Kamberi, I. A. & McCann, S. M. (1969). *In vitro* response of the rat pituitary to gonadotrophin-releasing factors and to ions. *Endocrinology* **85**, 1046–1056.

Wall, P. D. (1967). The mechanisms of general anesthesia. *Anesthesiology* **28**, 46–53.

Wallace, C. (1953). Observations on mammary development in calves and lambs. *J. agric. Sci., Camb.* **43**, 413–421.

Walters, E. & McLean, P. (1967). Effect of thyroidectomy on pathways of glucose metabolism in lactating rat mammary gland. *Biochem. J.* **105**, 615–623.

Ward, P. F. V. & Huskisson, N. S. (1966). The effect of mammary gland denervation on the fatty acid composition of goat's milk. *J. Dairy Res.* **33**, 43–49.

Warner, N. E., Reynolds, M. & Henning, C. E. (1968). A method for microscopy of the mammary gland in the living mouse. *Medna exp.* **18**, 151–155.

Waugh, D. & Hoeven, E. van der (1962). Fine structure of the human adult female breast. *Lab. Invest.* **11**, 220–228.

Weber, A. F., Kitchell, R. L. & Sautter, J. H. (1955). Mammary gland studies—I. The identity and characterization of the smallest lobule unit in the udder of the dairy cow. *Am. J. vet. Res.* **16**, 255–263.

Weber, A. F., Wyand, D. S. & Phillips, M. G. (1957). Studies of the incidence and morphology of accessory glandular tissue in the teat canal of the bovine mammary gland. *Am. J. vet. Res.* **18**, 761–763.

Weir, D. M. (editor) (1967). *Handbook of Experimental Immunology.* Oxford & Edinburgh: Blackwell.

Weller, C. P., Mishkinsky, J. & Sulman, F. G. (1968). Non-specificity of prolactin assay based on luteotrophic effect in mature mice. *J. Endocr.* **42**, 485–486.

Wellings, S. R. (1961). *Electron Microscopic Studies of the Mammary Gland of the C3H/Crgl Mouse during Pregnancy, Lactation, and Involution.* Ph.D. Thesis, University of California; quoted by Sekhri, Pitelka & DeOme (1967*b*).

— (1969). Ultrastructural basis of lactogenesis. In *Lactogenesis: the Initiation of Milk Secretion at Parturition*, edited by Reynolds, M. & Folley, S. J., pp. 5–25. Philadelphia: University of Pennsylvania Press.

Wellings, S. R. & DeOme, K. B. (1961). Milk protein droplet formation in the Golgi apparatus of the C3H/Crgl mouse mammary epithelial cells. *J. biophys. biochem. Cytol.* **9**, 479–485.

— (1963). Electron microscopy of milk secretion in the mammary gland of the C3H/Crgl mouse—III. Cytomorphology of the involuting gland. *J. natn. Cancer Inst.* **30**, 241–267.

Wellings, S. R., DeOme, K. B. & Pitelka, D. R. (1960). Electron microscopy of milk secretion in the mammary gland of the C3H/Crgl mouse—I. Cytomorphology of the prelactating and the lactating gland. *J. natn. Cancer Inst.* **24**, 393–421.

Wellings, S. R., Grunbaum, B. W. & DeOme, K. B. (1960). Electron microscopy of milk secretion in the mammary gland of the C3H/Crgl mouse—II. Identification of fat and protein particles in milk and in tissue. *J. natn. Cancer Inst.* **25**, 423–437.

Wellings, S. R. & Nandi, S. (1968). Electron microscopy of induced secretion in mammary epithelial cells of hypophysectomized-ovariectomized-adrenalectomized BALB/cCrgl mice. *J. natn. Cancer Inst.* **40**, 1245–1258.

Wellings, S. R. & Philp, J. R. (1964). The function of the Golgi apparatus in lactating cells of the BALB/cCrgl mouse. An electron microscopic and autoradiographic study. *Z. Zellforsch. mikrosk. Anat.* **61**, 871–882.

Wellings, S. R. & Roberts, P. (1963). Electron microscopy of sclerosing adenosis and infiltrating dust carcinoma of the human mammary gland. *J. natn. Cancer Inst.* **30**, 269–287.

Wells, P. N. T. & Evans, K. T. (1968). An immersion scanner for two-dimensional ultrasonic examination of the human breast. *Ultrasonics* **6**, 220–228.

Welsch, C. W., Negro-Vilar, A. & Meites, J. (1968). Effects of pituitary homografts on host pituitary prolactin and hypothalamic PIF levels. *Neuroendocrinology* **3**, 238–245.

Welsch, C. W., Sar, M., Clemens, J. A. & Meites, J. (1968). Effects of estrogen on pituitary prolactin levels of female rats bearing median eminence implants of prolactin. *Proc. Soc. exp. Biol. Med.* **129**, 817–820.

Westersten, A., Herrold, G. & Assali, N. S. (1960). A gated sine wave blood flowmeter. *J. appl. Physiol.* **15**, 533–535.

Wheeler, C. E., Cawley, E. P. & Curtis, A. C. (1953). The effects of topically applied hormones on growth, pigmentation and keratinization of the nipple and areola. *J. invest. Derm.* **20**, 385–399.

Wheelock, J. V. & Dodd, F. H. (1969). Non-nutritional factors affecting milk yield in dairy cattle. *J. Dairy Res.* **36**, 479–493.

Wheelock, J. V., Rook, J. A. F., Dodd, F. H. & Griffin, T. K. (1966). The effect of varying the interval between milkings on milk secretion. *J. Dairy Res.* **33**, 161–176.

Whitlock, D. G. & Perl, E. R. (1961). Thalamic projections of spino-thalamic pathways in monkey. *Expl Neurol.* **3**, 240–255.

Whittlestone, W. G. (1954). Intramammary pressure changes in the lactating sow—III. The effects of level of dose of oxytocin and the influence of rate of injection. *J. Dairy Res.* **21**, 188–193.

Wijmenga, H. G. & Molen, H. J. van der (1969). Studies with 4-^{14}C-mestranol in lactating women. *Acta endocr., Copenh.* **61**, 665–677.

Wilhelmi, A. E. (1961). Fractionation of human pituitary glands. *Can. J. Biochem. Physiol.* **39**, 1659–1668.

Willmer, J. S. & Foster, T. S. (1965). Restoration of hepatic and mammary gland hexosemonophosphate shunt activity in the adrenalectomized lactating rat by adrenal corticoids. *Can. J. Physiol. Pharmac.* **43**, 905–913.

Witten, D. M. (1969). *The Breast: an Atlas of Tumor Radiology*. Chicago: Year Book Medical Publishers.

Woessner Jr., J. F. (1969). The physiology of the uterus and mammary gland. In *Lysosomes in Biology and Pathology*, edited by Dingle, J. T. & Fell, H. B., vol. 1, chap. 11. Amsterdam, London: North-Holland Publishing Co.

Wolstenholme, G. E. W. & Cameron, M. P. (editors) (1962). Immuno-assay of hormones. *Ciba Fdn Colloq. Endocr.* **14**.

Wolthuis, O. L. (1963a). An assay of prolactin based on a direct effect of this hormone on cells of the corpus luteum. *Acta endocr., Copenh.* **42**, 364–379.

Wolthuis, O. L. (1963*b*). A new prolactin assay method; some experiments which provide arguments for its specificity. *Acta endocr., Copenh.* **42,** 380–388.

— (1963*c*). The effects of sex steroids on the prolactin content of hypophyses and serum in rats. *Acta endocr., Copenh.* **43,** 137–146.

Wood, P. D. P. (1969). Factors affecting the shape of the lactation curve in cattle. *Anim. Prod.* **11,** 307–316.

Wooding, F. B. P., Peaker, M. & Linzell, J. L. (1970). Theories of milk secretion: evidence from the electron microscopic examination of milk. *Nature, Lond.* **226,** 762–764.

Wood-Jones, F. & Turner, J. B. (1931). A note on the sensory characters of the nipple and areola. *Med. J. Aust.* **1,** 778–779.

Woods, W. H., Holland, R. C. & Powell, E. W. (1969). Connections of cerebral structures functioning in neurohypophysial hormone release. *Brain Res.* **12,** 26–46.

Wrenn, T. R., Bitman, J., DeLauder, W. R. & Mench, M. L. (1966). Influence of the placenta in mammary gland growth. *J. Dairy Sci.* **49,** 183–187.

Wright, A. D. & Taylor, K. W. (1967). Immunoassay of hormones. In *Hormones in Blood*, 2nd edn, edited by Gray, C. H. & Bacharach, A. L., vol. 1, chap. 3. London & New York: Academic Press.

Yalow, R. S. & Berson, S. A. (1969). Topics on radioimmunoassay of peptide hormones. In *Protein and Polypeptide Hormones*, edited by Margoulies, M., Excerpta Medica International Congress Series No. 161, pp. 36–44.

Yamashita, K. (1967). Electron microscopic observations on the anterior pituitary of the crab-eating monkey (*Macaca irus*). *Okajimas Folia anat. jap.* **43,** 299–323.

Yanai, R. & Nagasawa, H. (1969). Quantitative analysis of prolactin by disc electrophoresis and its relation to biological activity. *Proc. Soc. exp. Biol. Med.* **131,** 167–171.

Yanai, R., Nagasawa, H. & Kuretani, K. (1968). Disc electrophoretic analysis of growth hormone and prolactin in the anterior pituitary of mouse. *Endocr. jap.* **15,** 365–370.

Yokoyama, A. (1956). Milk-ejection responses following administration of 'tap' stimuli and posterior pituitary extracts. *Endocr. jap.* **3,** 32–38.

Yokoyama, A., Halász, B. & Sawyer, C. H. (1967). Effect of hypothalamic deafferentation on lactation in rats. *Proc. Soc. exp. Biol. Med.* **125,** 623–626.

Yokoyama, A. & Ôta, K. (1965). The effect of anaesthesia on milk yield and maintenance of lactation in the goat and rat. *J. Endocr.* **33,** 341–351.

Yokoyama, A., Shinde, Y. & Ôta, K. (1969). Endocrine control of changes in lactose content of the mammary gland in rats shortly before and after parturition. In *Lactogenesis: the Initiation of Milk Secretion at Parturition*, edited by Reynolds, M. & Folley, S. J., pp. 65–71. Philadelphia: University of Pennsylvania Press.

Yoshinaga, K., Hawkins, R. A. & Stocker, J. F. (1969). Estrogen secretion by the rat ovary *in vivo* during the estrous cycle and pregnancy. *Endocrinology* **85**, 103–112.

Young, R. L., Bradley, E. M., Goldzieher, J. W., Myers, P. W. & Lecocq, F. R. (1967). Spectrum of nonpuerperal galactorrhea: report of two cases evolving through the various syndromes. *J. clin. Endocr. Metab.* **27**, 461–466.

Young, S. & Nelstrop, A. E. (1969). The use of immunofluorescence to detect milk proteins in lactating mammary glands of rats. *J. Endocr.* **45**, 613–614.

— (1970). The detection by immunofluorescence of casein in rat mammary glands. *Br. J. exp. Path.* **51**, 28–33.

Younglai, E. V. & Solomon, S. (1969). Neutral steroids in human pregnancy: isolation, formation and metabolism. In *Foetus and Placenta*, edited by Klopper, A. & Diczfalusy, E., pp. 249–298. Oxford & Edinburgh: Blackwell.

Zaks, M. G. (1962). *The Motor Apparatus of the Mammary Gland.* 1st English edn, edited by Cowie, A. T. Edinburgh & London: Oliver & Boyd.

Zarrow, M. X., Denenberg, V. H. & Anderson, C. O. (1965). Rabbit: frequency of suckling in the pup. *Science, N.Y.* **150**, 1835–1836.

Zarrow, M. X., Grota, L. J. & Denenberg, V. H. (1967). Maternal behaviour in the rat: survival of newborn fostered young after hormonal treatment of the foster mother. *Anat. Rec.* **157**, 13–17.

Zarzycki, J. (1964). An electron-microscopic study on the origin of collagen fibers in the mammary gland. *Folia morph.* **23**, 205–212.

Zarzycki, J., Peryt, A., Klubińska, B., Zak, K. & Hajac, T. (1969). Experimental histochemical studies of the process of resorption of the secretion in the mammary gland of the guinea-pig. *Folia histochem. cytochem.* **7**, 365–378.

Ziegler, H. & Mosimann, W. (1960). *Anatomie und Physiologie der Rindermilchdrüse.* Berlin & Hamburg: Paul Parey.

Zotikova, I. N. (1955). Vliyanie nervnoĭ sistemȳ na sekretsiyu i vȳvedenie moloka u beloĭ mȳshi. *Trudȳ Inst. Fiziol. I. P. Pavlova* **4**, 63–67.

— (1962). Rol' éfferentnoĭ innervatsii molochnoĭ zhelezȳ v regulatsii sekretsii molochnogo zhira y beloĭ mȳshi. *Dokl. Akad. Nauk SSSR* **142**, 204–207.

Ultrastructure

To the references listed in Table 1.1 can be added a study on the rat mammary gland by Richards & Benson (1971a, b).

As the apical plasma membrane of the alveolar cell envelops the fat globule (pp. 28–31) it acquires a thick layer of adsorbed or bound material which is apparently neutral lipid derived from the fat globule (Keenan, Olson & Mollenhauer, 1971). The presence of plasma membrane enzymes has been demonstrated on the surface of the milk fat globule (Patton & Trams, 1971).

The evidence that the Golgi cisternal membranes merge with the plasma membrane when the vesicles rupture and discharge their protein granules into the alveolar lumen (p. 31) is further discussed by Keenan, Saacke & Patton (1970). These authors also note that in the udder of the lactating cow there occur alveoli composed of non-secretory cells constituting 10–20% of the parenchyma. In no alveolus, however, was there observed a mixture of secretory and non-secretory cells, i.e. in any one alveolus all the cells are either fully secretory or dormant. The presence of these immature alveoli are difficult to explain but this synchronization of cellular activity suggests that some type of communication exists between the cells of an alveolus.

There is now evidence that the lactose may accumulate with proteins in the secretory vesicles of the Golgi apparatus and be discharged together into the alveolar lumen (Keenan, Morré & Cheetham, 1970).

Bässler (1970) has reviewed the morphology of the hormone induced structural changes in the mammary gland as revealed in particular by electron microscopic and histochemical studies. Considerable attention is paid to the periductal or intralobular connective tissue—the mantle tissue—and to its behaviour and function in normal mammogenesis and in mastopathies. The ultrastructural features of the region of contact of the mammary parenchyma and the mantle tissue—the epithelial stromal junction —has been described and its role in the transport of materials to and from the epithelium discussed by Ozzello (1970).

Filaments or fibrils may be observed in proliferating alveolar cells and Bässler (1970) warns against confusing such cells with the myoepithelial cells.

The alveoli of the mammary gland of the lactating mouse as displayed by the scanning electron microscope have been described by Nemanic & Pitelka (1971). Some alveoli may be confluent with adjacent alveoli and have several exits; the microvilli are particularly numerous at the apical junctions of the alveolar cells so that the borders between cells are delineated by bands of microvilli. Shallow craters are present on the cell surface which indicate the site of fat globules in the process of excretion—the globules having ruptured during the alcoholic dehydration used in preparing the specimen.

Cytochemistry
Immunoglobulin-producing cells

Immunoglobulin-producing cells have been detected in the mammary glands of sheep, after the infusion of antigen, by staining the tissues with specific antisera conjugated with fluorescein isothiocyanate. The precise location of these cells in the connective tissue within and between lobules indicate that they are identical with the pyroninophil mast cells (Lee & Lascelles, 1970).

Iron. Subcellular fractionation of the mammary gland of the lactating rat 6 hr after an intravenous injection of ^{59}Fe shows that the iron is located in the supernatant fraction probably associated with caseinogen inside the Golgi vacuoles (Loh, 1970).

Jordan & Morgan (1970) have postulated that the main specific function of the milk transferrin in the rabbit lies in the defence of the mammary glands against bacterial infection.

CELLS IN MILK

Colostrum. Richards & Benson (1971c) have noted discrepancies between the distribution of macrophage-like cells as seen in electron-microscopic preparations and the distribution of macrophages as revealed by vital staining under light microscopy in regressing mammary glands. In view of their observations the possibility that some alveolar cells become phagocytic (pp. 39–41) cannot be excluded. The origin of the colostral corpuscles therefore remains in doubt.

Milk. A cyclic variation has been observed in the somatic cell content of human milk which corresponded to the periodicity of the menstrual cycle (Whittlestone, 1970).

ADDENDUM 2

PROLACTIN AND RELATED MAMMOTROPHIC HORMONES

Primate prolactin

Since Chapter 2 was written the existence of primate prolactin as a hormone distinct from primate GH has been established. Observations similar to those first reported by Forsyth (pp. 68, 132) of the occurrence of high lactogenic activity in the blood of lactating women while the levels of HGH were negligible have been made by Frantz & Kleinberg (1970) and by Turkington (1972*b*); this lactogenic activity can, moreover, be inactivated by an antiserum to ovine prolactin but not by an antiserum to HGH (Frantz, 1972). A similar lactogenic activity is frequently present in the blood of patients with galactorrhoea, including that associated with tranquillizing therapy (Frantz & Kleinberg, 1970; Forsyth, Besser, Edwards, Francis & Myres, 1971; Forsyth & Myres, 1971; Frantz, 1972). These observations establish that a lactogenic hormone other than HGH or HCS occurs in human blood.

The secretion by human pituitary tissue cultured *in vitro* of a lactogenic hormone distinct from HGH, as first reported by Pasteels (see p. 68, also Pasteels, 1972*b*), has been confirmed by Friesen and his colleagues (Friesen, Guyda & Hardy, 1970; Friesen, Belanger, Guyda & Hwang, 1972) and by Greenwood (1972). Likewise the secretion of a similar lactogenic hormone by monkey pituitary tissue when cultivated *in vitro*, as previously reported by Nicoll and his colleagues (p. 68; Nicoll, 1972), has also been confirmed (Guyda & Friesen, 1971; Friesen *et al.*, 1972). By gel filtration techniques and affinity chromatography prolactin, both human and monkey, has been isolated virtually free from GH from culture media and homogenates. As a result, radioimmunoassays have now been developed for assaying primate prolactin (Guyda & Friesen, 1971; Friesen *et al.*, 1972; Greenwood, 1972) and the immediate requirement is the setting up of a standard preparation of human prolactin so that assays in different laboratories can be placed on a comparable basis.

Chemistry of mammotrophic hormones

HGH. The primary structure of HGH as shown on Fig. 2.2, p. 60, is now known to be incorrect (see Niall, 1971; Niall, Hogan, Sauer, Rosenblum & Greenwood, 1971; Li, 1972). The so-called tryptophan sequence, positions 17 to 31 inclusive as shown on Fig. 2.2 has after Phe_{31} two extra residues—leucine and arginine— and this whole sequence should be inserted between the positions 76 and 77 shown in Fig. 2.2. On renumbering, this tryptophan sequence now comprises positions 77 to 93 inclusive (Ile_{77} Ser_{78} . . . Glu_{90} Phe_{91} Leu_{92} Arg_{93}). A further correction is the transposing of Pro_{128} and Gly_{130} (as numbered in Fig. 2.2.) so that these become Gly_{130} and Pro_{132} in the revised sequence. HGH therefore consists of 190 amino acid residues not 188 as stated on p. 59.

HCS. The primary structure of HCS has now been determined. It is a protein of 190 amino acids with valine and phenylanine as NH_2-terminal and COOH-terminal residues respectively. Its single tryptophan residue is located at position 85; there are six methionine residues occupying positions 14, 64, 95, 124, 169 and 178. There are two disulphide bridges forming two loops, one between residues 53 and 164, the other between 181 and 188. The number of residues, the positions of the single tryptophan residue (85) and of the two disulphide bridges are thus the same as in the revised sequence of HGH. Indeed the primary structure of the two hormones is remarkably similar; 160 of the amino acid residues occupy identical positions while amino acid pairs related through highly favoured codon substitutions occupy all but two of the remaining positions (see Niall *et al.*, 1971; Li, 1972;

Sherwood, Handwerger & McLaurin, 1972). While there is clear evidence that the complete integrity of the molecules is not necessary for the biological activities of HGH and HCS authors diverge on the effects which particular chemical modifications have on the biological and immunological activities of the molecules (see also Beck & Catt, 1971). In view of the close homologies between these two hormones and their homologies with sheep prolactin, Niall *et al.* (1971) postulate that these hormones have arisen from a shorter primordial peptide through gene duplication and that one or more of the internally homologous regions of HGH, HCS or sheep prolactin may prove to possess the structural requirements for mammotrophic activity (see Niall, 1971; Niall *et al.*, 1971).

Sheep prolactin. Studies by Aloj & Edelhoch (1970) on the properties of sheep prolactin and bovine growth hormone which depend on structure suggest that the conformations of sheep prolactin and bovine growth hormone are homologous.

Mammotrophins of non-primate placentae

Goat. Evidence of the occurrence of a mammotrophic hormone in the goat placenta has recently been reported by Buttle & Forsyth (1971) who detected high lactogenic activity in the blood of pregnant goats by bioassay when radioimmunoassays for pituitary prolactin indicated that prolactin levels in the blood were very low. This lactogenic activity is likely to be of placental origin since secretory activity is induced in mouse mammary explants co-cultured with pieces of goat placentome (Forsyth, 1972). The appearance of this hormone in the blood of the goat about mid pregnancy coincides with the onset of intensive lobulo-alveolar growth in the mammary gland (p. 110).

Rat. Rat chorionic mammotrophin has potent luteotrophic effects on the corpus luteum of the rat but if the luteal cells are deprived of trophic hormones for 48 hr then rat chorionic mammotrophin exerts a luteolytic action similar to that exhibited by sheep prolactin in the same circumstances (Matthies & Lyons, 1971).

Mode of action of prolactin

Prolactin is said to interact with cell membrane receptors; it apparently does not have to enter the cell since Sepharose-prolactin beads exhibit the activities of free prolactin in stimulating nuclear

RNA synthesis in mammary epithelium preparations (Turkington, 1970). The subsequent biochemical changes within the cell leading to the synthesis of casein are discussed by Turkington (1972*a*).

Immunological studies

The presence of proteins which are immunologically and electrophoretically related to HCS have been demonstrated in extracts prepared from term placentae of monkey, rat, dog, pig, horse, sheep, rabbit and cow, in declining order of similarity (Gusdon, Leake, Van Dyke & Atkins, 1970). Rabbits actively immunized against HCS when delivered of live pups failed to lactate and their mammary glands were said to be underdeveloped; a possible neutralization of rabbit pituitary and/or placental lactogen by HCS antibodies is postulated (el Tomi, Crystle & Stevens, 1971).

An extensive study of the immunochemical relatedness of growth hormone in pituitary extracts from various vertebrate species has been reported by Hayashida (1970) in which it is shown that the growth hormones are separable into general immunochemical categories which closely correspond to the respective phylogenetic classes from which the species originate.

Methods of assay

Raud & Odell (1971) observing discrepancies between potency estimates of prolactin activity as determined by the systemic pigeon crop-sac bioassay and a specific radioimmunoassay, re-investigated the specificity of the crop-sac assay and obtained evidence that in *crude* bovine pituitary extracts a substance other than prolactin could stimulate the crop sac; this substance appeared to be ACTH or some associated material. It is not known whether this material acts directly or through the release of lactogenic hormones.

Further organ culture techniques in addition to that of Brumby & Forsyth (pp. 72–73) for the bioassay of lactogenic activity in blood have been described by Frantz & Kleinberg (1970) and by Turkington (1972*b*). Both use pregnant mouse mammary explants; in the former the secretory response is assessed by the visual scoring of histological sections of the explants, in the latter by measuring casein synthesis. The use of suitable antisera to identify the lactogenic hormone (see p. 132) is proving a valuable adjunct in such bioassasys.

As noted above radioimmunoassay methods for human and monkey prolactins are now available. Radioimmunoassays for rat prolactin (p. 77) are discussed in some detail by Neill & Reichert (1971).

Cellular origin

In the primate, anterior pituitary prolactin cells have now been clearly distinguished from those which secrete GH by histological and by fluorescent antibody techniques (Herbert & Hayashida, 1970; Pasteels, 1972*a*). By electron microscopy prolactin cells can be recognized by the irregular shape of their granules; the formation and release of these granules can, moreover, be readily ascertained (Pasteels, 1972*a*).

Comparative and evolutionary aspects

Nicoll & Bern (1972) have recorded over 80 different physiological actions claimed for prolactin among the vertebrates. These can be classified into one or more of several different categories, e.g. reproduction, water and electrolyte balance, growth effects, effects on integumentary (ectodermal) structures, and synergism with steroid hormones or effects on organs which are also influenced by steroids. It may be noted that only the mammary gland is affected by all these categories of action. Nicoll & Bern regard prolactin as the pituitary hormone which did not become committed to a few specific processes but which is used to regulate physiological processes that are peculiar to different vertebrate groups.

ADDENDUM 3

MAMMARY GROWTH

Methods of studying mammary growth

Radiographic techniques. Further to the references given on p. 86 an atlas of mammography displaying the roentgenography of all phases of breast development has now been published (Gershon-Cohen, 1970).

Organ culture studies (p. 121)

Rivera (1971) has reviewed culture techniques as applied to the mammary gland and has discussed the assessment of mammary development *in vitro*.

Mammary growth in foetus

The *in vivo* analysis of the hormonal basis for the sexual dimorphism in the development of the mammary gland in the foetal mouse (see pp. 95–100) has been fully confirmed by Kratochwil (1971) in *in vitro* studies. Mammary rudiments from 13-day foetuses cultured in medium free from hormones followed the female pattern of growth whereas in the presence of testosterone or of a co-culture of foetal testis the rudiments, whether from male or female foetuses, assumed the male pattern of growth. The effect of androgens is therefore a direct effect on the mammary rudiment.

Ceriani, Pitelka, Bern & Colley (1970) have described the histology and ultrastructure of the mammary rudiments of the 17-day rat foetus and of the new-born rat. In the former the rudiment is a solid cord of cells surrounded by a basal lamina and sheath of mesenchymal cells, the ultrastructure being characteristic of undifferentiated foetal tissue. At birth the gland consists of a branching system of ductules in which there is a lumen. The epithelium has lost its foetal characteristics, cells bordering the lumen have numerous microvilli and are tightly joined by junctional complexes. Some fat droplets are present in the cells, the Golgi apparatus is abundant but not sensibly active in protein synthesis and there is a moderate amount of rough endothelial reticulum. Ceriani *et al.* (1970) also studied the response of the 17-day mammary rudiments to organ culture in medium (a) free of hormones (b) containing insulin (I) (c) containing I + prolactin (P) and (d) containing I + P + aldosterone (A). In the absence of hormones the epithelium proliferated but showed no organized pattern of growth and the basal lamina and the connective tissue sheath disappeared. With the addition of insulin the rudiment showed some branching, lumina appeared and the enveloping stroma was well developed. I + P in the medium improved ductal organization and some fat droplets appeared in the cells. With the three hormones I + P + A the explanted rudiments came to resemble the mammary glands of new-born rats and the Golgi vacuoles often contained protein granules. Thus while some cell proliferation in the absence of hormones can occur in the cultured mammary gland from the foetal rat, histological organization of the duct system and organelle differentiation within the parenchymal cells require the presence of insulin, prolactin and aldosterone. The foetal mammary gland can thus respond to suitable hormonal stimulation *in vitro* in a fashion that foreshadows its adult functions: it synthesizes fat and a casein-like protein.

Post-natal mammary growth

In a detailed study on DNA synthesis and cell proliferation (p. 109) in mouse mammary gland Bresciani (1971) has observed that the fraction of cells engaged in DNA synthesis is very low in the ductal epithelium throughout development, but higher in the end buds and alveoli; during pregnancy the fraction drastically increases both in the alveolar and ductal epithelium.

Substantial lobulo-alveolar growth can be induced in mouse mammary glands cultured *in vitro* by the addition to the medium of insulin, adrenal steroids, ovarian steroids, prolactin and growth hormone provided the mice are pre-treated with ovarian steroids (see p. 121). Singh, DeOme & Bern (1970) have now determined the minimum pre-treatment periods and the minimum hormone levels in the culture medium required for seven strains of mice. After pre-treatment it was noted that ovarian hormones were not required in the culture medium. In one strain (BALB/cCrgl) after pre-treatment lobulo-alveolar development can be induced in a medium containing insulin, prolactin and aldosterone (Singh & Bern, 1969), i.e. in the absence of growth hormone; thyroxine if present in the medium in low concentrations had a synergistic effect on lobulo-alveolar growth but at higher levels it was antagonistic.

Some confusion can arise over the terms *mammary growth* and *differentiation*. As used with reference to *in-vivo* and to many *in-vitro* studies (e.g. Singh *et al.*, 1970) the terms comprise extension and branching of the mammary duct system and the formation of lobules of alveoli, i.e. a *morphological* differentiation of the parenchyma involving extensive cell proliferation (see above). For the induction of this type of growth and alveolar differentiation in the mammary glands of the rat and mouse, on a scale comparable to normal mammogenesis, prolactin and usually growth hormone are necessary whether the process is occurring *in vivo* (see pp.

115–117) or *in vitro* (p. 120, and above). These terms, however, may also be applied to the behaviour of mammary epithelium as observed in explants of alveolar tissue from pregnant mice *in vitro* when, in the presence of insulin alone, the alveolar cells divide into daughter cells after which little further proliferation occurs; these daughter cells (or possibly only one of them—see Turkington, Majumder & Riddle, 1971) in the presence of insulin + cortisol then undergo a process of organellar differentiation which permits them to respond to prolactin with the synthesis of milk protein (see pp. 156–160). Explants of mammary ducts from virgin mice will show a similar response to insulin (see Addendum 4). This is clearly a different use of the terms 'mammary growth' and 'alveolar differentiation', the cells divide but once, the differentiation is towards function not morphology and the hormonal requirements are different. It is therefore essential to indicate clearly the type of mammary growth and alveolar differentiation being considered otherwise discussion of hormonal requirements leads only to confusion. It may be noted that insulin alone does not stimulate cell division in rat mammary explants; in this species prolactin must also be added to the medium for cell proliferation to occur (Dilley, 1971).

Oral contraceptives and mammary growth

Leis (1970) reviewing the literature finds no reliable evidence to indicate that oestrogen-progestogen contraceptives have any deleterious effect on the breast. There is, however, general agreement that if any adverse change is detected in the breast while a patient is taking contraceptive pills they should be discontinued.

Levels of hormones in blood during pregnancy

Oestrogen. In pregnant sheep (gestation: 138–148 days) the levels of total unconjugated oestrogens in the blood were less than 5 pg/ml. plasma until about one month before parturition when they increased slowly reaching 20–40 pg/ml. some 5 days before parturition. On the day of parturition, or on the previous day, peak concentrations of 75–411 pg/ml. were observed. No oestrogens could be detected in the blood on the day after parturition (Challis, 1971).

Progesterone. Levels of progesterone in the peripheral blood of the cow during pregnancy have been reported by Donaldson, Bassett & Thorburn (1970); values of 4–6 ng/ml. plasma occurred in early pregnancy increasing to a maximum of 7–8 ng/ml. at about 240 days; the levels declined 2–3 weeks before calving.

In pregnant sheep (gestation: 146–152 days) there was a gradual increase in progesterone levels to about day 140 when levels of 10–20 ng/ml. were noted, thereafter levels fell to 2 ng/ml. at parturition (Fylling 1970).

In pregnant goats Blom & Lyngset (1971) observed a gradual rise in the peripheral blood levels of progesterone reaching a maximum of 33 ng/ml. at 90 days; thereafter the levels declined to 7 ng/ml. before parturition. These values are considerably higher than those previously reported (p. 131).

Prolactin and HCS. In pregnant women Friesen *et al.* (1972) observed that prolactin and HCS increase progressively in the serum to reach levels of 200 ng/ml. and 8 μg/ml. respectively. In pregnant monkeys no consistent increase in prolactin was observed but occasional high values were noted.

ADDENDUM 4

MILK SECRETION

Measurement of milk yield

Dilution techniques using a marker such as polyethylene glycol can be used to determine the volume of the milk pool within the mammary gland. The recent introduction of [141]cerium and ^{14}C-labelled polyethylene glycol as markers facilitates this determination (Snipes & Lengemann, 1970).

Composition of milk

Changes in composition may occur while milk is held in the alveoli (p. 136) but the milk stored in the ducts and cisterns apparently remains unchanged for long periods by virtue of the

impermeability of these structures to the main soluble constituents of milk (Linzell & Peaker, 1971).

Two further species may be added to Table 4.1 (p. 141), namely
Dall sheep (Cook, Pearson, Simmons & Baker, 1970) and the
snowshoe hare (Baker, Cook, Bider & Pearson, 1970).

The constitutent fatty acids of the milk fats of some 106 species,
representing 14 orders of mammals, have now been investigated;
the recent study by Glass & Jenness (1971) gives references to
earlier investigations.

Cytology of lactogenesis

Further to the ultrastructural studies of induced lactogenesis
(pp. 149–151) Fiddler, Birkinshaw & Falconer (1971) have described the changes occurring in the alveolar epithelium in response
to the intraduct injection of prolactin in the pseudopregnant
rabbit; after 48 hr the cells have developed an extensive rough
endoplasmic reticulum with cisternae, the Golgi apparatus is
hypertrophied and the vesicles contain secretory granules. The
lactose content of the tissue begins to rise on the 3rd day and
increases steeply during the 4th and 5th days after the injection.
The production of casein-like proteins begins on the 3rd day.

Initiation of milk secretion

Chadwick (1971) has confirmed an earlier observation that
ACTH can induce lactogenesis in the pseudopregnant rabbit.
He also noted that treatment with ACTH or with adrenal steroids
increases the sensitivity of the mammary gland of the pseudopregnant rabbit to intraductally injected prolactin. In view of these
observations he considers it likely that adrenal steroids are normally
involved in lactogenesis in the rabbit.

It has been suggested that in pregnant mice lactose synthesis is
initiated at the end of gestation by a stimulation of the synthesis
of α-lactalbumin thereby completing the lactose synthetase unit
(p. 155). Recent studies in this laboratory by Jones (1971) cast
doubt on the validity of this concept since the effective concentration of α-lactalbumin within the Golgi apparatus does not change
greatly at the time of parturition and certainly not enough to
account for the massive increase in lactose synthesis. In the goat
not only are both components of lactose synthetase present in the
mammary gland by mid pregnancy but they function to produce

a high level of lactose (Jones, unpublished). Why, while both components are present in the mouse mammary gland during the second half of pregnancy, they should remain non-functional is yet to be determined.

Functional differentiation of alveolar cells (see also Addendum 3)

When explanted *in vitro*, the alveolar cells from pregnant mice are initially sensitive to insulin and divide into daughter cells (pp. 156–160), on the other hand explants of mammary epithelium from virgin mice are initially insensitive but, after a few days in culture, they acquire sensitivity to the hormone comparable to that of the pregnancy tissue. This phenomenon has been studied and discussed by Friedberg, Oka & Topper (1970). Apart from the fact that the acquisition of insulin sensitivity is a consequence of removal of the tissue from the animal little is known of the mechanisms involved. The observations, however, may have relevance to the changing sensitivities of target tissues under physiological conditions and the selectivity of hormone actions.

Effects of hormones on established lactation

Insulin. A study by Martin & Baldwin (1971*a*) on rats made diabetic with alloxan and maintained through pregnancy and lactation by daily injections of insulin has confirmed that insulin is essential for the maintenance of lactation in the rat (p. 165). Observations on the shift in metabolite patterns induced in the mammary glands of lactating rats after the injection of an anti-insulin serum suggests that the influence of insulin on the mammary gland is mediated through its effects upon the redox state of free nicotinamide adenine nucleotides, effects possibly exerted by a reduction in activity of the electron transport system (Martin & Baldwin, 1971*b*).

In vitro studies with insulin bound to Sepharose indicate that insulin need not enter the alveolar cell to effect its action but can interact with cell membrane receptors (Turkington, 1970).

Ovarian hormones

Bruce & Ramirez (1970) have shown a direct inhibitory effect of oestrogen on milk secretion in rats by placing small implants in the mammary tissue; similar implants of oestrogen into the pituitary increased milk yield.

Further studies have appeared on the effects of oral contraceptives on lactation (p. 166). Lynestrenol if administered to rats for some days before and after parturition will completely inhibit the onset of milk secretion but lactation is normal if the administration is discontinued after delivery (Kurcz, Nagy, Kiss & Halmy, 1970). When lynestrenol is given during lactation, i.e. with continuation of the suckling stimulus, the degree of inhibition depends on the dose and the time after delivery, depression of milk yield occurring more readily in the early post delivery period. On stopping the treatment the milk yields quickly recover as judged by the growth of the litter. In this study on rats large doses (5–20 mg/day) of lynestrenol were required to obtain the effect.

In lactating women norethisterone ethanate (200 mg every 84 days) or medroxyprogesterone acetate (150 mg every 90 days) had no deleterious effects on lactational performance (Karim, Ammar, el Mahgoub, el Ganzoury, Fikri & Abdou, 1971). In clinical trials of lynestrenol + mestranol (Lyndiol 2.5), ethinyl oestradiol, and mestranol, a significant depression of milk yields was noted with Lyndiol 2.5 but not with the other two steroids (Borglin & Sandholm, 1971).

Oestrogen-progesterone or oestrogen-testosterone combinations did not aid in the suppression of milk secretion in ewes which had lost their lambs in early lactation (Young & Clarke, 1971).

Regression and involution of the mammary gland

A study of the ultrastructural changes occurring in the mammary glands of the lactating rat after premature weaning has been made by Richards & Benson (1971*a, b, c*). Of particular interest are their observations on the retardation of mammary regression by injections of various hormones and drugs. Prolactin alone maintained the ultrastructural integrity of the alveoli to a significant degree but the best preservation was obtained with prolactin + ACTH. Thus despite the non-removal of milk from the mammary gland the alveolar cells can retain, at least for a time, their normal ultrastructure if suitable and adequate hormonal stimuli are provided.

Excretion of drugs in milk

Cyclophosphamide appears in human milk within an hour of administration (Wiernik & Duncan, 1971).

ADDENDUM 5

Nursing and suckling behaviour in the bovine have been studied during the first eight hours post partum by Selman, McEwan & Fisher (1970*a, b*). The mechanics of suckling behaviour by the human infant were analysed by Kron & Litt (1971) in which the infant's oral apparatus was considered as a hydraulic pump. However, since precautions were taken to avoid the occurrence of positive pressure in the apparatus, and only negative sucking pressures were permitted to occur, the physiological significance of the results must remain in question (see p. 196).

The release of oxytocin in response to suckling and handmilking in the goat has now been investigated more extensively in this laboratory by A. S. McNeilly (1971) (see pp. 206, 252). A major feature of this more recent work is that whereas the earlier work, which had shown a lack of effect of handmilking in triggering oxytocin release, had been carried out during the long, declining phase of lactation, McNeilly (1971) found that handmilking was a more effective stimulus for the release of oxytocin in early, than in late, lactation. McNeilly (1971) concludes that, in the lactating goat:-oxytocin may be released at any time during the suckling or milking procedure; the release is not preferentially associated with any one particular component stimulus but rather with the total sum of stimuli associated with suckling or milking; neither of the two stimuli, suckling or handmilking, are more effective than the other in evoking oxytocin release; there is extreme variability in the release of oxytocin, both between animals and between individual suckling or milking episodes in the same animal; there is a greater probability of a release of oxytocin occurring in response to handmilking in early, than in late, lactation; and, finally, there is a greater probability of a release of oxytocin occurring before the start of suckling than before the start of handmilking.

ADDENDUM 6

Further evidence for direct involvement of the paraventricular nuclei in the milk-ejection reflex was presented by Ôba, Ôta & Yokoyama (1971) who showed that implants of atropine in these nuclei blocked the reflex. The ascending pathway of the milk-ejection reflex has now been investigated in the midbrain of the goat (Knaggs, McNeilly & Tindal, unpublished work) and was found to lie in the extreme lateral tegmentum, as it does in the small laboratory animals.

Grosvenor & Mena (1971) found that a period of time must elapse following a suckling-induced release of prolactin in the lactating rat before suckling can again effect release of the hormone. This was also observed when prolactin release was blocked during the initial suckling by injection of purified hypothalamic extract, which suggested a central inhibition of release during the refractory period.

Direct evidence for secretion of prolactin by pituitary grafts, and the enhancement of prolactin release by oestradiol and by hypothalamic lesions was presented by Chen, Amenomori, Lu, Voogt & Meites (1970) who reported on serum prolactin levels in hypophysectomized, ovariectomized rats bearing 0, 1, 2 or 4 anterior pituitaries (AP) under the kidney capsule at various periods after transplantation. Rats with no AP transplants had barely detectable levels of serum prolactin, rats with one AP transplant had levels similar to those of oestrous rats (120 ng/ml. serum), those with two AP transplants had 170 ng/ml. serum, while those with four AP transplants had values of 250 ng/ml. serum, which is similar to that seen during lactation (280 ng/ml.). Also, injection of oestradiol benzoate increased the level of serum prolactin in animals bearing AP transplants, and bilateral lesions in median eminence or anterior hypothalamus of ovariectomized rats caused significant increases in the serum prolactin level from a control value of 20 to 125 and 85 ng/ml., respectively. Similarly, median eminence lesions in the rat were reported to elevate circulating prolactin levels by Bishop, Krulich, Fawcett & McCann (1971).

In addition to raised circulating prolactin levels, there was also an increased incidence of mammary tumours in Sprague-Dawley rats after placement of bilateral lesions in the median eminence (Welsch, Nagasawa & Meites, 1970). In this connexion, the growth of carcinogen-induced mammary tumours can be suppressed by ergocornine (Nagasawa & Meites, 1970), which inhibits prolactin secretion by a direct action on hypophysial cells (Pasteels & Ectors, 1970).

The release of prolactin in response to milking in the cow and goat has been investigated further by Johke (1970). In the cow, release was greatest in the early stage of lactation and decreased progressively with advancing lactation. Prolactin release also occurred in response to feeding in the cow, although this was believed to be a conditioned release associated with the milking routine. In addition, sham-milking of heifers and virgin goats caused release of prolactin, as did a variety of non-specific stimuli, including venepuncture (see pp. 272–274). This latter aspect is emphasized by Raud, Kiddy & Odell (1971) who point out that the radioimmunoassay of bovine blood samples taken by venepuncture may give misleading results since the stress of the procedure will itself cause elevation of circulating prolactin levels. Fell, Beck, Blockey, Brown, Catt, Cumming & Goding (1971) reported a rise in blood prolactin level from a basal value of approximately 5 ng/ml. to 15–30 ng/ml. during suckling and machine milking in the cow. In the ewe, blood prolactin levels were significantly higher during pro-oestrus (49 ng/ml.) and day 1 of oestrus (40 ng/ml.) than during day 2 of oestrus (11 ng/ml.), metoestrus (15 ng/ml.) or dioestrus (14 ng/ml.) (Reeves, Arimura & Schally, 1970).

MacLeod, Fontham & Lehmeyer (1970) presented evidence that dopamine inhibited release of prolactin from the pituitary gland *in vitro* and suggested that catecholamines may have a physiological role to play in the control of prolactin secretion. Indeed, the administration of α-methyl-meta-tyrosine or α-methyl-para-tyrosine, drugs which inhibit catecholamine activity, caused a rapid release of prolactin in the rat (Lu, Amenomori, Chen & Meites, 1970). The effect of dopamine on prolactin release *in vitro* was shown to be dose-dependent, low doses of dopamine (2–40 ng/ml. incubation medium) were ineffective whereas 80–640 ng dopamine/ml. medium decreased prolactin release (Koch, Lu & Meites, 1970). Injection of dopamine into the third ventricle of the rat increased the level of prolactin-inhibiting activity in pituitary stalk plasma (Kamberi, Mical & Porter, 1970). In more recent work it was found that injection into the third ventricle of the rat of 1·25 or 2·5 μg dopamine caused plasma prolactin levels to fall to 42% of pre-injection levels after 30 min. Higher doses of dopamine were less effective, while adrenaline and noradrenaline were only effective at the 100 μg level (Kamberi, Mical & Porter, 1971). None of the drugs were effective when perfused into the pituitary or into the stalk median eminence region, which indicated that they must have been acting through the mediation of the hypo-thalamus. However, the fact that prolactin levels were not reduced further than 42% by dopamine, and the absence of a dose-response relationship *in vivo*, is in general agreement with the finding that implants of catecholamines in the median eminence of the lactating rabbit did not suppress lactation completely, and hence could not have blocked the release of prolactin completely (Shani, Knaggs & Tindal, 1971), which might suggest a supporting, or intermediary, rather than a cardinal role for catecholamines in the prolactin-release mechanism.

Grosvenor, Mena, Maiweg, Dhariwal & McCann (1970), in a continuation of earlier studies, concluded that the increased blood level of prolactin after suckling in the rat stimulates the re-accumu-lation of prolactin in the pituitary, possibly by means of a hypo-thalamic factor. In a related study, this group concluded that the lactational response of the rat mammary gland to prolactin is optimal only if the gland is stimulated periodically by the hormones released by suckling (Grosvenor, Maiweg & Mena, 1970).

Further evidence for nervous connexions between mammary gland and brain being non-essential for the maintenance of lac-tation in the rabbit was provided by Beyer & Mena (1970), since lactogenesis occurred in rabbits which had been spinal sectioned during pregnancy, and milk secretion continued at a reduced rate for several days. Circulating levels of prolactin in the pseudopregnant rat, measured by radioimmunoassay, were depressed by median eminence implants of prolactin (Voogt & Meites, 1971) and pseudopregnancy was terminated. Injection of hypothalamic extract into rats on the morning of pro-oestrous or oestrus depressed serum prolactin levels. When hypothalamic extract was injected into lactating rats before a suckling episode, the extract did not prevent the release of prolactin in response to suckling (Amenomori & Meites, 1970), in contrast to the blocking effect of purified hypothalamic extract (Grosvenor & Mena, 1971).

REFERENCES TO ADDENDA

Aloj, S. M. & Edelhoch, H. (1970). Conformational similarity of ovine prolactin and bovine growth hormone. *Proc. natn. Acad. Sci. U.S.A.* **66,** 830–836.

Amenomori, Y. & Meites, J. (1970). Effect of a hypothalamic extract on serum prolactin levels during the estrous cycle and lactation. *Proc. Soc. exp. Biol. Med.* **134,** 492–495.

Baker, B. E., Cook, H. W., Bider, J. R. & Pearson, A. M. (1970). Snow-shoe hare (*Lepus americanus*) milk. I. Gross composition, fatty acid, and mineral constitution. *Can. J. Zool.* **48,** 1349–1352.

Bässler, R. (1970). The morphology of hormone induced structural changes in the female breast. *Ergebn. allg. Path. path. Anat.* **53,** 1–89.

Beck, C. & Catt, K. J. (1971). Effects of enzymatic and chemical digestion on the immunological reactivity of human chorionic somatomammotropin. *Endocrinology* **88,** 777–782.

Beyer, C. & Mena, F. (1970). Parturition and lactogenesis in rabbits with high spinal cord transection. *Endocrinology* **87,** 195–197.

Bishop, W., Krulich, L., Fawcett, C. P. & McCann, S. M. (1971). The effect of median eminence (ME) lesions on plasma levels of FSH, LH and prolactin in the rat. *Proc. Soc. exp. Biol. Med.* **136,** 925–927.

Blom, A. K. & Lyngset, O. (1971). Plasma progesterone levels in goats during pregnancy measured by competitive protein binding. *Acta endocr., Copenh.* **66,** 471–477.

Borglin, N-E. & Sandholm, L-E. (1971). Effect of oral contraceptives on lactation. *Fert. Steril.* **22,** 39–41.

Bresciani, F. (1971). Ovarian steroid control of cell proliferation in the mammary gland and cancer. In *Basic Actions of Sex Steroids on Target Organs,* edited by Hubinont, P. O., Leroy, F. & Galand, P., pp. 130–159. Basel: Karger.

Bruce, J. O. & Ramirez, V. D. (1970). Site of action of the inhibitory effect of estrogen upon lactation. *Neuroendocrinology* **6,** 19–29.

Buttle, H. L. & Forsyth, I. A. (1971). Prolactin concentration and lactogenic activity in the plasma of pregnant and lactating goats. *J. Endocr.* **51,** xxxiii–xxxiv.

Ceriani, R., Pitelka, D. R., Bern, H. & Colley, V. B. (1970). Ultrastructure of rat mammary-gland anlagen *in vivo* and after culture with hormones. *J. exp. Zool.* **174,** 79–99.

Chadwick, A. (1971). Lactogenesis in pseudopregnant rabbits treated with adrenocorticotrophin and adrenal corticosteroids. *J. Endocr.* **49**, 1–8.

Challis, J. R. G. (1971). Sharp increase in free circulating oestrogens immediately before parturition in sheep. *Nature, Lond.* **229**, 208.

Chen, C. L., Amenomori, Y., Lu, K. H., Voogt, J. L. & Meites, J. (1970). Serum prolactin levels in rats with pituitary transplants or hypothalamic lesions. *Neuroendocrinology* **6**, 220–227.

Cook, H. W., Pearson, A. M., Simmons, N. M. & Baker, B. E. (1970). Dall sheep (*Ovis dalli dalli*) milk. I. Effects of stage of lactation on the composition of the milk. *Can. J. Zool.* **48**, 629–633.

Dilley, W. G. (1971). Morphogenic and mitogenic effects of prolactin on rat mammary gland *in vitro*. *Endocrinology* **88**, 514–517.

Donaldson, L. E., Bassett, J. M. & Thorburn, G. D. (1970). Peripheral plasma progesterone concentration of cows during puberty, oestrous cycles, pregnancy and lactation, and the effects of undernutrition or exogenous oxytocin on progesterone concentration. *J. Endocr.* **48**, 599–614.

el Tomi, A. E. F., Crystle, C. D. & Stevens, V. C. (1971). Effects of immunization with human placental lactogen on reproduction in female rabbits. *Am. J. Obstet. Gynec.* **109**, 74–77.

Fell, L. R., Beck, C., Blockey, M. A. de B., Brown, J. M., Catt, K. J., Cumming, I. A. & Goding, J. R. (1971). Prolactin in the dairy cow during suckling and machine milking. *J. Reprod. Fert.* **24**, 144–145.

Fiddler, T. J., Birkinshaw, M. & Falconer, I. R. (1971). Effects of intraductal prolactin on some aspects of the ultrastructure and biochemisty of mammary tissue in the pseudopregnant rabbit. *J. Endocr.* **49**, 459–469.

Forsyth, I. A. (1972). Use of a rabbit mammary gland organ culture system to detect lactogenic activity in blood. In *Lactogenic Hormones*, edited by Wolstenholme, G. E. W. & Knight, J., Ciba Foundation Symposium No. 130. Edinburgh & London: Churchill Livingstone (in press).

Forsyth, I. A., Besser, G. M., Edwards, C. R. W., Francis, L. & Myres, R. P. (1971). Plasma prolactin activity in inappropriate lactation. *Brit. med. J.* **3**, 225–227.

Forsyth, I. A. & Myres, R. P. (1971). Human prolactin. Evidence obtained by the bioassay of human plasma. *J. Endocr.* **51**, 157–168.

Frantz, A. G. (1972). Physiological and pathological secretion of human prolactin studied by *in vitro* bioassay. In *Lactogenic Hormones*, edited by Wolstenholme, G. E. W. & Knight, J., Ciba Foundation Symposium No. 130. Edinburgh & London: Churchill Livingstone (in press).

Frantz, A. G. & Kleinberg, D. L. (1970). Prolactin: evidence that it is separate from growth hormone in human blood. *Science, N.Y.* **170**, 745–747.

Friedberg, S. H., Oka, T. & Topper, Y. J. (1970). Development of insulin-sensitivity by mouse mammary gland *in vitro*. *Proc. natn. Acad. Sci. U.S.A.* **67**, 1493–1500.

Friesen, H., Belanger, C., Guyda, H. & Hwang, P. (1972). The synthesis and secretion of placental lactogen and prolactin. In *Lactogenic Hormones*, edited by Wolstenholme, G. E. W. & Knight, J., Ciba Foundation Symposium No. 130. Edinburgh & London: Churchill Livingstone (in press).

Friesen, H., Guyda, H. & Hardy, J. (1970). Biosynthesis of human growth hormone and prolactin. *J. clin. Endocr. Metab.* **31**, 611–624.

Fylling, P. (1970). The effect of pregnancy, ovariectomy and parturition on plasma progesterone level in sheep. *Acta endocr., Copenh.* **65**, 273–283.

Gershon-Cohen, J. (1970). *Atlas of Mammography*. Berlin, Heidelberg, New York: Springer-Verlag.

Glass, R. L. & Jenness, R. (1971). Comparative biochemical studies of milk. VI. Constituent fatty acids of milk fats of additional species. *Comp. Biochem. Physiol.* **38B**, 353–359.

Greenwood, F. C. (1972). Radioimmunoassay of human prolactin. In *Lactogenic Hormones*, edited by Wolstenholme, G. E. W. & Knight, J., Ciba Foundation Symposium No. 130. Edinburgh & London: Churchill Livingstone (in press).

Grosvenor, C. E., Maiweg, H. & Mena, F. (1970). Effect of nonsuckling interval on ability of prolactin to stimulate milk secretion in rats. *Am. J. Physiol.* **219**, 403–408.

Grosvenor, C. E. & Mena, F. (1971). Evidence for a refractory period in the neuroendocrine mechanism for the release of prolactin. *Endocrinology* **88**, 355–358.

Grosvenor, C. E., Mena, F., Maiweg, H., Dhariwal, A. P. S. & McCann, S. M. (1970). Effect of hypothalamic extracts and exogenous prolactin on reaccumulation of prolactin in the pituitary of the lactating rat after suckling. *J. Endocr.* **47**, 339–346.

Gusdon, Jr., J. P., Leake, N. H., Van Dyke, A. H. & Atkins, W. (1970). Immunochemical comparison of human placental lactogen and placental proteins from other species. *Am. J. Obstet. Gynec.* **107**, 441–444.

Guyda, H. J. & Friesen, H. G. (1971). The separation of monkey prolactin from monkey growth hormone by affinity chromatography. *Biochem. biophys. Res. Commun.* **42**, 1068–1075.

Hayashida, T. (1970). Immunological studies with rat pituitary growth hormone (RGH). II. Comparative immunochemical investigation of GH from representatives of various vertebrate classes with monkey antiserum to RGH. *Gen. comp. Endocr.* **15**, 432–452.

Herbert, D. C. & Hayashida, T. (1970). Prolactin localization in the primate pituitary by immunofluorescence. *Science, N.Y.* **169**, 378–379.

Johke, T. (1970). Factors affecting the plasma prolactin level in the cow and the goat as determined by radioimmunoassay. *Endocr. jap.* **17**, 393–401.

Jones, E. A. (1971). Studies on the particulate lactose synthetase of mouse mammary gland and the role of α-lactalbumin in the initiation of lactose synthesis. *Biochem. J.* (in press).

Jordan, S. M. & Morgan, E. H. (1970). Plasma protein metabolism during lactation in the rabbit. *Am. J. Physiol.* **219**, 1549–1554.

Kamberi, I. A., Mical, R. S. & Porter, J. C. (1970). Prolactin-inhibiting activity in hypophysial stalk blood and elevation by dopamine. *Experientia* **26**, 1150–1151.

— (1971). Effect of anterior pituitary perfusion and intraventricular injection of catecholamines on prolactin release. *Endocrinology* **88**, 1012–1020.

Karim, M., Ammar, R., el Mahgoub, S., el Ganzoury, B., Fikri, F. & Abdou, I. (1971). Injected progestogen and lactation. *Br. med. J.* **1**, 200–203.

Keenan, T. W., Morré, D. J. & Cheetham, R. D. (1970). Lactose synthesis by a Golgi apparatus fraction from rat mammary gland. *Nature, Lond.* **228**, 1105–1106.

Keenan, T. W., Olson, D. E. & Mollenhauer, H. H. (1971). Origin of the milk fat globule membrane. *J. Dairy Sci.* **54**, 295–299.

Keenan, T. W., Saacke, R. G. & Patton, S. (1970). Prolactin, the Golgi apparatus, and milk secretion: brief interpretative review. *J. Dairy Sci.*, **53**, 1349–1352.

Koch, Y., Lu, K. H. & Meites, J. (1970). Biphasic effects of catecholamines on pituitary prolactin release *in vitro*. *Endocrinology* **87**, 673–675.

Kratochwil, K. (1971). *In vitro* analysis of the hormonal basis for the sexual dimorphism in the embryonic development of the mouse mammary gland. *J. Embryol. exp. Morph.* **25**, 141–153.

Kron, R. E. & Litt, M. (1971). Fluid mechanics of nutritive sucking behaviour: the suckling infant's oral apparatus analysed as a hydraulic pump. *Med. biol. Engng* **9**, 45–60.

Kurcz, M., Nagy, I., Kiss, Cs. & Halmy, L. (1970). Suppressive effect of lynestrenol on lactation. *Acta med. hung.* **27**, 137–144.

Lee, C. S. & Lascelles, A. K. (1970). Antibody-producing cells in antigenically stimulated mammary glands and in the gastro-intestinal tract of sheep. *Aust. J. exp. Biol. med. Sci.* **48**, 525–535.

Leis, Jr. H. P. (1970). The pill and the breast. *N.Y. St. J. Med.* **70**, 2911–2918.

Li, C. H. (1972). Chemistry of lactogenic hormones. In *Lactogenic Hormones*, edited by Wolstenholme, G. E. W. & Knight, J. Ciba Foundation Symposium No. 130. Edinburgh & London: Churchill Livingstone (in press).

Linzell, J. L. & Peaker, M. (1971). Permeability of mammary ducts in the lactating goat. *J. Physiol., Lond.* **213**, 48–49P.

Loh, T-T. (1970). Iron in the lactating mammary gland of the rat. *Proc. Soc. exp. Biol. Med.* **134**, 1070–1072.

Lu, K. H., Amenomori, Y., Chen, C. L. & Meites, J. (1970). Effects of central acting drugs on serum and pituitary prolactin levels in rats. *Endocrinology* **87**, 667–672.

MacLeod, R. M., Fontham, E. H. & Lehmeyer, J. E. (1970). Prolactin and growth hormone production as influenced by catecholamines and agents that affect brain catecholamines. *Neuroendocrinology* **6**, 283–294.

McNeilly, A. S. (1971). *A Study of Blood Levels of Oxytocin in the Goat in Relation to Stimuli associated with the Reproductive Cycle.* Ph.D. thesis, University of Reading.

Martin, R. J. & Baldwin, R. L. (1971*a*). Effects of alloxan diabetes on lactational performance and mammary tissue metabolism in the rat. *Endocrinology* **88**, 863–867.

— (1971*b*). Effects of insulin and anti-insulin serum treatments on levels of metabolites in rat mammary glands. *Endocrinology*, **88**, 868–871.

Matthies, D. L. & Lyons, W. R. (1971). Luteotrophic and luteolytic effects of rat chorionic mammotropin. *Proc. Soc. exp. Biol. Med.* **136**, 520–523.

Nagasawa, H. & Meites, J. (1970). Suppression by ergocornine and iproniazid of carcinogen-induced mammary tumors in rats; effects on serum and pituitary prolactin levels. *Proc. Soc. exp. Biol. Med.* **135**, 469–472.

Neill, J. D. & Reichert, Jr. L. E. (1971). Development of a radioimmunoassay for rat prolactin and evaluation of the NIAMD rat prolactin radioimmunoassay. *Endocrinology* **88**, 548–555.

Nemanic, M. K. & Pitelka, D. R. (1971). A scanning electron microscopic study of the lactating mammary gland. *J. Cell. Biol.* **48**, 410–415.

Niall, H. D. (1971). Revised primary structure for human growth hormone. *Nature New Biology* **230**, 90–91.

Niall, H. D., Hogan, M. L., Sauer, R., Rosenblum, I. Y. & Greenwood, F. C. (1971). Sequences of pituitary and placental lactogenic and growth hormones: evolution from a primordial peptide by gene reduplication. *Proc. natn. Acad. Sci. U.S.A.* **68**, 866–869.

Nicoll, C. S. (1972). Secretion of prolactin and growth hormone by adenohypophyses of rhesus monkeys *in vitro*. In *Lactogenic Hormones*, edited by Wolstenholme, G. E. W. & Knight, J. Ciba Foundation Symposium No. 130. Edinburgh & London: Churchill Livingstone (in press).

Nicoll, C. S. & Bern, H. A. (1972). On the actions of prolactin among the vertebrates: is there a common denominator? In *Lactogenic Hormones*, edited by Wolstenholme, G. E. W. & Knight, J. Ciba Foundation Symposium No. 130. Edinburgh & London: Churchill Livingstone (in press).

Ôba, T., Ôta, K. & Yokoyama, A. (1971). Inhibition of milk-ejection reflex in lactating rats by systemic administration and intracerebral implantation of atropine. *Neuroendocrinology* **7**, 116–126.

Ozzello, L. (1970). Epithelial-stromal junction of normal and dysplastic mammary glands. *Cancer, N.Y.* **25**, 586–600.

Pasteels, J. L. (1972*a*). Morphology of prolactin secretion. In *Lactogenic Hormones*, edited by Wolstenholme, G. E. W. & Knight, J. Ciba

Foundation Symposium No. 130. Edinburgh & London: Churchill Livingstone (in press).

— (1972*b*). Tissue culture of human hypophyses: evidence of a specific prolactin in man. In *Lactogenic Hormones*, edited by Wolstenholme, G. E. W. & Knight, J. Ciba Foundation Symposium No. 130. Edinburgh & London: Churchill Livingstone (in press).

Pasteels, J. L. & Ectors, F. (1970). Mode d'action de l'ergocornine sur la sécrétion de prolactine. *Archs. int. Pharmacodyn. thér.* **186,** 195–196.

Patton, S. & Trams, E. G. (1971). The presence of plasma membrane enzymes on the surface of bovine milk fat globules. *FEBS Lett.* **14,** 230–232.

Raud, H. R., Kiddy, C. A. & Odell, W. D. (1971). The effect of stress upon the determination of serum prolactin by radioimmunoassay. *Proc. Soc. exp. Biol. Med.* **136,** 689–693.

Raud, H. R. & Odell, W. D. (1971). Studies of the measurement of bovine and porcine prolactin by radioimunnoassay and by systemic pigeon crop-sac bioassay. *Endocrinology,* **88,** 991–1002.

Reeves, J. J., Arimura, A. & Schally, A. V. (1970). Serum levels of prolactin and luteinizing hormone (LH) in the ewe at various stages of the estrous cycle. *Proc. Soc. exp. Biol. Med.* **134,** 938–942.

Richards, R. C. & Benson, G. K. (1971*a*). Ultrastructural changes accompanying involution of the mammary gland in the albino rat. *J. Endocr.* **51** (in press).

— (1971*b*). Structural changes associated with inhibition of involution of the mammary gland in the albino rat. *J. Endocr.* **51** (in press).

— (1971*c*). Involvement of the macrophage system in the involution of the mammary gland in the albino rat. *J. Endocr.* **51** (in press).

Rivera, E. M. (1971). Mammary gland culture. In *Methods in Mammalian Embryology*, edited by Daniel, J. C., pp. 442–471. San Francisco & Reading: Freeman.

Selman, I. E., McEwan, A. D. & Fisher, E. W. (1970*a*). Studies on natural suckling in cattle during the first eight hours post partum. I. Behavioural studies (dams). *Anim. Behav.* **18,** 276–283.

— (1970*b*). Studies on natural suckling in cattle during the first eight hours post partum. II. Behavioural studies (calves). *Anim. Behav.* **18,** 284–289.

Shani, J., Knaggs, G. S. & Tindal, J. S. (1971). The effect of noradrenaline, dopamine, 5-hydroxytryptamine and melatonin on milk yield and composition in the rabbit. *J. Endocr.* **50,** 543–544.

Sherwood, L. M., Handwerger, S. & McLaurin, W. D. (1972). The structure and function of human chorionic somatomammotrophin (placental lactogen). In *Lactogenic Hormones*, edited by Wolstenholme, G. E. W. & Knight, J. Ciba Foundation Symposium No. 130. Edinburgh & London: Churchill Livingstone (in press).

Singh, D. V. & Bern, H. A. (1969). Interaction between prolactin and thyroxine in mouse mammary gland lobulo-alveolar development *in vitro. J. Endocr.* **45,** 579–583.

Singh, D. V., DeOme, K. B. & Bern, H. A. (1970). Strain differences in response of the mouse mammary gland to hormones *in vitro*. *J. natn. Cancer Inst.* **45**, 657–675.

Snipes, M. B. & Lengemann, F. W. (1970). Determination of contained-milk volume of the mammary gland of the goat by [141]cerium and ^{14}C-PEG-4000. *J. Dairy Sci.* **53**, 1596–1602.

Turkington, R. W. (1970). Stimulation of RNA synthesis in isolated mammary cells by insulin and prolactin bound to Sepharose. *Biochem. biophys. Res. Commun.* **41**, 1362–1367.

— (1972*a*). Molecular biological aspects of prolactin. In *Lactogenic Hormones*, edited by Wolstenholme, G. E. W. & Knight, J. Ciba Foundation Symposium No. 130. Edinburgh & London: Churchill Livingstone (in press).

— (1972*b*). Measurement of prolactin activity in human serum by the induction of specific milk proteins *in vitro*: results in various clinical disorders. In *Lactogenic Hormones*, edited by Wolstenholme, G. E. W. & Knight, J. Ciba Foundation Symposium No. 130. Edinburgh & London: Churchill Livingstone (in press).

Turkington, R. W., Majumder, G. C. & Riddle, M. (1971). Inhibition of mammary gland differentiation *in vitro* by 5-bromo-2'-deoxyuridine. *J. biol. Chem.* **246**, 1814–1819.

Voogt, J. L. & Meites, J. (1971). Effects of an implant of prolactin in median eminence of pseudopregnant rats on serum and pituitary LH, FSH and prolactin. *Endocrinology* **88**, 286–292.

Welsch, C. W., Nagasawa, H. & Meites, J. (1970). Increased incidence of spontaneous mammary tumors in female rats with induced hypothalamic lesions. *Cancer Res.* **30**, 2310–2313.

Whittlestone, W. G. (1970). Periodicity in the cell content of human milk. *N.Z. med. J.* **72**, 113–114.

Wiernik, P. H. & Duncan, J. H. (1971). Cyclophosphamide in human milk. *Lancet* **i**, 912.

Young, N. E. & Clarke, J. D. (1971). Drying-off ewes in early lactation. *Vet. Rec.* **88**, 80–82.

INDEX